PINEAL
CHEMISTRY

Publication Number 894

AMERICAN LECTURE SERIES

A Publication in

The **BANNERSTONE DIVISION** *of*

AMERICAN LECTURES IN LIVING CHEMISTRY

Edited by

I. NEWTON KUGELMASS, M.D., Ph.D., Sc.D.

Consultant to the Departments of Health and Hospitals
New York City

□□□ PINEAL □□□ CHEMISTRY

□ □

IN CELLULAR AND PHYSIOLOGICAL MECHANISMS

□ □

By

W.B. Quay, Ph.D.

Professor, Neuroendocrinology Section, Biomedical Unit,
Waisman Center on Mental Retardation and Human Development,
Endocrinology–Reproductive Physiology Program and
Department of Zoology, University of Wisconsin
Madison, Wisconsin

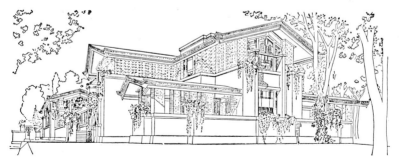

CHARLES C THOMAS • PUBLISHER
Springfield • Illinois • U.S.A.

Published and Distributed Throughout the World by
CHARLES C THOMAS • PUBLISHER
BANNERSTONE HOUSE
301–327 East Lawrence Avenue, Springfield, Illinois, U.S.A.

With THOMAS BOOKS *careful attention is given to all details of
manufacturing and design. It is the Publisher's desire to present books
that are satisfactory as to their physical qualities and artistic possibilities
and appropriate for their particular use.* THOMAS BOOKS *will be true
to those laws of quality that assure a good name and good will.*

Printed in the United States of America

BB-14

FOREWORD

OUR LIVING CHEMISTRY SERIES was conceived by the Editor and Publisher to advance the newer knowledge of chemical medicine in the cause of clinical practice. The interdependence of chemistry and medicine is so great that physicians are turning to chemistry, and chemists to medicine in order to understand the underlying basis of life processes in health and disease. Once chemical truths, proofs and convictions become foundations for clinical phenomena, key hybrid investigators clarify the bewildering panorama of biochemical progress for application in every day practice, stimulation of experimental research, and extension of postgraduate instruction. Each of our monographs thus unravels the chemical mechanisms and clinical management of many diseases that have remained relatively static in the minds of medical men for three thousand years. Our new Series is charged with the *nisus élan* of chemical wisdom, supreme in choice of international authors, optimal in standards of chemical scholarship, provocative in imagination for experimental research, comprehensive in discussions of scientific medicine, and authoritative in chemical perspective of human disorders.

Dr. Quay of Madison, Wisconsin gives the pineal its rightful place among the endocrine glands after twenty centuries of speculation about its phylogenetic roots. It is an end organ of the peripheral sympathetic system, conveying photic and other stimuli to it. It is a regulator of regulators, never acting directly on peripheral target organs. It bears distinctive operational mechanisms of optimal metabolic activity and chemical rhythmicity, with marked sensitivity to environmental control. The chemical story of the pineal gland is presented in terms of the static or morphological and the dynamic or physiological. For the organic chemist the main focus of atten-

v

tion is the structure and configuration of pineal components while for the biochemist, the main problems evolve from the behavior and function of these substances in the organized systems of the pineal gland. Both static and dynamic chemical knowledge is so clearly unraveled as to make the comprehensive review a great fascination to read and reread for complete understanding, correlation, and criticism of the heterogeneous world literature on the pineal.

Whoever started out toward the unknown pineal consented to venture alone in his philosophic probing. Much of the experimental research was conceptual e.g., the search for a concept to explain a chance observation or exploit a new technique, or the effort to validate a concept serendipitously derived by devising proper experiments. Every dream of every worker dashed itself against the great mystery like a wasp against a window and no one ventured to open the window until the wealth of new material unfolded with all its stimulating potentialities in the last decade. And the best of these integrations is vested in this contribution with the viewpoint of an impartial scholar to make an impact on the better understanding of function and behavior in health and disease.

"Research, though toilsome, is easy;
Imagination, though delightful, is difficult."

I. Newton Kugelmass, M.D., Ph.D., Sc.D., Editor

PREFACE

NO ORGAN OF DEBATED function in the human body has passed through such a complex structural remodeling during evolution as the pineal gland. Recent electron microscopic and cytochemical studies in many laboratories, nevertheless, support the belief that the mammalian pineal's chief characteristics are those of an endocrine gland. Even more significant, however, in the current rapid expansion of pineal research are the exciting discoveries of pineal chemical individuality, high levels of metabolic activity, profound chemical rhythmicity and exquisite sensitivity to environmental control. Confirmed now in different laboratories, these findings disparage the time worn presumption that the mammalian pineal is a vestigial organ lacking functional significance. More directly significant for the emerging denouement are the recently demonstrated physiological and chemical interactions involving the pineal gland. Indeed, chemical techniques and chemical results comprise the *sine qua non* both in today's exponential phase of pineal research and in tomorrow's applications of its results to problems in physiology and medicine.

A comprehensive and detailed analysis of all aspects of pineal chemistry has not been published previously. The present monograph reviews mammalian and human pineal chemistry with emphasis on physiological correlations and interpretations. It is written with the intent that research progress made with diverse techniques and by different laboratories be objectively reported, evaluated and integrated. Relevant scientific literature has been reviewed for this book including most of that published through the first half of 1972. The intended readers are biomedical scientists and others who wish either detailed knowledge or summary evaluations of pineal composition and its significance. The latter may be gained readily from the last chapter and from the concluding section of each of the other chapters.

Current investigators of the pineal gland and its importance in physiology and neurobiology soon appreciate that remarkable, fundamental and exciting developments have occurred within the last ten years. Many of these, however, are either not known to, or appreciated by, workers in related areas. It is hoped that this review and integrative analysis will increase general understanding of the potential of pineal research in our endeavors to reveal the body's adaptive mechanisms in health and disease.

ACKNOWLEDGMENTS

THE AUTHOR'S LABORATORY investigations on pineal composition and function have been supported in part at different times by research grants from the National Institutes of Health, U.S. Public Health Service, and the National Science Foundation, by a research fellowship from the Netherlands Organization for the Advancement of Pure Research (Z.W.O.) and by research professorships from the Adolph C. and Mary Sprague Miller Institute for Basic Research in Science, University of California, Berkeley. I am grateful for this aid, and also for the hospitality, encouragement and help extended by colleagues and hosts at various times during these studies. In this connection I wish to thank particularly Richard M. Eakin and Morgan Harris of the Department of Zoology, University of California, Berkeley; J. Ariëns Kappers, Director of the Central Institute for Brain Research, Amsterdam; and Julius Axelrod, National Institute of Mental Health, Bethesda. Other colleagues to whom I am grateful for collaborations and important discussions, include Joseph T. Bagnara, Edward L. Bennett, Sheila Guth, Franz Halberg, Johan F. Jongkind, Geoffrey C.T. Kenny, David Krech, R.K. Meyer, Robert Millar, Norman C. Negus, Nello Pace, Charles L. Ralph, Russel J. Reiter, Aristeo Renzoni, Mark R. Rosenzweig, Lewis I. Smart, Nora G. Smiriga, Robert C. Stebbins, Paola S. Timiras, Joseph T. Velardo and others.

It is a pleasure to acknowledge as well, the help and stimulation of many students and assistants whose work with me related to pineal or brain chemistry. Among these are Peter C. Baker, Rodger L. Bick, Gerard F. Brewer, George F. Buletza Jr., Dale D. Feist, D. Frank Ferguson, Mohammad A. Hafeez, Erwin H. Hesselberg, Tad D. Kelley, Gloria M. Lew, Edward L. Orr, John Y.-K. Pun, Daniel C. Wilhoft and Joseph Wong.

The preparation of this book has been aided by the office assistance of Helen S. Dawson, Karen Mendelsohn, Robin Quate and Catherine Tse. The final rendition of the illustrations has been favored by the skill and patience of Emily Reid. To these and others, I am most sincerely grateful.

W. B. QUAY

ABBREVIATIONS

ACh	Acetylcholine
AChE	Acetylcholinesterase
ADP	Adenosine diphosphate
AMP	Adenosine monophosphate
ATP	Adenosine triphosphate
c-AMP	Cyclic 3′,5′-adenosine monophosphate
ChAc	Choline acetyltransferase
ChE	Cholinesterase
COMT	Catechol-O-methyltransferase
CPM	Counts per minute (radioactivity)
DA	Dopamine (3,4-dihydroxyphenylethylamine)
DD	Continuous darkness
DNA	Deoxyribonucleic acid
DOPA	3,4-Dihydroxyphenylalanine
DPM	Disintegrations per minute (radioactivity)
GABA	γ-Aminobutyric acid
HCG	Human chorionic gonadotropin
5-HIAA	5-Hydroxyindole-3-acetic acid
HIOMT	Hydroxyindole-O-methyltransferase
HNMT	Histamine-N-methyltransferase
5-HT	5-Hydroxytryptamine (serotonin)
5-HTP	5-Hydroxytryptophan
hypx	Hypophysectomized
ip	Intraperitoneal
iv	Intravenous
LD	Standardized daily light-dark cycles twenty-four hours long
LL	Continuous light
M	Molar
MAO	Monoamine oxidase
MFB	Medial forebrain bundle
5-MIAA	5-Methoxyindole-3-acetic acid

5-MT	5-Methoxytryptamine
NE	Norepinephrine
6-OHDA	6-Hydroxydopamine
pCPA	*p*-Chlorophenylalanine
PNMT	Phenylethanolamine-*N*-methyltransferase
ppm	Parts per million
RNA	Ribonucleic acid
S.A.	Specific activity
SAH	S-Adenosylhomocysteine
SAMe	S-Adenosylmethionine
T	Tryptophan

CONTENTS

xiii

PINEAL
CHEMISTRY

□ □

Chapter One

DEVELOPMENT

INTRODUCTION

THE PINEAL GLAND, or epiphysis cerebri as it is sometimes known, develops from the roof of the brain.
The site of pineal development in vertebrates is consistently a median region at the posterior end of the diencephalon and just anterior to the posterior commissure. In mammals
the pineal primordium or anlage is at first a single shallow
evagination.[321, 402, 517] It appears early in the embryonic phase
of human development, at about thirty-three days after
ovulation,[698] or when the embryo has a crown-rump length
of 6–7 mm.[462] Its anterior base is crossed by the habenular
commissure and its posterior base is crossed by the posterior
commissure. The cells of the primordium proliferate first from
the rostrodorsal wall and later from the caudal or posterior
wall, forming, according to some authors, transient anterior
and posterior anlagen or developmental divisions.[462,517]
However, indications of such divisions are soon lost in human
pineals and at least most other mammalian species. The
neuroepithelial proliferations forming the pineal consist of
cords and follicles of cells invested by embryonic mesoderm.
The neuroepithelial cells of the pineal give rise to the
parenchymal cells and spongioblasts of the organ, and the
embryonic mesoderm or meningeal mesenchyme gives rise
to the stromal tissue, which consists of connective tissue and
contained blood vessels. Figure 1 summarizes the developmental origins of these cell types and their usual descendants
within mammalian pineals.

3

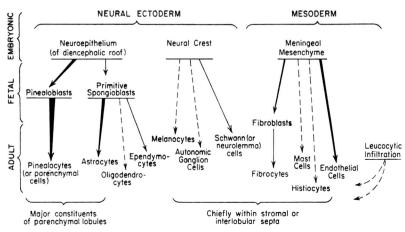

Figure 1. Developmental origins of cells found in mammalian pineals. This schematic summary represents a combination of classical views concerning the derivation of various ectodermal and mesodermal cells[122,536] with views concerning specifically pineal histogenesis.[462,786] Relative thicknesses of the arrows for cellular descents are intended to reflect approximately the relative numbers of cells of each kind. Dashed arrows signify origins of cells that are present only variably, according to present knowledge.

    The pinealocyte or pineal parenchymal cell is the cell type of greatest interest since it is unique to the pineal and usually comprises the majority of the cells within the organ. Early cytological studies of these cells were never able to agree on ages at which they were either fully differentiated or most active metabolically. As we shall see in later chapters, studies of developmental changes in pineal biochemistry and metabolism indicate that the specific activities of these cells are low or not notable until a few days or weeks after birth in the usually studied laboratory species of small mammals. Similar quantitative metabolic or biochemical studies have not been made of pineals from primate infants. Nevertheless, on the basis of cytological evidence and extrapolation of maturation and life span data from laboratory species it is likely that full differentiation and activity of the human pineal are attained within a period of a few months or several years after birth. The cytological evidence here referred to is that available so far largely in qualitative terms for human fetal

and infant pineals. Pinealocyte cytoplasmic, nuclear and nucleolar hypertrophy combined with nuclear creasing, folding
and pleomorphism are mammalian pineal cytological characteristics suggestive of attainment of full differentiation and
activity. In comparable degrees they are observed in postnatal
pineals of man and laboraory species. Acquisition of these
characteristics by pinealocytes of the species studied in most
detail, the rat, corresponds roughly in time to the acquisition
of full metabolic and biochemical activity within the pineal.
Still needed, however, are quantitative and more explicitly
correlative studies of pinealocyte cytology, differentiation and
metabolism in mammals including man.

DEVELOPMENTAL PATTERNS

Rat

Mammalian pineal development is known best in the
laboratory rat. Prenatal morpho- and histogenesis of the rat
organ have been investigated particularly by Sugiura,[947] Gardner[305] and Kappers.[460] Kappers provides from staged embryos
(15, 16, 17, 18, 19 days), newborn and 1 week old rats photomicrographs of excellent quality and with remarkable detail.
Many features and events in the morphogenesis of the rat
pineal and contiguous structures may be appreciated best
by referring to these illustrations.

A comprehensive outline of the stages and events in the
development and maturation of the rat's pineal organ is provided in Table I. This is derived from the results of many
investigators and embodies the most convincing and broadly
based proof for any mammalian species that pineal maturation
is postnatal, and that pineal-specific biochemical activity
begins several weeks postnatally. In a further condensation
of the information presented here, we can say that the rat's
pineal gland has three major developmental and maturational
phases: (1) morphogenesis, (2) cellular proliferation, and (3)
cellular hypertrophy and differentiation. These overlap to
some extent but can be assigned the following approximate
periods respectively: (1) twelfth day of embryonic life until

TABLE I
Developmental Stages of the Rat Pineal Organ.*

Age (days)	Events
Embryonic & Fetal:	
12–14½	First appearance of shallow epiphyseal evagination.
14½–16	Rapid dorsocaudal elongation of the now tubular organ; appearance of mantle and marginal layers outside of the germinative neuroepithelium; differentiation of primitive spongioblasts and (?) pinealoblasts.
16–17	Proliferation of parenchymal cords and follicles from the distal and dorsal walls of the epiphyseal evagination.
17–18	Appearance of perivascular connective tissue septa between the parenchymal cords and follicles; pinealoblasts and daughter cells show different degrees of differentiation and enlargement and form perivascular palisades.
19—a few hours after birth (21–23 days)	Rapid growth by cellular proliferation; compaction of the organ with resulting reduction or loss of follicular structure; growth of sympathetic nerve fibers (presumptive nervi conarii) to dorsal and distal edges of pineal.
Postnatal: 0–3	Precipitous fall in mitotic activity and beginning of growth phase due to pinealocyte hypertrophy; penetration of pineal by sympathetic nerve fibers followed by their ramification and the occurrence of their catecholamine-containing terminals around blood vessels and among clusters of parenchymal cells; increased consolidation of a distinct connective tissue (meningeal) capsule around the organ.
3–7	Reduction of the recessus pinealis and gradual separation of the body of the pineal from the recessus as dorsal and distal attachments are maintained with the floor of the confluens sinuum; development of histochemically detectable indoleamine fluorescence in pinealocytes with levels of 5-hydroxytryptamine about 50 percent of adult values; beginning of appearance of sparse degenerating cells of unknown significance.
1–2 weeks	Reduction of mitotic activity to trace levels nearly equivalent to those of the adult; continuation of pinealocyte differentiation and hypertrophy; rapid rise in pineal content of monoamine oxidase and 5-hydroxytryptophan decarboxylase, with the former reaching adult level and the latter attaining approximately 50 percent of the adult level; 5-hydroxytryptamine content rises to adult level; hydroxyindole-O-methyltransferase becomes detectable and rises to about 10–30 percent of the adult level.
2–3 weeks	Pinealocyte hypertrophy continues; rapid increase in and attainment of adult levels by 5-hydroxytryptophan decarboxylase.
3–5 weeks	Pinealocyte hypertrophy continues; attainment of adult levels by hydroxyindole-O-methyltransferase.
9–12 weeks	Gradual cessation of growth and parenchymal hypertrophy.

* Data derived from references[151,161,213,305,425,432,460,498,585,588 323,825,947,1021,1102]

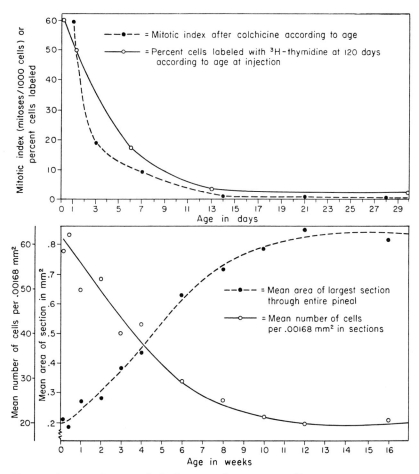

Figure 2. Top. Postnatal decline in the rat pineal's mitotic activity, as studied by two methods. Data for mitotic index after colchicine from Quay and Levine[825] and for percent cells labeled with ^{3}H-thymidine from Wallace *et al.*[1021]

Bottom. Postnatal changes in pineal cross-sectional area and mean number of cells per unit area (replotted from Quay and Levine[825]).

birth; (2) sixteenth day of embryonic life until a few days after birth; (3) birth until nine to twelve weeks later.

Quantitative analyses of postnatal developmental changes in rat pineal mitotic activity have been made by use of two radically different techniques (Fig. 2, top). Quay and Levine in 1957[825] reported changes in pineal mitotic activity revealed by injection of colchicine, which interrupted mitoses and allowed an accumulation of mitotic figures during the timed postinjection period. Recently Wallace and co-workers[1021] reported changes in pineal proliferative activity revealed by injection of tritiated ($= {}^3H$) thymidine and quantitative autoradiography. The results of the two studies are essentially in agreement, as far as the timing of the postnatal fall in the mitotic activity and the low adult levels are concerned (Fig. 2, top). The results of either method may be imperfect, however, as a basis for calculation of absolute mitotic activity at any particular time without additional studies. The investigation using colchicine employed mitotic counts in pineals fixed during the morning, eighteen hours after the injection of colchicine during the previous afternoon. It has been shown subsequently by Quay and Renzoni[826] that maximal mitotic activity, at least in the adult rat pineal, occurs near midday, the time of day not included in the period of mitotic arrest and analysis in the previous study. Furthermore, as a mitotic arrest drug or stathmokinetic agent for some kinds of cells, colchicine is suboptimal in its properties. Thus, in some tissues following colchicine, arrested metaphases may degenerate prior to fixation or the metaphase arrest may be incomplete.[238,960] Although colchicine has been found to come close to meeting the basic requirements of a stathmokinetic agent in studies of intestinal mitoses,[960] its degree of success may possibly be different in the case of the pineal. Further studies of its actions on pineal and other neuroectodermal cells are needed, along with evaluation of other arrest agents that may be closer to the ideal in their actions and effectiveness in these tissues.

The autoradiographic technique for detecting and counting mitotic cells also depends upon certain assumptions the validity of which has not been tested for the pineal and which has been questioned in the case of some other kinds of mammalian cells. It is assumed that: (1) a single injection of ${}^3H$-thymidine remains available in the animal for a limited time; (2) that only those cells in the S *phase* (DNA synthetic phase prior to division) at the time of injection will take and retain the radiochemical; and (3) that DNA is metabolically stable to the extent that the incorporated ^{3}H-thymidine is lost only when the cell divides and half of its thymidine is passed to each daughter cell. Wallace and coworkers[1021] believed that their value of 60 percent labeled cells in pineals of rats 120 days after injection of neonates with tritiated thymidine provided an underestimation of the real pineal mitotic activity. This was based on consideration of two possible factors: (1) loss of label through time as a result of supposed repeated cell divisions and label dilution; and (2) incomplete representation of mitotic cells due to the likelihood of only some of the cells being in the S (DNA synthetic) phase during exposure to the single injection of ^{3}H-thymidine. However, some other possibilities may be cited, and these may be interpreted as possibly leading to an overestimation of pineal mitotic activity. In organs, including the brain, in which mitoses are either very rare or practically absent, Pelc[726] has shown with adult mice killed at different times after injection of ^{3}H-thymidine, significant numbers of labeled cell nuclei. He suggested that in such tissues of adults, cells may periodically renew their DNA by a process whose nature and details are still unknown. Study of the possibility of tritiated thymidine being taken up by neuronal mitochondria has shown a less than 1 percent labeling of these axons.[563] Another potential source of concern is the effect of the radiation on the living cells. While doses (0.05–0.10 μc/g) usually adequate for autoradiography have not been found to produce any detectable radiation injury, there is no independent proof that there may not be caused some as yet unappreciated perturbation of cell proliferation, according to Cronkite and co-workers.[182] It may be noted that the rats in the pineal autoradiography study by Wallace *et al.*[1021] received intraperitoneal injections of ^{3}H-thymidine at a dose level of 10.0 μc/g body weight. Thus for a variety of technical reasons, some of which we have noted above, it is possible that estimates of pineal mitotic activity are apt to be slightly low if based solely on the results from application of colchicine and possibly either low or high if based solely on labeling with tritiated thymidine.[164,340,727]

Obviously needed are additional studies of the effects, temporal relations and turnover of tritiated thymidine, particularly in relation to the responses and fates of specific cell types.

At this stage of our review of pineal development and maturation in the rat, it may be appropriate to note a transitory kind of cellular degeneration that occurs between three days and three weeks after birth.[825] During this period, scattered and sparse cells in the pineals of untreated, as well as colchicine-injected animals, are involved in a peculiar process of degeneration. The nucleus of each degenerating cell is connected to that of a normal cell by a slender strand of material. The cytoplasm of the ovoid degenerating cells is clear and the nucleus is progressively more pyknotic in the older animals up to two or three weeks postnatally. By a few weeks later such cells are undetectable, having been resorbed or phagocytized. Such closely timed cellular deaths are a normal occurrence in embryonic tissue systems. Although far fewer in relative numbers, these transient degenerating pineal cells resemble superficially transient degenerating cells in spinal cord and ganglia of chick embryos, as described by Hamburger and Levi-Montalcini.[366,554] Similar phenomena have been described in spinal ganglia of diverse vertebrates including man and in the frog retina.[324] This process in the ganglia coincides with the differentiation of early neuroblasts and in the retina coincides with the differentiation of the three primary cell layers. In the rat pineal also, this process seems to occur during the period of histogenesis and differentiation of major types of neuroectodermal cells. The ontogenetic significance of these abortive cells and the inductive, humoral or other agents possibly responsible for them remain unknown. Reviews by Glücksmann[324] and Saunders[887] may be consulted for additional information.

Continued postnatal growth of the rat pineal through the agency principally of increase in size of the parenchymal cells was noted by Izawa.[432] He found that between the ages of twenty and one hundred fifty days the number of parenchymal cells per unit area decreased one third, while the weight of the pineal nearly doubled. Although the number of neuroglial cells increased during this period, they comprised only from about 2 to 12 percent of the cells, and microscopically it was evident that most of the pineal growth was due to parenchymal cell hypertrophy. A subsequent quantitative analysis of these events in the postnatal rat pineal was presented by Quay and Levine and is reproduced in modified form in Figure 2 (bottom). Essentially similar results and plots of rat pineal growth and cell density have been published subsequently by other investigators. [152,866,1021] At nine to twelve weeks after birth the size of the parenchymal cells, the cell density and the size of the pineal are shown to have attained adult values (Figure 2, bottom).

Postnatal growth of the rat pineal has been studied also on the basis of changes in pineal weight.[213,432] In these studies, plots of pineal weight according to age suggest fluctuations or departures from a smooth linear or curved line for mean values. Des Gouttes[213] showed falls in pineal weights at six to seven, ten to eleven and sixteen to nineteen days and primarily rising weights at the other intervals. Izawa[432] found a dip in pineal weights between thirty and sixty days. These fluctuations have not been confirmed as yet by other investigators and are not reflected to any statistically significant degree in the available data on pineal mitoses and growth in linear dimensions. Some doubt surely remains concerning the age dependency of these fluctuations in mean pineal weights until confirmatory studies are made. The quantitative and statistical evidence presented for the fluctuations is as yet incomplete and possible contributions of other biological factors such as differences in litter size and precise time of autopsy within the daily photoperiod, are still open to speculation.

Commonly agreed upon, however, is the attainment of adult or plateau levels in pineal size, weight, cytology and chemistry by nine to twelve weeks after birth. As we shall see in later chapters the chemistry and metabolism of the pineal in adult and older rats are consistent with the belief in continued pineal activity or function through adult life. Published reports relevant to possible changes in cell numbers and cytological *structures* in older rats are still rather subjective and unsupported by quantitative analyses. Various environmental factors and experimental treatments have been shown to be capable of modifying pineal volume or weight in postnatal and in adult rats. But, no study has provided any evidence of either a significant, experimentally produced increase in pineal cell numbers in the adult, or a significant decline in pineal cell numbers in old age or after experimental manipulations. On the basis of presently available data, it is possible to account for changes in pineal size in adult rats primarily by volumetric changes within its individual cellular and tissue constituents rather than by changes in its numbers of pinealocytes or other cell types. The early postnatal decline in mitotic activity, the extremely low mitotic activity in the adult and the lack of either regenerative capacity or nonmalignant hyperplastic responses in the adult suggest that the mammalian pineal, and particularly its population of parenchymal cells, resembles the central nervous system and its neurons in its greatly attenuated capacity for adult growth by increase in number of cells.

Izawa[432] noted that pineal weights from his rats were slightly less in females than in males when compared as absolute weight, but they were slightly greater (3.4%) in females when compared in proportion to body weight. He found a 2.6 percent greater female pineal weight in relation to body weight in the data from another investigator. However, Quay and Levine were unable to find any sexual differences in pineal growth measurements, nor any significant pineal changes that could be correlated with puberty. Furthermore, no significant differences in pineal mitotic activity were found in: (1) eight week old males, castrates and normals, some of each injected daily for four days with 5.0 mg testosterone; (2) four week old males and females, some of which were injected daily for four days with 17β-estradiol; and (3) littermates sixty days old, some of which received multiple injections of 17β-estradiol starting either five or twenty-five days after birth.[825]

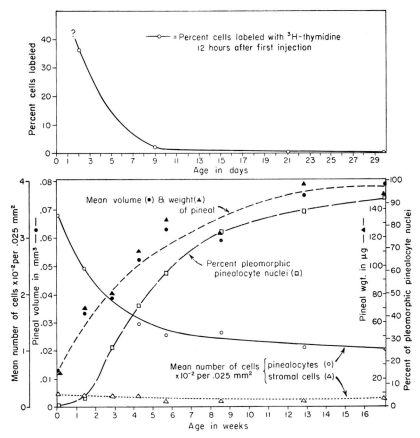

Figure 3. Top. Postnatal decline in the mouse pineal's mitotic activity, as revealed by autoradiography following injection of ^{3}H-thymidine (data from Dill and Walker[220]).

Bottom. Postnatal changes in mouse pineal characteristics (data from Ito and Matsushima[428]).

Mouse

Pineal development and growth in laboratory mice (*Mus*) have been studied during the postnatal period and show temporal patterns of change very similar to those described for the laboratory rat (*Rattus*), as might be expected for this closely related murine rodent (Fig. 3). The postnatal mitotic activity, studied recently by Dill and Walker[220] using the autoradiographic method, shows the same rapid decline. There is a suggestion, however, that the final fall of mouse

pineal mitotic activity to trace or adult levels may lead by
several days that of the rat pineal (compare top portions of
Fig. 2 and 3). More data are needed in order to verify this.
But, if we look at the mouse pineal's postnatal volumetric and
cytologic changes, as recently described by Ito and Matsushima,[428] we find additional evidence for a possible but
slight precocity in differentiation and maturation (compare
bottom portions of Fig. 2 and 3). Additional points of interest
in the normal development of the mouse pineal shown in
Figure 3, bottom, are: (1) increasing pleomorphism of
pinealocyte nuclei; (2) relative constancy of stromal cell density as the size of the organ increases; and (3) a suggestion
of growth stasis between forty and sixty days. Nuclear
pleomorphism in pinealocytes takes the form of nuclear
creasing, folding and general irregularity in shape. Analogous
nuclear transformations have been described as well in a great
many other kinds of secretory cells in animals. Especially
when supported by cytochemical and other kinds of evidence,
such nuclear pleomorphism in glandular cells may be diagnostic of a differentiated and functionally active state. Nuclear
pleomorphism in adult pinealocytes is common in numerous
kinds of mammals,[84] but quantitative study of its development
is apparently limited to that recently presented by Ito and
Matsushima[428] for the laboratory mouse.

Relative constancy of stromal cell density during pineal
growth is probably another general characteristic of the early
postnatal life of mammalian pineals of different species.
Notable too in the mouse pineal, as well as in those of mammals of greater body size, is an estimated 10 percent final
concentration of stromal cells in the fully differentiated adult
organ.

A stasis in the mouse pineal growth near or following the
time of puberty has been suggested and is indicated in Figure
3 by the plotted means for pineal volume and weight.[428] Since
the supporting data are still statistically and biologically
inconclusive, the curve describing pineal growth in Figure
3 is smoothed and does not follow a course from one mean
to the next. It does remain within the limits of the standard
deviations, however. Added evidence for a possible gonadal

effect on pineal growth has been provided more recently, however, by Ito and Matsushima.[430] Gonadectomy at thirty-five days, especially of female mice, led to a 20 percent increase in pineal volume over controls at 120 days of age. Described also was a highly significant and 37 percent decrease in mouse pineal volume by 120 days after hypophysectomy at ninety days. Both volumetric effects are believed, on the basis of cell density measurements, to be due to changes in the size of the pinealocytes rather than in their numbers.[430] Daily injections for one to five days of "estrogen" ($4\mu g$) and/or progesterone (1.25 mg) to adult ovariectomized mice failed to provoke pineal mitoses detectable by the autoradiographic method.[220]

Domesticated Species

Non-laboratory domesticated species of mammals of larger body size have not been sufficiently studied by quantitative methods to trace the development and maturation of the pineal. This is inspite of the fact that the life span, some features of pineal histology and certain other biological characteristics of these animals come closer to those of man than to do those of laboratory rats and mice. Early and detailed descriptions of the morphogenesis of the pineal in a number of different species are available.[384,518,986-988] Available studies of pineal histogenesis in these species are often less helpful, being without measurements and without essential evidence for some of the inferences which were made. [445,620] Even in the case of pineal mitotic activity, there is very little precise information. Comments such as those by Bargmann,[84] that in the epiphysis of a four week old dog numerous mitoses were found, indicate at least that postnatal mitotic activity occurs. Quantitative data for pineal growth in domesticated larger mammals is largely limited to postnatal weight changes. Study of pineal weight in 153 sheep and 110 cattle by Santamarina and Venzke[883] revealed attainment of adult pineal weights in two year old sheep and two to three year old cattle (Tables II and III). Possible differences correlated with sex, reproductive activity or castration are suggested by the data for some age groups, but inconsistencies and extreme

Pineal Chemistry

TABLE II
Postnatal weight changes in sheep pineals (mg)*.

Age Group (years)	Females Non-pregnant	Females Pregnant	Males Normal	Males Castrate
1	56.50 ± 12.30	——	——	72.81 ± 28.84
2	95.40 ± 27.32	——	96.64 ± 27.07	101.90 ± 40.38
3	78.33 ± 44.27	98.73 ± 11.21	102.96 ± 40.28	103.32 ± 15.24
4	86.00 ± 18.38	84.76 ± 20.61	87.37 ± 45.78	——
4–11	79.10 ± 25.82	——	——	64.26 ± 23.25

* Data from Santamarina and Venzke.[883]

TABLE III
Postnatal weight changes in cattle pineals (mg)*.

Females Age (years)	Normal	Males Age (years)	Normal	Males Age (years)	Castrate
5/12	78.50 ± 32.38	5/12	79.69 ± 37.61		——
1–2	133.80 ± 24.60	½–1½	160.50 ± 33.90	7/12–1⅓	96.50 ± 21.45
2	161.69 ± 39.58		——		——
3	274.50 ± 78.27		——		——
4	261.37 ± 95.77	2–6	174.00 ± 53.71	2–5	160.50 ± 74.91
5	262.00 ± 88.63		——		——
6	193.66 ± 62.53		——		——
7	178.00 ± 46.69		——		——
8	229.27 ± 73.92		——		——
10–11	238.00 ± 72.83	10	318.00		——

* Data from Santamarina and Venzke.[883]

individual and probable breed variation weaken these suggestions, as far as the available data are concerned. Thus, for example, in castrated male sheep, pineal weights ranged from 22 to 214 mg. Microspically the pineals of older sheep and cattle included some that appear on cytological and structural grounds to be as active as those of two to three year olds.[325,883]

Man

Surprisingly and unfortunately, quantitative data on human pineal development is limited to morphological descriptions of early stages and weights and grosser histological features in postnatal and usually considerably advanced ages. Pineal embryonic and fetal morphogenesis in man was reviewed briefly earlier in this chapter. Original articles can be consulted for details.[65,317,321,323,389,402,517,697,698] Adult form and nearly adult size of the pineal are evident in the newborn. But, information on mitotic activity is lacking. Also deficient is quantitative information about human pineal characteristics around the time of birth and the first months of postnatal life. Cytological descriptions of infants' pineals suggest that pinealocyte differentiation may extend postnatally from a few months to several years, with complete differentiation by five to seven years after birth.[1018] This is in harmony with recent findings concerning enzyme activities in human pineals, which are considered in detail in later chapters. No significant differences in levels of pineal enzyme activity occur between the three to twelve year old and older age groups when hydroxyindole-O-methyltransferase, monoamine oxidase and histamine-N-methyltransferase are measured.[1075]

The only published anatomical measurements which may be related to human pineal growth and maturation are pineal weights from miscellaneous autopsies. Most commonly cited are the sets of weights published over forty years ago by Uemura and Berblinger.[104,993] The 210 weights resulting from pooling their data reveal an approximately 40 percent increase between the first and seventh decades and a subsequent marked decrease (Fig. 4, top). Profound individual variation and irregularity or inconsistency, as far as sexual differences are concerned, provide the other major impressions obtainable from the data. A more recent study based on 147 autopsies confirmed correlation of pineal weight with age, but failed to find correlations with body weight, brain weight, sex or color.[853] There is general agreement that pineal weights are similar in children and in the elderly.[104,188,853,993] Some question may be warranted, however, concerning the age-relatedness of the larger and heavier pineals of the late adult years. Cystic enlargement sometimes occurs.[151] Furthermore, a significant number of the larger pineals during these years occur in patients with malignancies (Fig. 4, bottom).[853] The attach-

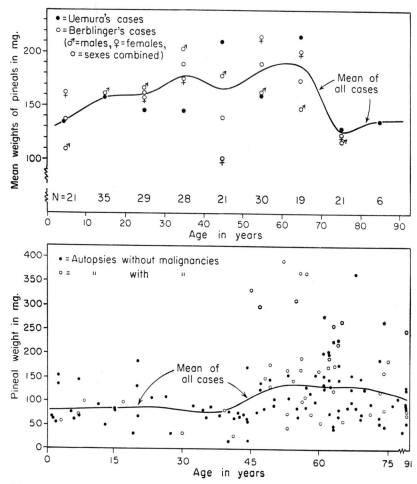

Figure 4. Top. Mean weights of 210 human pineals according to decade of life (N = number of cases per decade; data from Uemura,[993] and Berblinger[104]).

Bottom. Distribution of individual human pineal weights according to age and presence or absence of malignancies of all kinds at death (data from Rodin and Overall[853]).

ment of any cause and effect relationship to this circumstance is premature at this time. Rodin and Overall[853] have discussed some of the possibilities, including: (1) individuals with large pineals are some susceptible to malignancy; and (2) malignancy in some manner affects pineal function. Periodic attempts to attribute some antitumor potency to the pineal have not been confirmed or encouraged by recent experimental assays.[457] Future gathering of human autopsy data relevant to possible correlations of pineal weight with age and other factors should value the provision of data on life habits and specific therapy in the premortem period, and also the possible contributions of edema and secondary metastases to pineal increases in size or weight. Metastasis to the pineal is not uncommon. Numerous cases have been reported in detail. In these, tissue sources were diverse and clinical signs of intracranial lesions often absent.[364,701,706] A famous example of a large human pineal is one that weighed 1.0 gram and was derived from a seventy-five year-old man.[84] Return to the original description of the case, however, reveals that the pineal may have been augmented by metastasis from a lung carcinoma.[98]

CONCLUSIONS

1. Pineal morphogenesis occurs during embryonic and fetal life.

2. Proliferation of pinealocytes, or pineal-specific parenchymal cells, drops rapidly after birth.

3. Significant postnatal pineal growth to adulthood and old age is mainly by pinealocyte hypertrophy and secondarily and variably by increase in glial and stromal tissues or their products.

4. Neither significant increase in pinealocyte numbers nor pineal regeneration has ever been demonstrated in any adult mammal. In this regard mammalian pineal growth and regenerative capacities are like those of the central nervous system.

5. Pinealocyte differentiation and attainment of adult pineal size and biochemical characteristics occur during a postnatal period of several weeks to several months or years depending on the species. These processes of differentiation and maturation are complete near the time of puberty in laboratory rodents and possibly in sheep and cattle. But, in man they antedate puberty by many years.

6. There is still no consistent or statistically significant evidence that any phase of pineal development in any mammal is affected directly and specifically by gonadal or reproductive activities.

7. Regressive phenomena in mammalian pineals are of two kinds: (a) sparse cellular degeneration during the histogenetic phase of pineal development, observed in the rat; and (b) reduction of pineal weight in old age to the mean levels of infants or subadults, but without loss of biochemical capacities. Both phenomena have their counterparts in other active regions or derivatives of the nervous system, and their pineal occurrence is not inconsistent with pineal functional activity throughout adult life.

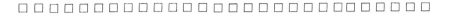

Chapter Two

ANATOMY

BASIC RELATIONS AND STRUCTURE

Anatomical Relations

MAMMALIAN PINEALS are median and compact organs. They usually lie close to their point of origin between the habenular and posterior commissures (Fig. 5). This is the situation in man, dog, sheep, cattle and many others. However, in some but not all kinds of rodents variable amounts of the pineal body become drawn out from the roof of the diencephalon during development, perhaps due to an early and firm meningeal attachment of the pineal in these species to what is destined to become the floor of the sinus rectus and confluens sinuum. In the laboratory rat this leads to a complete separation of the pineal body from the roof of the diencephalon, but for a few aberrant loops of nerve fibers from the habenular and posterior commis-sures.[460,463-465] In this species the detached and relatively superficial position of the organ appears made to order for study of the effects of pineal removal (= pinealectomy). In a number of other rodent species an appreciable amount of pineal tissue may remain at the basal intercommissural position and an additional amount may be strung out either continuously or discontinuously between the basal and distal sites.[767,786] Thus, pinealectomy performed in a manner analogous to that sufficient for laboratory rats (*Rattus norvegicus*) will be incomplete in such species. There is evidence, however, that cytologically and physiologically the distal and basal portions of the pineal in these species are not exactly equivalent.[767,786] Although pinealocytes occur in

21

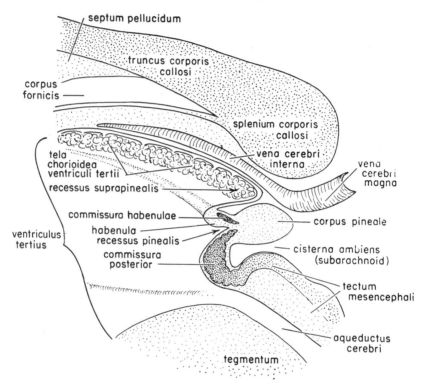

Figure 5. Anatomical relations of a human and generally typical mammalian pineal as seen in a sagittal section of the brain.

both portions, cytological response to environmental photoperiod is more notable in the distal one, at least in the only species (*Peromyscus leucopus*) studied in this regard.[767]

Close anatomical relations between pineal and the third ventricle occur in many mammals. This comes about through the agency primarily of two posterior and median projections of the third ventricle, the recessus pinealis between the commissures and at or near the place of the embryonic epiphyseal evagination, and the recessus suprapinealis or dorsal sac anterior and dorsal to the habenular commissure. Both of these diverticula are quite modest in size in man. This is seen in Figure 5 and can be appreciated, as well, in lateral view x-ray ventriculograms of the pineal region. Even among primates, however, there is pronounced variation from one species to another in the sizes of these ventricular extensions and their degree and extensiveness of union with the pineal.[518,804,810,950] Neither functional significance nor pathways for supposed pineal secretory activity have been demonstrated for these ventricular relations of the pineal in mammals. In all adult mammals at least the majority of the pinealocytes are remote from any extension of, or secretory pathway to, the third ventricle.

Pineal innervation in mammals is exclusively autonomic. With the possible exception of some of the fibers in some kinds of lower primates, this autonomic innervation is currently believed to be entirely sympathetic.[466,542] Studies, especially by LeGros Clark[542] and Kappers[460,463,464] have demonstrated that the pineal nerve fibers originating from the habenular and posterior commissures are merely aberrant loops passing through the organ and lacking synaptic relations enroute (Fig. 6), with the possible exception of a few basal commissural fibers having synaptic relations with ependymal structures near or on the recessus pinealis.[409,542,1093]

Mammals, unlike vertebrates of several other Classes, have no sensory or afferent nerve fibers from the pineal extending into the central nervous system. According to most of the recent research on the subject all of the mammalian pineal's nerve fibers are efferent in relation to the nervous system and innervate pineal vasculature and parenchymal cells. These fibers are mostly, if not entirely, sympathetic postganglionic axons from the plexus caroticus internus and the ganglion cervicale supericus (superior cervical sympathetic ganglion) (Fig. 6). This conclusion is supported by the degeneration of the fibers following superior cervical ganglionectomy, usually studied in the rat, and by the histochemical and biochemical results we shall review in later chapters concerning monoaminergic and cholinergic transmitters and enzyme systems. In various kinds of monkeys and related lower primates, but not in man or anthropoids or other mammalian groups, there are large numbers, up to two thousand, of neuron cell bodies within the pineal.[369,509,542,558] The most common interpretation of these at this time is that they are peripherally

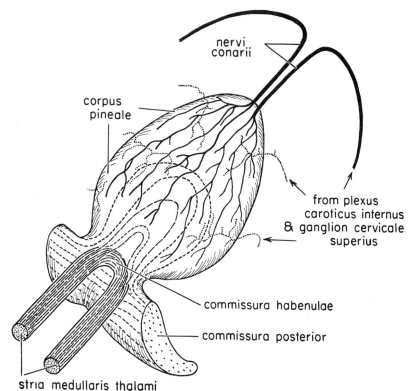

nervi conarii

corpus pineale

from plexus caroticus internus & ganglion cervicale superius

commissura habenulae

commissura posterior

stria medullaris thalami

Figure 6. Anatomical relations and sources of the pineal nerve fibers found in most mammals, including man.

placed sympathetic postganglionic multipolar neurons contributing to pineal efferent innervation.[463-466] Furthermore, it might be noted that the possibility of additional intracranial distributions of such cell bodies along the sympathetic fibers and plexuses to the pineal region remains open since systematic or complete microscopic study of these has never been accomplished. This possibility is supported by Mitchell's[645] review and research concerning the intracranial extremities of the sympathetic trunks. He suggested that the true cranial extremities of the sympathetic trunks are within the skull in relation to a cranial ganglion impar and that the nervi and plexus caroticus internus, with their contained groups of discrete ganglion cells, are not postganglionic fibers of the superior cervical ganglion but are at least in part a cephalic segment of a preganglionic and sympathetic trunk distribution.

An alternative interpretation of pineal innervation in monkeys has been presented by Kenny[480] who studied the effects of sectioning the greater superficial petrosal nerve in two animals. From apparent degenerative changes within the pineal neuropil and nervus conarii, he concluded that the nerve cells and preganglionic fibers, in these structures respectively, belong to the parasympathetic division of the autonomic nervous system. More extensive and detailed supporting studies are needed, however, in order to substantiate this interpretation.

Nevertheless, whatever their sources may be, the nerve fibers distributing and ramifying within the pineal are of two anatomical categories. A diffuse and perhaps primitive system found in all species consists of small fibers accompanying blood vessels (dotted fibers in Fig. 6). A variably consolidated and apparently derived system is found in some mammals, including rodents and primates. This consolidated fiber system enters the posterior pole of the organ when the pineal is basal in position, as it is in man and other primates. It forms a median nervus conarii. A presumably homologous consolidated fiber system enters bilaterally the posterolateral corners of the organ, when the pineal is distal in position as it is in the laboratory rat. In this case we have paired nervi conarii. According to the results of unilateral superior cervical ganglionectomy on these fibers within cat pineals, innervation of the pineal is primarily homolateral with the exclusion of only a few crossing fibers.[856] In animals having a single and median nervus conarii the portion of the nerve distal to the pineal lies within or adjacent to the wall of the straight sinus (Fig. 8).[460,542] At a further point in animals with a single nervus conarii there is presumably a bifurcation at which bilateral portions of the nerve fuse, having ascended from each side within the tentorium cerebelli, the dense layer of supporting tissue between the cerebellum and the cerebral hemispheres. In animals like the rat, having paired nervi conarii, the bilateral passage of the nerves from tentorium to the pineal is shorter and more direct.

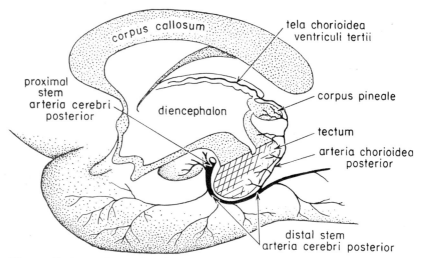

Figure 7. Arterial supply of the pineal from the arteria cerebi posterior (adapted from Kaplan and Ford[459]).

Blood is supplied to the pineal by small arteriolar branches from offshoots of the posterior choroid arteries (= arteria chorioidea posterior). Two posterior choroid arteries branch off from the posterior cerebral artery (= arteria cerebri posterior) lateral to the cerebral peduncle (Fig. 7). The lateral one of the two posterior choroid arteries supplies the choroid plexus of the lateral ventricle within the cerebral hemisphere of that side, and the medial one of the posterior choroid arteries supplies the choroid plexus of the roof of the third ventricle and dorsal sac and, in addition, the pineal organ and neighboring tissues.[542,569,1014] There is no specific pineal artery or even any specific group of pineal arteries or arterioles. A scattered and variable distribution of small penetrating arterioles over the pineal's connective tissue capsule appears to be the general rule for mammals. These do not extend far within the organ, but within a short distance lead into a capillary or sinusoidal capillary plexus. The arterioles supplying the pineal are not accompanied closely by veins or venules, and do not appear to be involved in the kind of portal supply system connecting the hypothalamus with the hypophysis.

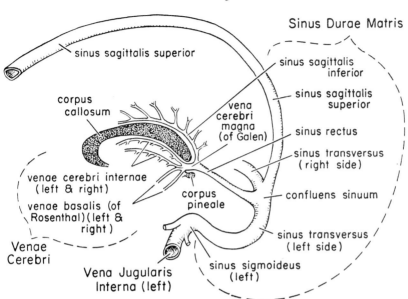

Figure 8. Anatomical relations of the human pineal to the deep cerebral veins (venae cerebri) and the dural venous sinuses (sinus durae matris).

Blood within the pineal is contained by the capillaries and venules which are of microscopic size but numerous. These drain into larger venules that course beneath the capsule of the organ before passing through the adjacent meningeal tissue and eventually into the larger veins or dural venous sinuses of the vicinity.[1014] In man this means into the great cerebral vein (= vena cerebri magna of Galen, Fig. 8) and thence through the sinus rectus, confluens sinuum, sinus transversus, sinus sigmoideus and internal juglar vein. Thus, as on the arterial side, the venous side of pineal vasculature is represented by several or numerous small vessels of variable exact position and number. Vascular variability in the pineal region characterizes as well the anatomical relations of the larger veins and sinuses. This can be seen both in comparisons between different kinds of laboratory mammals,[97,1014] and within a single species such as man.[403,440,569] Angiographic studies employing x-rays have been of the greatest value in demonstrating variations in the vascular patterns of the human pineal region. Diagnosis and localization of tumor masses of the pineal region by deflection or distortion in the courses of the major vessels of the region were the primary interests in such studies.[440,569] However, application of pineal region angiographic analysis to future studies of pineal chemistry *in vivo* is worthy of consideration. Perhaps only by cannulation of pineal blood supply and drainage can we appraise pineal metabolism *in vivo* and its chemical additions to the blood passing through it. Such studies have not yet been reported.

The pineal has a critical anatomical position in relation to intracranial venous drainage. At least in man and some other mammals, it lies close to the union of the outflow from the deep cerebral veins with the median and deep dural venous sinuses (Fig. 8). Pineal tumors often restrict or divert this venous outflow by compression of the great cerebral vein or adjacent parts of the venous system against the splenium of the corpus callosum (Fig. 5).[97,569] Although little is known about the normal dynamic controls of venous pressure and flow in these deep vessels, there is no consistent or good evidence that the pineal has any direct physical action in this system normally. Speculations have been made to the effect that the pineal or a neighboring arachnoid structure[542] may have a valvular or pressure dependent role in regulation of venous blood flow in this region. These ideas are contradicted by extensive angiographic evidence,[440] but remain to be tested directly by appropriate experimentation.

Histology and Cytology

Pineal cellular contents and major tissue constituents have been outlined already to a limited degree in our description of pineal development above and in Figure 1. It is important to realize that some knowledge of pineal histology and cytology is necessary in order to understand and evaluate information on pineal chemistry. The chemistry of any particular pineal is a function of the relative numbers and activities of its cells and the distribution and quantitative relations of its major tissue types. Quantitative differences of these kinds occur between different species and, in at least some species, occur according to age. Qualitative differences according to species or age are more subtle and difficult to establish. The major pineal tissue divisions of neuroectodermal parenchymal lobules and mesodermal stromal connective tissue and capsule occur throughout mammals (Fig. 1).[786] There are, however, species and sometimes individual differences in the relative quantitative distribution of these and other tissue categories within the pineal. Thus, human pineals, as well as those of many other species, have a greater number and percent composition of myelinated nerve fibers in the more basal region (Fig. 6). This would be reflected in chemical analyses of basal, as compared with distal, portions of pineal bodies. This basal region of greater nerve fiber content is not sharply defined but rather in this and other internal differences in pineal tissue composition presents a gradient. In no way does the mammalian pineal present functional divisions like a *pars nervosa* and *pars glandularis*, such as occurs in the hypophysis.[860] A different kind of functional differentiation of basal and distal parts of the pineal occurs in some rodents in which cellular response to photoperiod is most notable in the distal part.[767]

Besides the basal to distal gradient in pineal composition there is often a cortical to medullary gradient. A subcapsular cortical zone can be noted on the basis of greater relative content of neuroglial cells and stromal elements and lesser relative content of pinealocytes, as compared with deeper or medullary parts of the organ. This histological gradient is perhaps most easily recognized in some adult ungulates and lagomorphs but can be recognized in examples from other groups including primates. Some cytological evidence has been found, too, showing that in the laboratory rat cortical and medullary pinealocyte populations may differ at least statistically in their degree of response to light and twenty-four hour rhythmic changes.[781,826] In this case, the more central or medullary pinealocytes show the greater change following continuous light or during daily twenty-four rhythms.

Ultrastructure

Studies using electron microscopy have provided two major kinds of information relevant to pineal chemistry, (1) demonstration of localization of chemical constituents or processes at the subcellular or macromolecular level within pineal tissue, and (2) provision of clues concerning origins, fates and functional relations of the chemical products of the pinealocytes. Ultrastructural cytochemical studies for the localization of pineal compounds represent extensions of both light microscopical cytochemical and more purely biochemical investigations. They will be considered in later chapters in connection with particular classes of pineal compounds. The second kind of electron microscopical information relevant to pineal chemistry, on the basis of it being more simply ultrastructural and descriptive, comes up for consideration both in this introductory and essentially anatomical review chapter and in the final synthesis of information supporting concepts of pineal function and physiology.

The most important pineal feature for both light and electron microscopical studies is the pinealocyte or pineal parenchymal cell. This importance is based on the premise that whatever is most specific and distinctive in pineal chemistry and function must reside in cells of this category. A typical pinealocyte is diagrammed in Figure 9. It should be emphasized that this is a composite representation of cells of the category. Such cells have significant structural differences in different kinds of mammals,[429,879,903,1026] and may consist of more than one subtype and show differences according to previous treatment and age. Diverse opinions have been expressed concerning the relative degree of structural resemblance between pinealocytes and basic neuroectodermal cell types, especially neuroglia, sensory cells and neurons. Electron microscopy has strengthened the evidence for sensory and neuronal resemblances and at least in some species for an endocrine secretory activity. Like neuronal cells, pinealocytes often have two or more cellular or cytoplasmic processes, numerous subsurface cytoplasmic cisterns, microtubules, vesicles of various descriptions, organelles for active oxidative metabolism and protein synthesis and at least portions of structures usually associated with synaptic contacts in central nervous or retinal tissues. The cytoplasmic processes sometimes include shorter and thinner members

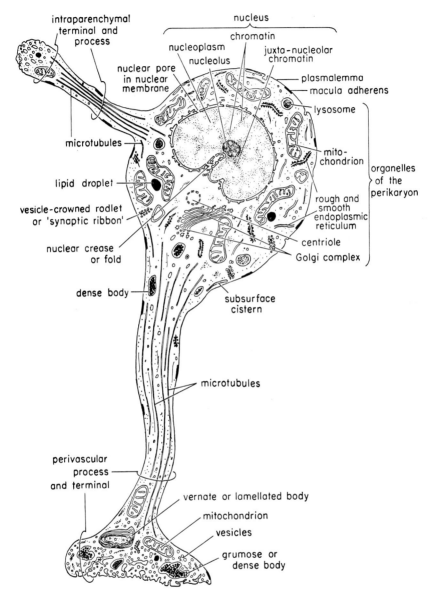

Figure 9. Composite diagram of a typical mammalian pinealocyte. Some liberties have been taken with the relative sizes of some of the organelles and the representations of various systems of membranes, which are actually double or more complex than shown.

that terminate within the extracellular space within the cluster of parenchymal cells, and longer and thicker members that terminate within or close to the perivascular space surrounding many of the pineal capillaries.[37, 39,854,1026,1056] Evidence for pinealocyte secretory activity and the nature of its secretion precursors is most sharply focused within the large and club or foot-shaped terminals of these perivascular cytoplasmic processes (Fig. 9). Vesicles and grumose or dense bodies are the structures within the processes that are most frequently cited as possible containers of materials to be released or secreted. In some kinds of mammals, and perhaps especially in laboratory rats and mice, the perivascular terminals of the pinealocyte processes end freely in a perivascular space. A thin basal lamina separates this space from the capillary endothelial cell. As in many endocrine glands, the capillary endothelium of the pineal in these same species has thinned areas and fenestrations,[344,347,348,429,643] again suggestive of modification to facilitate passage of secretion into the capillary blood stream. In some other kinds of mammals, the perivascular terminals of the pinealocytes are covered by cytoplasmic processes of the astrocytic glial cells and endothelial fenestration is apparently less common. This is the case for the primate pineals that have been investigated in detail with the electron microscope.[1026]

Other intercellular relations of the pinealocytes are of great functional interest as well. Of these, the possible synaptic contacts are of the greatest concern currently. Within the parenchymal lobules, or clusters of pinealocytes, sympathetic terminals are seen to innervate the pinealocytes.[24,37,1026] The pattern and details of this innervation at the ultrastructural level are not yet worked out. Tantalizing but incomplete evidence exists for some sort of synapse-like relationship between nominal pinealocytes.[37,407,1026] Clusters of cytoplasmic vesicles near the plasmalemma and the *synaptic ribbons* or vesicle-crowned rodlets are such bits of enigmatic evidence (Fig. 9). More often seen are junctional contacts of a presumably more purely structural or supportive type, such as the macula adherens or desmosome (Fig. 9).

CONCLUSIONS

1. Mammalian pineals are median dorsal intracranial organs, but their exact anatomical positions and relations in the adult vary according to genus or species, within primates as well as most other groups.

2. Pineal innervation in mammals is thought to be exclusively autonomic and to consist largely of postganglionic sympathetic fibers from intracranial or superior cervical ganglia bilaterally. No afferent or sensory fibers from the pineal to the nervous system in mammals are known. Intrapineal fibers from habenular and posterior commissures are believed to be merely aberrant loops without synaptic contacts within the organ.

3. Pineal blood supply is by small and variable arteriolar branches of offshoots from the posterior choroid arteries. Within the organ are numerous capillaries and venules. The latter drain into larger venules that course beneath the capsule, and from these blood passes into variable and larger veins that traverse the adjacent meningeal tissue and eventually lead into the larger veins or dural venous sinuses of the vicinity.

4. Within the organ there are sometimes regional differences in quantitative characteristics, relative proportions and apparent responsiveness in tissue and cell components. However, these internal compositional differences are always in the form of subtle gradients, peripheral to central and proximal (basal) to distal, rather than as well defined subdivisions.

5. Electron microscopic studies affirm the uniqueness and probable primary functional significance of the pinealocyte or pineal parenchymal cell category. While showing some ultrastructural resemblance to neuronal and sensory cells, it has the modifications and attributes of a metabolically active endocrine secretory cell. The perivascular terminals of these cells contain grumose or dense bodies and diverse vesicles either or both of which may possibly contain precursors of hormonal secretion.

6. Intercellular relations within the pineal are complex.

Although the electron microscope confirms sympathetic innervation of the pinealocytes and reveals presynapse-like structures within nominal pinealocytes, the organization and dynamics of these are poorly understood.

Chapter Three

INORGANIC CONSTITUENTS

TRACE ELEMENTS

INORGANIC CONSTITUENTS of pineal glands have been studied by pathologists for many years. Such work, nevertheless, has depended largely on qualitative and not always chemically specific techniques and has focused primarily on the pineal concretions (corpora arenacea) and pigment inclusions. Results that have been obtained for the inorganic composition of the pineal concretions are presented in a subsequent section of this chapter, and those that relate particularly to pigment inclusions appear for the most part in Chapter Thirteen.

Scarcely begun is the application of newly perfected and highly sensitive methods for the analysis of trace elements in tissues, including pineal and brain. One such method, neutron activation analysis, has been used recently by Wong and Fritze[1061] with very interesting results. Comparisons of these results with earlier ones based on other methods, and considerations of their possible metabolic and general biochemical meanings, are the chief concerns in the following paragraphs.

Copper

Cattle and pig pineals have relatively high concentrations of copper when compared to different brain regions of the same animals (Table IV). These tabulated and recent results based on neutron activation analysis are lower, however, as far as brain regions are concerned, than those reported previously for the same general regions of human brain, as studied by the colorimetric diethyldithiocarbamate method of Eden and Green.[186,973] It is not known how much of this

TABLE IV
Concentrations of Cu in pineals and brain regions (μg/g dry weight)*.

Region (N) =	Calves (3 mos. old) (1–4)	Cows (2+ years old) (2)	Pig (3 mos. old) (1)
Pineal	19, 21, 25, 42	7.8, 8.6	22
Hippocampus	13	8.9 ± 0.7, 11 ± 2	19 ± 1
Cerebellum (gray matter)	8.2	———	———
Thalamus	7.2 ± 0.1	4.0	9.8
Cerebral Cortex (gray matter)	7.0 ± 1.8	———	———
Midbrain	6.2 ± 0.1	4.4	11
Medulla Oblongata	5.9	4.0	12
Pons	5.9, 7.3, 7.5, 11	2.7 ± 0.5	6.9 ± 1.1
Cerebral Cortex (white matter)	4.8 ± 0.7	2.5	———
Spinal Cord	3.7	———	———
Cerebellum (white matter)	3.3 ± 0.8	———	———

`* Data from Wong and Fritze.[1061]

difference is due to species differences in copper concentration in the brain and how much is due to technical factors. It is known that at least in the liver, the organ of the main reserve of copper, sheep and cattle have higher concentrations than man, pigs, horses and various laboratory animals.[600] Much of the early work and the recent results are in general agreement, nevertheless, that brain copper concentrations are higher in gray matter than in white.[179,186,973,976,1061] The results in Table IV suggest, furthermore, that with the possible exception of the cow hippocampus, diverse brain regions are exceeded by the pineal in copper content. This may be the result in part of the particular selection of brain regions for comparison. Higher contents have been found in the substantia nigra (59.9 μg/g) and locus caeruleus (201.1 μg/g) by the colorimetric procedure.[973,976,1025] Even with allowances for the general lower values (Table IV) reported from the neutron activation method, the value for the locus caeruleus clearly exceeds what might be expected from the pineal by the same colorimetric analytical technique.

Copper is likely to be a functional constituent within all living cells.[600] Its occurrence in specific protein fractions and enzymes in brain is of the greatest interest.[299] This situation may be true possibly of related tissues as well. The high copper content shared by pineal, substantia nigra and locus caeruleus is likely to be based on similarities in contents of copper-containing proteins and enzymes. While further discussion about these compounds in brain tissue is possible, very little can be reported as yet about them in the pineal.

TABLE V
Concentrations of Mn in pineals and brain regions (μg/g dry weight)*.

Region (N) =	Calves (3 mos. old) (1–4)	Cows (2+ years old) (2)	Pig (3 mos. old) (1)
Pineal	2.9, 2.9, 3.2, 3.3	2.2, 2.2	4.2
Cerebellum (gray matter)	2.9	———	———
Hippocampus	1.7	1.4 ± 0.1, 1.6 ± 0.1	1.5 ± 0.2
Thalamus	1.6 ± 0.1	1.0	0.8
Cerebral Cortex (gray matter)	1.3 ± 0.3	———	———
Midbrain	1.2 ± 0.1	1.2	1.2
Medulla Oblongata	1.2	0.9	1.0
Pons	1.0, 1.2, 1.3, 1.3	0.6 ± 0.1, 0.7 ± 0.1	0.7 ± 0.1
Cerebellum (white matter)	1.2 ± 0.3	———	———
Spinal Cord	1.1	———	———
Cerebral Cortex (white matter)	0.7 ± 0.1	0.6	———

* Data from Wong and Fritze.[1061]

Manganese

This trace element also shows a relatively high concentration in the pineal as compared with diverse brain regions (Table V). In this table the manganese content of cattle and pig brains, as measured by the neutron activation method, appears to be close to what has been reported earlier in human and rabbit brain by other methods.[287,299,341] A relatively still higher pineal manganese concentration was found in rabbits by a catalytic microchemical method[286] (pineal 15 p.p.m. in dried tissue; brain 1.6 p.p.m.)[287] By this method, manganese contents of a large variety of rabbit organs were compared. After long bone, the tissues with the greatest manganese contents, in descending order were pituitary (2.4 p.p.m. in fresh tissue), pineal (2.3 p.p.m.), lactating mammary gland (2.2 p.p.m.), liver (2.1 p.p.m.) and so on with many others. In another study it was found that of ocular tissues from oxen, the retina was especially rich in manganese (0.10–0.32 p.p.m. in fresh tissue; 0.82–2.6 p.p.m. in dried tissue).[288] Very little of this was dialysable, and a smaller amount occurred in a fraction containing the photoreceptor cells than occurred in the rest of the retina.

Manganese is indispensable in the mammalian body and is of vital significance for the activity of a number of enzymes. Speculative generalities might be offerred to account for its levels and significance in the pineal gland. But, facts are lacking concerning its chemical associations in this organ.

TABLE VI

Concentrations of Zn in pineals and brain regions (μg/g dry weight)*.

Region (N) =	Calves (3 mos. old) (1–4)	Cows (2+ years old) (2)	Pig (3 mos. old) (1)
Pineal	80, 95, 102, 112	87, 93	72
Hippocampus	70	52 ± 3, 64 ± 3	49 ± 2
Cerebral Cortex (gray matter)	66 ± 10	————	————
Cerebellum (gray matter)	51	————	————
Thalamus	39 ± 1	21	21
Midbrain	36 ± 1	22	26
Medulla Oblongata	39	27	18
Pons	30, 32, 32, 33	16 ± 1, 24 ± 1	17 ± 3
Cerebral Cortex (white matter)	20 ± 2	21	————
Cerebellum (white matter)	19 ± 4	————	————
Spinal Cord	16	————	————

* Data from Wong and Fritze.[1061]

Zinc

Pineal zinc concentrations also are high as compared with those of diverse parts of the brain (Table VI) and, indeed, are high in comparisons with many other organs or tissues. The results for brain zinc contents shown here from the work of Wong and Fritze[1061] and based on neutron activation analysis are comparable in general levels with those obtained by Hu and Friede[412] using atomic absorption spectroscopy. The latter study did not include pineal but contained a topographically more detailed sampling of the brain. In this survey the human Ammon's horn, a subdivision of the hippocampal formation, had a zinc content distinctly greater than what had been observed in cattle and pig pineals by Wong and Fritze.[1061] Combined histochemical and electron microscopic studies of zinc in Ammon's horn show that it is concentrated within the giant boutons or terminations of mossy fibers that synapse with the apical dendrites of the pyramidal cells.[371] Zinc is present in a number of metalloenzymes, but its chemical relations are known neither in Ammon's horn nor in the pineal.

Iron

Iron has been reported in the pineal both as occurring in a free state and in bound forms.[91,761,876,941] The latter include iron-containing pigments and concretions which are primarily of histological and pathological concern and iron-containing enzymes which are of great metabolic importance. Iron-containing pigments have been studied by histochemical techniques and will be reviewed in the chapter on pineal pigments. Chemical analyses revealing iron in pineal concretions will be discussed in the section concerning these structures. Quantitative studies of pineal iron in other chemical associations have not yet appeared.

Other Elements

Calcium and magnesium within the pineal have been studied as components of concretions but not in the rest of the tissue. Molybdenum, iodine, cobalt, aluminum, barium, chromium, titanium, silver, nickel, mercury, strontium and lead are all worthy of analysis in this organ, but published reports have not appeared. A deficiency also exists in published data on levels of nontrace elements, such as sodium and potassium in the pineal.

UPTAKE OF INORGANIC COMPOUNDS

Pineal uptake from the blood stream *in vivo* of various compounds has been investigated by a variety of methods and for quite diverse reasons. The categories of compounds so studied include inorganic salts, dyes, fluorescein-tagged proteins, amines, drugs and radioactive tracers. The organic and macromolecular categories here listed will be considered in later chapters except as they may be relevant to interpretations here of the uptake of inorganic materials.

Studies comparing the blood-tissue barrier systems in pineal, brain and other organs were made by Wislocki and Leduc (1952)[1054] and by Dempsey and Wislocki (1955)[206] using silver nitrate as a vital "stain." Rats were given drinking water containing 1.5 grams of silver nitrate per liter for nine to fifteen months. Fixed tissue sections were examined by light and electron microscopy. Unlike various other parts of the central nervous system, the choroid plexuses, area postrema, intercolumnar tubercle, neurohypophysis and pineal had depositions of silver when so treated. However, in all of these structures the silver was deposited in the basement membrane around the capillary endothelium, in and upon connective tissue cells and fibers forming a loose pericapillary sheath, and in an outer membrane separating this sheath from the parenchymal cells. This demonstrated the less restrictive barrier system in these particular structures as compared with the great majority of brain regions, which failed to show silver deposits. Further evidence of the permeability of pineal capillaries was provided by intraperitoneal injection of trypan blue and its subsequent microscopic localization solely within pineal macrophages and not in the parenchymal cells nor in the connective tissue spaces.[170;1054] Indications that the chemical nature of the dye and the route of injection are significant for the uptake pattern have been provided by more recent studies. Feldberg and Fleischhauer[267] perfused bromophenol blue from the lateral ventricle to the aqueduct of anesthetized cats and found staining throughout the brain's central gray matter and the pineal body, but none in the hypophysis. Klatzo and co-workers[492] conjugated fluorescein isocyanate with bovine albumin (fraction V) and bovine gamma globulin (fraction II) and perfused these materials from the cat lateral ventricle to the lumbar subarachnoid space. The distributions of the fluorescent protein conjugates were studied by fluorescence microscopy. Fluorescein-labeled albumin was found to have penetrated the periventricular gray matter of the brain, and especially in the hypothalamus and in the pineal. Some of the pineal cells were reported to have an intense fluorescence, but no fluorescein-labelled albumin had penetrated the anterior or posterior lobes of the hypophysis.

Alkali metal isotopes

Pineal uptake of radioactive isotopes of rubidium (^{86}Rb) and potassium (^{42}K) has been used in calculations of its blood flow.[326,328] This is one of a series of methods based on physiological principles of exchanges between blood and tissues, blood flow patterns through tissues, and use of an inert but freely diffusible substance as a tracer.[481] ^{86}Rb and ^{42}K are used frequently as such tracers since an almost infinite sink is provided for them by the most frequently studied tissues, such as cardiac and skeletal muscles, and since their exchange between capillary blood and such tissues is a process limited by the rate of local blood flow.[1052] Studies on pineal blood flow by Goldman and co-workers[326,328] have used a variation of Sapirstein's method based on uptake of ^{86}Rb or ^{42}K. The method follows the assumption that the quantity of ^{86}Rb or ^{42}K taken up by an organ is proportional to its blood flow and that the organ has the same extraction ratio toward the labeled, circulating isotope as the body as a whole during the first minute after intravenous injection. In such conditions the ratio between organ uptake and body uptake is equal to the ratio between organ blood flow and cardiac output. However, if, as with brain, the organ fails to retain the isotope after initial delivery, the blood flow is considered to be open to underestimation by this method. When, as with pineal, the organ is non-homogeneous in that the isotope is rejected by one compartment and taken up by another, an initial peaking of the organ's isotope content will be followed by a lower steady state or plateau (Fig. 10). Five seconds after injection of ^{86}Rb solution into a chronically catheterized femoral vein in an anesthetized (pentobarbital) rat, 0.0085 percent of the cardiac output, or 8 percent/gram was found to perfuse or be contained in the pineal. Subsequently the pineal content of ^{86}Rb fell to a plateau (Fig. 10). No sexual differences in this behavior were found in the rats used. A similar plateau (at 3.5 percent/gram) was found between fif-

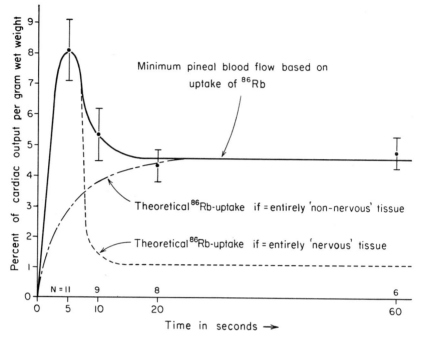

Figure 10. Minimum pineal blood flow in relation to cardiac output in 185–225 gram rats based on fractional uptake of [86]Rb (means ± standard errors; (N) = numbers of animals; data of Goldman and Wurtman[328]).

teen and sixty seconds after injection of [42]K in another strain of rats at rest and without anesthesia.

The results (Fig. 10) were interpreted as suggesting that the pineal is a two-compartment system. The first compartment quickly loses its isotope content, within about ten seconds, either through rejection, as in brain, or through shunting by means of arteriovenous anastomoses, although the latter are not known to exist in the organ. The second compartment extracts or captures the ^{86}Rb and retains it for a minute or longer, as in non-nervous tissues, such as thyroid or heart. Neither structural limits nor correlates of these two theoretical pineal compartments are as yet known.

On the basis of the pineal's plateau level of ^{86}Rb content in relation to cardiac output determined in a separate but comparable group of animals, Goldman and Wurtman[328] estimated minimum pineal blood flow in anesthetized rats to be 2 ml/minute/gram. On the basis of the pineal's peak level of ^{86}Rb content and experience with similar peaks in nervous tissue, they estimated the true blood flow to be at least 4 ml/minute/gram. They concluded that the "minimum rate of rat pineal blood flow per g. exceeds that of most endocrine organs, equals that of neurohypophysis and is surpassed only by that of the kidney."[328] However, it had been shown earlier that the blood content of the rat pineal is only a fifth that of the hypophyseal anterior lobe and a third that of the neurohypophysis.[772] Therefore, it might be concluded that either or both the flow rate or ^{86}Rb extractive capacity of the pineal are high as compared with other endocrine and parenchymal organs. Without additional studies of these processes, however, and especially by other methods and indicators, exact interpretation of the pineal data seems insecure at this time. The complexity and organ-specific peculiarities of results of the ^{86}Rb-uptake method have been experimentally explored and demonstrated in the case of some of the larger organs,[300,956] but have not been critically appraised in the case of the pineal.

Application of the ^{86}Rb-uptake method to studies of possible physiological controls of the pineal has shown that ten days after either bilateral superior cervical ganglionectomy or section of the cervical sympathetic trunk, pineal fractional blood flow or ^{86}Rb uptake was reduced by one-third, and compensatory vasomotor response to pressor quantities of norepinephrine or vasopressin was lost.[326] The fact that results by this method may not be necessarily diagnostic of relative level of functional activity is brought out by application of the method to studies of pituitaries autotransplanted to beneath the kidney capsule. After this procedure the grafted pituitary's fractional ^{86}Rb uptake or minimum blood flow increased to more than three times normal, although there was demonstrated reduction in its size, weight and functioning.[327] This seeming paradox, however, is likely to be due to the overriding effects of trauma or tissue pathology on capillary permeability and physiology within such grafts.

TABLE VII
^{131}I uptake by pineals and thyroids of adult rats on an iodine-deficient diet for about two weeks. Results are expressed as percents of the injected dose of $1.5\mu c$ ^{131}I injected intraperitoneally. Eighteen to twenty animals were killed at each time after injection.

Organ	Percent ^{131}I uptake at:	
	1 hour	24 hours
Pineals (pooled	0.002%	$\pm$ 0.000%
Thyroids (means & ranges)	6.4% (2.3–10.4%)	32% (26–44%)

Isotopic Iodine

Pineal uptake of ^{131}I in both normal and hypophysectomized rats was studied by Reiss, Badrick and Halkerston.[838] One hour after intravenous injection of $2\mu c$ of ^{131}I, radioactivity counts/minute/tissue weight were higher in the pineal than the studied parts of brain and several parenchymal organs, with the exception of the thyroid gland. This general relationship was true also in hypophysectomized animals, but the activity then averaged somewhat greater in the pineal and was markedly reduced in the thyroid. Pineal radioactivity from uptake of ^{131}I was much less than that of the thyroid in normal animals, and it was variable and not significantly greater than that of blood in both normal and hypophysectomized animals. In an unpublished study, Rosenberg and Quay failed to find marked pineal uptake or retention of ^{131}I in adult rats (Table VII). It can be concluded that the pineal does not appear to have a specific and highly active uptake such as that of the thyroid, but that it may possibly have a transient low level uptake relatively greater than that in brain and some other organs. The kinetics and study of such a pineal uptake, however, require an experimental approach and analysis entirely distinct from that usually employed in studies of iodine uptake by the thyroid.

Better evidence exists for appreciable pineal uptake of ^{131}I-labeled thyroid hormones.[284,285]

^{32}P-phosphate

A remarkably high *in vivo* uptake of ^{32}P-labeled inorganic phosphate ($Na_2 HPO_4$) was discovered by Borell and Örström (1945)[128] to occur in the rat pineal, especially in comparisons with different parts of the brain. Contemporary interpretation of such uptake emphasized a close correspondence between it and metabolic rate. Thus, brain was considered to have a lower rate than we now know to be true from a variety of other methods. This was due to the fact that access to intravascular phosphate by most brain tissue regions is normally severely limited by the so-called blood-brain barrier. This barrier, in a gross sense, is much less in the pineal, the choroid plexuses of the brain ventricles, the hypophysis and some hypothalamic nuclei. Although ^{32}P-phosphate is experimentally rapidly taken up by brain *in vivo* from cerebrospinal fluid or intracisternal injection, this is not considered to be a normally significant route for brain phosphate uptake.[3] Inspite of the blood-brain phosphate barrier and the low significance of the cerebrospinal fluid as an exchange route, the central nervous system has a very active phosphorus metabolism. The gist of these considerations, as far as the pineal is concerned, is that relative uptake or retention of ^{32}P-phosphate from the blood stream may not necessarily be indicative of a particular level of either metabolism in general or of phosphorus metabolism in particular.

Uptake of ^{32}P-phosphate by the pineal, as well as by other organs, has been expressed usually in terms of relative specific activity. Specific activity (S. A.) is the amount of radioactivity per unit amount of substance and may be given in a variety of ways, such as counts per minute per micromole (CPM/μmole), millicuries per milligram (mc/mg), disintegrations per minute per millimole (DPM/mmole) and others; thus:

$$\text{S. A. of an organ} = \frac{\text{amount of radioactivity}}{\text{total amount of P}}$$

Relative specific activity (R. S. A.) is calculated with some standard as a reference, such as a diluted sample of the isotope injected or the specific activity of another and possibly metabolically more stable organ from the same animal; thus:

$$\text{R. S. A. of an organ} = \frac{\text{Specific activity of the organ}}{\text{radioactivity (CPM) of a diluted standard solution}}$$

or
$$= \frac{\text{specific activity of the organ} \times 100}{\text{specific activity of a standard organ.}}$$

TABLE VIII

Calculation of relative (^{32}P) specific activity by Borell and Örström[129]

Organ	Radioactivity (impulses per min.)	Total Phosphorus Content (μg)	Specific Activity	Relative Specific Activity
Cerebellum	130	2280.0	0.058	1
Pineal	137	71.5	1.92	33
Blood	800	149.0	5.35	92

The calculation of R. S. A. by Borell and Örström used the cerebellum as a standard, with an arbitrary value of 100[128] or 1.00[129] (Table VIII). Total and radioactive P contents of weighed, pooled tissue samples were determined following complete digestion in sulfuric acid and hydrogen peroxide.[128]

TABLE IX

Total phosphorus contents (as percent of wet weight), specific activities (S. A.) and relative specific activities (R. S. A.) of rat pineal, hypophyseal lobes, brain parts and whole blood.* Animals used in determination of S. A. and R. S. A. were killed (decapitated) 40 minutes after intraperitoneal injection of 0.03–0.04 mc of ^{32}P-sodium phosphate in 1 ml of 5 percent glucose.

Part	Total P	S. A.	R. S. A.
Whole blood	—	19.90 ± 4.35	40.50 ± 6.60
Pineal	0.94	8.20 ± 1.80	26.50 ± 5.50
Choroid plexus	0.92	3.27 ± 0.71	11.20 ± 2.80
Hypophyseal ant. lobe	0.59	2.14 ± 0.42	8.60 ± 1.20
Hypophyseal post. lobe	1.31	2.61 ± 0.53	7.90 ± 1.40
Habenula	—	1.10 ± 0.27	2.68 ± 0.48
Tuber cinereum			
ant. part	0.31	0.39 ± 0.05	1.12 ± 0.15
cent. part	—	0.62 ± 0.12	2.72 ± 0.46
post. part	0.38	0.48 ± 0.11	1.20 ± 0.14
Mammillary bodies	0.40	0.58 ± 0.14	1.49 ± 0.95
Olfactory lobe	0.33	0.41 ± 0.08	1.30 ± 0.17
Medulla oblongata	0.40	0.46 ± 0.10	1.02 ± 0.23
Cerebellum	0.35	0.33 ± 0.05	1.00 − fixed
Thalamus	0.38	0.31 ± 0.07	0.78 ± 0.12
Telencephalon	0.31	0.31 ± 0.06	0.76 ± 0.13
Pons	0.42	0.28 ± 0.02	0.72 ± 0.17
Corpora quadrigemina	0.37	0.27 ± 0.01	0.69 ± 0.07

* Data from Borell and Örström[128,129]

The total phosphorus content of the rat pineal was found to be high, but much more notable were the specific and relative specific activities (Table IX). A high level of pineal uptake of ^{32}P-phosphate was not limited to the rat, since other mammalian species also showed this characteristic (Table X). Phosphate uptake in pineal and other organs, as studied by Borell and Örström, was usually determined forty minutes after intraperitoneal injection of the isotope. If one examines their data for the time course of specific activity changes, it is seen that while pineal specific activity was high in relation to choroid plexus, hypophyseal lobes and parts of brain, it was low in relation to whole blood (Fig. 11). It is also seen (Fig. 11) that there was a greater per cent reduction in pineal specific activity between forty and 145 minutes after injection than in specific activity of choroid plexus or hypophyseal anterior lobe. Examination of the labeling of fractionated pineals forty and 130 minutes after injection showed that most of the radioactivity in the pineal even at forty minutes was in bound fractions and that active turnover occurred in these fractions (Table XI). The turnover was greatest among the phosphorylated derivatives revealed through brief hydrolysis. These were thought to represent intermediates in carbohydrate metabolism, while the components of the fraction precipitated by trichloroacetic acid were thought to represent phospholipids and nucleic acids. It is likely that the free phosphate fraction was overestimated and the fraction freed by ten minute hydrolysis was underestimated in these results (Table XI). This inference is made on the basis of the extreme lability in the reported conditions of many of the expected phosphate esters, such as creatine phosphate, ribose-1-phosphate, acetyl phosphate and others.[337]

Tissue content of ^{32}P-phosphate and its derivatives after intravascular or intraperitoneal administration is the net result of several different factors and general processes and can not be equated uncritically with level of tissue metabolic activity. Four oversimplified categories of factors and processes can be offered in order to facilitate conceptualization: (1) local vascular permeability to phosphate, (2) uptake of phosphate by means of both active and passive processes, (3) tissue binding of phosphate primarily in the course of synthesis of phosphorylated metabolic intermediates, and (4) turnover in relation to bound and unbound phosphate and its passage between cellular, extracellular and intravascular

TABLE X

Relative specific activities in diverse mammalian species (forty min.?) after intraperitoneal injection of ^{32}P-phosphate.* The specific activity of the cerebellum is used as a reference standard for each.

| Species | Number of Animals | Pineal | Organs Hypophysis | | Blood |
			Ant. Lobe	Post. Lobe	
Rat	36	26.5	8.6	7.9	40.5
Guinea pig	3	8.7	—	—	147.0
Rabbit	15	49.5	47.0	35.5	81.0
Pig	1	3.0	1.5	4.9	—
Cat	5	40.5	—	—	134.0

* Data from Borell and Örström.[129]

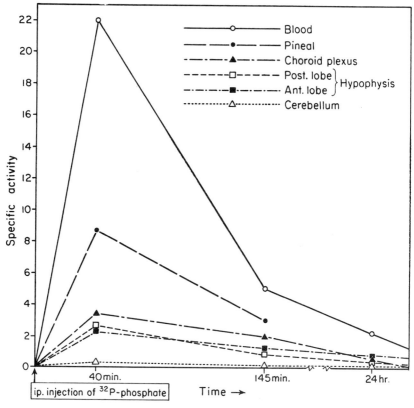

Figure 11. Specific activities of different organs from rats at different times after injection of ^{32}P-phosphate (modified from Borell and Örström[129]).

TABLE XI

Turnover of labeled phosphate fractions in rat pineal and blood as shown by two sampling times after intraperitoneal injection of ^{32}P-phosphate.*

^{32}P-fraction	Pineal Radioactivity	%	Blood Radioactivity	%
	at 40 minutes:			
Free phosphate	357	35	3450	90
Total organically bound phosphate	667	65	398	10
Released by ten minute hydrolysis	463	45	110	3
Residual fraction	167	17	240	6
Precipitated by trichloroacetic acid	37	3	48	1
	at 130 minutes:			
Free phosphate	40	28	2320	43
Total organically bound phosphate	103	72	3080	57
Released by ten minute hydrolysis	14	10	1330	25
Residual fraction	62	43	1550	29
Precipitated by trichloroacetic acid	27	19	198	3

* Data from Borell and Örström.[129]

compartments. The importance of local vascular permeability to phosphate for the uptake or exchange of ^{32}P-phosphate has been shown most clearly for the central nervous system. Trauma of many sorts leads to a prompt and often long lasting increase in the permeability of the blood-brain barrier to ^{32}P-phosphate and an increased isotope concentration in the affected region.[68, 69] The fact that the studies of pineal uptake of ^{86}Rb showed the presence of an impermeable compartment, like nervous tissue, along with a permeable compartment, suggests the possibility that pineal ^{32}P uptake or exchange may to some, but a lesser, degree be affected by capillary permeability changes. Direct experimental proof of this possibility is, however, lacking for the pineal. Likewise, nothing has been done with experimental analysis of transport mechanisms or cellular-compartmental localizations of labeled phosphate within the pineal. Results showing the levels of binding and turnover of ^{32}P are still largely limited to those of Borell and Örström (Table XI). Nearly all of the subsequent studies of ^{32}P uptake by the pineal provide data representing only gross content of ^{32}P at particular times after administration but without information as to chemical fractions or turnover.

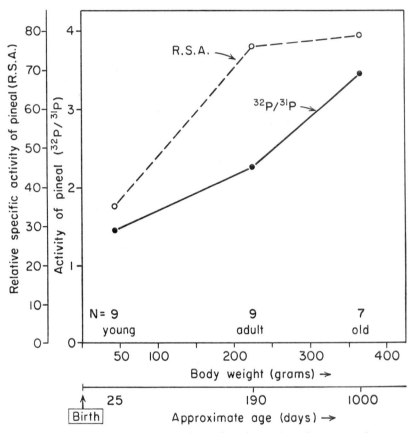

Figure 12. Age changes in pineal uptake of ^{32}P-phosphate in male Wistar rats under identical conditions. Twenty-four hours after intraperitoneal injection of 0.1 μc ^{32}P per gram body weight the animals were exsanguinated and the pineals removed for measurement of radioactivity. Relative specific activities were calculated as percents of radioactivity per mg of pineal to injected radioactivity per mg body weight of the animals (results from De Martino *et al*[204]).

De Martino, *et al.*[203,204] and Cassano, *et al.*[152] showed that pineal content of [32]P 24 hours after injection was greater in adult and old male rats than in young ones (Fig. 12). This is perhaps surprising in view of the more usual pattern with age in different organs, in which the specific activity of the organ's phosphorus decreases, partly because with age decreased turnover of phosphorus usually occurs.[387] The results of De Martino, *et al.* and Cassano, *et al.*[152,203,204] also serve to show that comparisons of pineal uptake or binding of ^{32}P may differ according to whether specific or relative specific activities are used (Fig. 12). Although the dosage of isotope may be adjusted to body weight, this does not insure that the relative distribution, uptake, turnover and binding will be comparable in a specific organ of a series of animals if there are age or physiological differences leading to increased or decreased sequestrations in other parts of the body. Thus, it is difficult without additional kinds of information about body distribution and turnover of ^{32}P to interpret the difference between pineal R. S. A. and ^{32}P/^{31}P ratio in comparing adult and old rats, such as those in Figure 12. Complementing these data from male Wistar rats are earlier data from female Long-Evans and other strains provided by Brewer and Quay.[135] Pineal ^{32}P content in relation to that of cerebellum (R. S. A.) was measured 30 to 40 minutes after intraperitoneal injection of 75–95 μc ^{32}P-phosphate. An increase with age comparable to that shown for male rats in Figure 12 occurred in females from immaturity to adulthood (50–230 days old), but a reduction occurred in old females, but whose ages were not precisely known.

Pineal uptake of ^{32}P in prepubertal rats has been studied by Roth primarily in relation to changes with time of day and exposure to light (Table XII).[865,866] Males injected and killed during the daily period of darkness had a pineal uptake averaging 75 percent greater than that of comparable animals injected and killed during the period of light, and there was no overlap in the individual values between the two groups. Moreover, no difference occurred in the circulating blood levels of ^{32}P of the two groups at the times of autopsy, and the ambient temperature did not fluctuate by more than 3° during the day-night experiment. The hypophyseal posterior lobe, but not the anterior lobe, showed a significant nocturnal rise in uptake also (Table XII). In a related experiment with female prepubertal rats, food and water were withheld for eight hours prior to injection, and individual animals were injected at different times over an extensive period either

TABLE XII

Pineal and hypophyseal specific activities (c.p.m./μg phosphorus) according to time of day and exposure to light.* Prepubertal male and female (26 days old, 65 grams) rats were killed and analyzed two to two and one-half hours after intraperitoneal injection with 50 μg (males) or 40 μg (females) of ^{32}P. Daily photoperiod for males was from 8:00–20:00 (LD 12:12) and for females from 5:00–18:00 (LD 13:11).

Illumination & Time of Injection	N	Pineal	Hypophysis	
			Posterior	Anterior
Males:				
In light 4+ hrs. 12:00–12:30	18–19	238 ± 28	123 ± 20	74 ± 12
In darkness 4+ hrs. 24:00–3:00	17–18	391 ± 23	172 ± 23	79 ± 14
Significance of difference:		P < 0.001	P < 0.001	N. S.
Females†:				
In light 5:00–13:00	14	232 ± 46	95 ± 16	63 ± 12
In darkness 18:00–2:00	14–15	391 ± 134	147 ± 49	59 ± 12
Significance of difference:		P < 0.01	P < 0.01	N. S.

* Data of Roth.[865,866]

† Counts were multiplied by 1.2 to allow comparisons with the data from males.

during the light or the dark phase. Results similar to those from the males were obtained (Table XII). Furthermore, it was noted that the uptake rose rapidly during the first three to four hours after the lights were extinguished and then began a decline which extended through the remaining portion of the dark phase and into the first part of the light phase.[866] This pattern, along with the pineal-^{32}P fractionation studies by Borell and Örström (Table XII), suggests that an increased rat pineal phosphorus metabolism is associated with the daily onset of darkness. This is especially interesting in relation to the sensitivity of some of the pineal's enzymatic and synthetic activities to phosphorylated intermediates and the apparent augmentation of these same activities promptly following the daily onset of darkness. These relationships and data supporting them will be discussed in later chapters.

Experimental studies on factors possibly regulating rat pineal uptake of ^{32}P *in vivo* have failed to delineate any clear relationship beyond that of the day-night difference just discussed (Table XIII). For some treatments, such as blinding, the data are too meager for any decision. For others, such

TABLE XIII

Experiments to modify rat pineal uptake of ^{32}P *in vivo*.

Procedures*	Results†	References
Blinding (1 week)	≟ or n. s.?	129
Hypophysectomy (hypx)		
2 μc ^{32}P iv 40 min.	↑	838
+ ACTH 100 min.	≟ normal	838
250 μc ^{32}P ip 150 min.		
♂s hypx (6–7 weeks)	≟ or n. s.	913
♂s hypx 2 mo., thymectomized 4 mo.	≟ hypx	913
♂s hypx 2 mo., 6x 1 mg chlorpromazine	≟ hypx	565
10 μc ^{32}P/100 g ip 24 hrs.	≟ controls	152
Adrenalectomy (adnx)		
250 μc ^{32}P ip 150 min.		
3 days postoperation	≟ sham & (↑?) normal	564
21 days postoperation	≟ normal	564
+ 6x 1 mg chlorpromazine ip daily	≟ or n. s. adnx	565
Ovariectomy (at 25–53 days)		
75–95 μc ^{32}P ip 30–40 min.		
21–60 days postoperation	≟ sham	135
+ 4x 2 or 4x 250 μg 17β-estradiol	≟ controls	135
+ 3x 5 mg progesterone	≟ controls	135
Orchidectomy		
10 μc ^{32}P/100 g 24 hrs.		
young	≟ normal	152
adult	≟ or n. s.?	152
old	≟ or n. s.?	152
Injections to intact animals		
young—old ♀ s, 4x 17β-estradiol,		
75–93 μc ^{32}P 30–40 min.	≟ controls	135
adult ♂s, 5 mg 5-HT ip 170 min. &		
300 μc ^{32}P 150 min.	≟ normal	567
adult ♂s, 1 or 4x 1 mg chlorpromazine/100 g,		
250 μc ^{32}P ip 150 min.	≟ normal	565
+ "acute stress" (pentobarbital 3 mg/100 g		
285 min., & 20% 3rd degree burn 270 min.)	↑ stress alone	565

* All times denote time of procedure prior to autopsy.

† ↑—significant increase; ≟—not modified; n. s.—not significant.

as hypophysectomy, available results are contradictory and are not resolvable with the data at hand. In view of the widespread effects of hypophysectomy and adrenalectomy on the uptake by other organs examined in the same studies, it is perhaps surprising that so little effect was registered by the pineal.[564,913] Among the treatments having no significant effects, ovariectomy and injections with female sex hormones,[135] are worthy of notice in relation to the often hypothesized physiological interrelation presumed for pineal and gonadotropic activities. Among the few treatments having effects, that involving thymectomy is obscure, as far as possible physiological explanations are concerned. The effect of chlorpromazine, manifest here (Table XIII) only in the case of acutely stressed animals, is interesting in relation to the results of numerous studies on the effect of this and related drugs on ^{32}P uptake and phospholipid metabolism by brain slices.[406] A major effect of chlorpromazine *in vitro* is an inhibition of oxidative phosphorylation, and its other metabolic effects also are largely inhibitory.[764] One of a number of other effects that may be pertinent to chlorpromazine's actions on the pineal is its inhibition of uptake of catecholamine by sympathetic nerves.[431] Nevertheless, simple or sure explanations of its effect on ^{32}P uptake by pineals of stressed rats can not be provided at this time.

Experimental studies using pineal tissue cultures will undoubtedly produce more meaningful results concerning the control and significance of pineal inorganic phosphate uptake. This is indicated by preliminary reports of increased pineal incorporation of ^{32}P into phospholipids when cultures are treated with catecholamines, propranolol and dibutyryl cyclic-AMP.[107,237]

CORPORA ARENACEA

Corpora arenacea (Fig. 13) are calcareous deposits or concretions. They are variable in occurrence within pineal glands of some species, as well as within parts of the brain and other tissues. They are known also as psammoma bodies, acervuli and brain sand. These pineal inclusions have had a long history in medical literature, especially that concerned with possible pathological and physiological correlations. Reviews of the older literature by Bargmann[84] and Heidel[374] and tabulations and references provided by Kitay and Altschule[490] can be consulted by interested readers. The best of now available evidence shows, however, that the classical research predilection for the pineal corpora arenacea was remarkably disparate in relation to their apparently slight biological or functional significance. Their appeal to early investigators probably derived partly from their being one of the few contents of the pineal that was easily analyzed in necropsy specimens and by the methods then available.

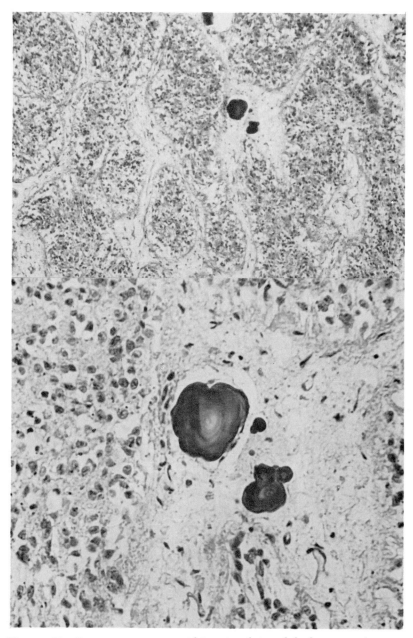

Figure 13. Corpora arenacea within pineal interlobular septa (seventy-seven year old woman, death due to cardiovascular disease and myocarditis). The same tissue section stained with acid alum hematoxylin and eosin is shown in low power above, and higher power below.

Their research appeal probably depended in part, too, on the hope or assumption that they might prove to be indicative of pathological processes of either systemic or pineal-dependent categories. Attempts have been made to use the corpora as evidence of pineal atrophy and involution in man in relation to age changes or disease states. As we shall see, the structure and composition of the corpora, along with their sites of origin, reveal their non-specific and generally benign nature, as far as most human pineal organs are concerned.[962] Furthermore, it will be seen that the presence or absence of corpora within particular human pineals is unrelated to levels of pineal-specific enzymatic activities.

Detection and Occurrence By Age and Species

Two kinds of methods have been used to detect corpora arenacea in pineal organs—microscopy and radiography. Microscopic examination of histological sections stained according to routine methods can reveal satisfactorily corpora several microns in diameter and larger. Corpora are usually intensely stained with acid alum hematoxylin (Fig. 13). They can be stained also by a great variety of other staining procedures.[84,517,560,748,876,1019] Alizarin red and the von Kóssa technique stain the corpora and suggest their content of calcium salts. The corpora are positive (stained red) by the periodic acid-Schiff procedure and are negative or weakly positive for acid mucopolysaccharides.[91,94,224] Fluorescence and polarized light microscopy have been employed also in their study.[94] Complete tally of the corpora arenacea within a pineal by microscopy requires examination of serial sections, since the corpora in some specimens may be rare and restricted to only one small location. More extensive and efficient appraisal is possible by radiological examination. Radiological localization of the human pineal gland by means of its calcareous corpora arenacea has been employed for many years. Radiological demonstration of displacement of the pineal *in vivo* from its normal position has been of diagnostic value where intracranial growths and spatial disturbances might be otherwise more difficult to detect or localize in a general way. Various methods or geometric coordinates have been proposed for the use of the pineal in radiological studies of intracranial displacements.[561,655] Radiological appraisal of pineal calcification or presence of concretions is not as sensitive a method as microscopy since very small, diffuse or few corpora arenacea may not be detected by the usual radiological methods.

Percentage occurrences of corpora arenacea in human pineal glands increase with age, according to the data of many investigators and according to either radiological or microscopic examinations.[84,374] There is, however, great individual variation at all ages in the occurrence or absence of these deposits.[34,962] Moreover, careful microscopic study shows that the pineal corpora arenacea are generally within the glial and connective tissue stroma rather than within the parenchymal lobules (Fig. 13).[152,201] Pinealocytes of normal appearance and having cytological characteristics suggesting an active metabolism are just as readily found in human pineals with numerous corpora arenacea as in those lacking corpora.[34,786] Worthy of notice, as well, is the fact that corpora arenacea and calcareous deposits can be at least as prevalent in other related or similar tissues, such as the choroid plexuses (Table XIV).[907] In these locations, however, they may be more diffuse and hence still allow radiological differentiation of the partially calcified pineal from other regions containing calcareous or radio-opaque deposits.

Corpora arenacea are found in the pineals of only certain few mammalian species. Most of these are ungulates, including cattle, horses, sheep, goats and pigs among domestic and the most often studied species.[84] Corpora arenacea have never been found in the much-studied laboratory rat,[305,432,786,947] nor in carnivores,[1007] insectivores, bats and primates, exclusive of man.[786,804,810,812,947] A satisfactory explanation for this species distribution never has been presented. Nevertheless, a possible clue may be suggested from the histological peculiarities of the pineal gland in man and ungulates. In both, the stroma and the interlobular tissue are prominent and become more so with age. Perhaps the development of the corpora arenacea is related to the consequences of stromal architecture and transport activities.

TABLE XIV

Percentage occurrences of corpora arenacea and calcareous deposits in human pineal glands and telencephalic choroid plexuses.*

Tissue & Procedure	Ages (years postnatal) Percent Occurrences								
Pineal Radiography	1–5	6–10	11–15	16–18	19	20	20–50	50–60	60+
Corpora	6.9%	17.1%	34.8%	44.1%	57.9%	68.8%	72.1%	78.0%	78.8%
Pineal Microscopy	1–5	6–10							
Corpora	42.6%	85.7%							
Choroid Plexus Microscopy			1–25				26–50	51–75	76+
Corpora			89%				93%	98%	100%
Stromal calcification			19%				81%	72%	100%

* Data of Lorenz (from Bargmann[84]), Heidel[374], Shuangshoti and Netsky.[907]

Structure and Chemistry

Concentric lamination is the most common and readily observed structural characteristic of pineal corpora arenacea when studied by the light microscope. It is, however, not invariable, and a remarkable variety of shapes, sizes and structural patterns can be found in a survey of human specimens.[34,84,829] When dried, fractured with a steel needle and observed with a dissecting microscope, each small section or concretion reveals a rather homogeneous whitish or tan core with no definite structural characteristics. No natural crystal faces can be found and no well-formed single crystals can be demonstrated. When studied under polarized light after blunt dissection and extraction with NaOH, the fragmented corpora show irregular dark bands in the shape of distorted Maltese crosses when viewed with crossed Nicol prisms as the crystals are rotated. This indicates that aggregates of very small microscopic crystals are present and that the crystals are more or less random in their orientation. They can be resolved only with electron microscopy because they range in size from about 100 to 1000Å.[224] They are needle-like in form, resembling such crystals obtained from calcified plaques in human aortae.[224]

Results from at least three laboratories and several methods concur in the assignment of the hydroxyapatite $(Ca_{10}(PO_4)_6$ $(OH)_2$ or $Ca_5(PO_4)_3OH)$ structure to the principal calcareous contents of the human pineal corpora arenacea.[27,224,829] After the organic material is extracted from pineal samples, the calcium and phosphorus contents of the inorganic material of the corpora can be determined, calcium by flame photometry and phosphorus by the acid molybdate method. In such analyses Earle[224] found a Ca/P ratio of 1.586, which is close to the calculated value (1.667) for hydroxyapatite. X-ray diffraction and x-ray fluorescence spectroscopy confirmed this identification and gave results similar to those obtained from bones and teeth. Some of the results, and especially gas generation upon treatment of the crystals with acid, indicated the presence also within the pineal corpora of carbonate apatite $(Ca_{16}(PO_4, CO_3, OH)_6 (OH)_2)$.[224] Histochemical studies suggest a variable presence of iron in the pineal corpora, particularly in the most superficial layers.[91,224,876] Magnesium also has been reported as a constituent.[876]

Sites and Mechanisms of Origin

Although a wide variety of sites has been suggested,[84,484,560] a primarily, if not exclusively, glial and stromal localization of the genesis of the pineal corpora arenacea appears likely.[152] This conclusion was originally most satisfactorily supported by del Rio Hortega[201] from his light microscopic studies of pineal sections stained by metallic impregnations. Recent work mostly supports but has not added much to this, inspite of the greater resolution now possible with the electron microscope. Most of the mammalian species whose pineals have been studied by electron microscopy do not show corpora arenacea, and electron microscopy of pineals from species that do, have had objectives other than tracing the origins of corpora arenacea.

The nucleation phenomenon required in the genesis of the corpora is not understood and has not been studied, as far as the pineal is concerned. Some parallels might be drawn, nevertheless, from studies of nucleation or apatite formation in solutions.[224] Apatites precipitated from neutral solutions are always poorly crystallized; co-precipitated impurities disturb the crystallization of apatite. If more carbonate is included, the apatite crystals become even more amorphous.

Physiological and Pathological Correlates

The possibility of correlating pineal calcification or content of corpora arenacea with particular physiological or pathological states or histories has excited medical interest for many years.[84] If any general conclusion or tentative indication can be drawn from the available information, it would be that either systemic or pineal cardiovascular disease or similarly compromising conditions are often concurrent with the formation of pineal corpora arenacea.

Such pineal calcification has long been thought to be unusually common when tumors are present in the pineal region.[569] This may be significant or useful, however, only in young patients, and there are contrary opinions about the correlation of radiologically visible pineal calcification and pineal tumors.[1020] In one study, greater pineal weight in patients with non-malignant, as compared to malignant, disease was suggested and was attributed to greater mineral content of the former.[961]

Various enzyme activities have been measured in human pineal specimens of different ages and varying in estimated presence or degree of calcification.[705,1075] No correlations were observed between enzyme activity levels and pineal calcification. The enzymes studied included monoamine oxidase (E.C. 1.4.3.4), N-acetylserotonin O-methyltransferase (E.C. 2.1.1.4; = "hydroxyindole O-methyltransferase"), histamine N-methyltransferase (E.C. 2.1.1.8) and aromatic L-amino acid decarboxylase (E.C. 4.1.1.26).

In recent as well as in early years, claims have been made for the correlation of pineal calcification through the accumulation of corpora arenacea with endocrinopathy.[490,740] Fradà and Micale,[289] from radiological studies of pineals in 120 women at ages within the fertile period, advanced the hypothesis that hyperfunction of the hypophyseal anterior lobe and problems in calcium metabolism at the time of pregnancy favor the appearance of pineal calcifications. Observations from other sources do not support this hypothesis. Godina[325] found that although pineal corpora arenacea increase with age in cattle, their increase could not be correlated with pregnancies. A tabulation by Pende[740] of the frequency of pineal calcification in 1121 cases of different "endocrinopathies" is difficult to evaluate, since ages are not specified and some of the associated behavior patterns (eg., "anomalie della libido e psicosessualità (ipererotismo, anerotismo, omosessualità, pervertimenti . . .") are uncertain in origin and relevance. While there possibly may be some kind of relation between pineal calcification and particular endocrinopathies, more clinical support and more sophisticated statistical methods are required in such investigations.

CONCLUSIONS

1. Copper, manganese and zinc are present in mammalian pineals in relatively high concentrations, as compared with most parts of the brain and many other organs. It is likely that their association within the pineal is, as in most other tissues, with specific protein fractions and enzymes.

2. Usually present, also, are iron, calcium, magnesium and phosphorus but in both bound and free forms and often associated with pigments (iron) or concretions known as corpora arenacea (calcium, phosphorus, magnesium and iron).

3. Pineal uptake from the blood of inorganic constituents has been used to evaluate the pineal's vascular barrier ($AgNO_3$), blood flow (^{86}Rb and [42]K) and possible metabolic relationships (^{131}I and ^{32}P).

4. Rat pineal uptake of ^{32}P inorganic phosphate is greater in adult than in young animals and is 75 percent greater at night than during the day. Results from numerous studies so far have failed to delineate any other consistent physiological relationships for relative uptake of ^{32}P by pineal glands.

5. Corpora arenacea are of common occurrence in human pineals and those of studied ungulate mammals. They are

probably glial and stromal in origin, as well as localization, and do not differ structurally or chemically from such deposits in a wide variety of other tissues. Their primary microcrystalline structure resembles that of an hydroxyapatite.

6. Although pineal corpora arenacea occur in greater frequency with age, they do not occur in all pineals from aged individuals, and their possible correlation with particular physiological or pathological states remains open to debate.

Chapter Four

LIPIDS

Pineal lipids have been studied through the use of four categories of methods: (1) separation and measurements by solubility; (2) tissue and cellular localization and estimation by histochemistry and light microscopy; (3) cellular and intracellular localization by electron microscopy; and (4) separation and measurement of structural kinds of lipid molecules by chromatography and other biochemical methods. The chemical specificity or chemical information imparted by the first three of these methods leaves much to be desired. But, results from the application of these methods to studies of mammalian pineals are especially helpful in defining lipid localizations and their quantitative changes with aging, pathology, and physiological or experimentally imposed conditions. In effect, the results on pineal lipid localizations and quantitative changes markedly improve our ability to interpret the significance of the molecular types of lipids detected and measured in the pineal by biochemical methods. It will be seen, also, that results from these different methods tend to be mutually supportive and to reinforce preliminary conclusions to be made concerning the regulation and significance of lipids within mammalian pineal glands.

SOLUBLE FRACTIONS
Technical and Comparative Differences

The term lipids is generally applied to substances which can be extracted from tissues by relatively non-polar, or *lipid* solvents, and which can be shown to have at least some of the physical properties of fats and oils. The percentage of either the wet or dry weight of pineal tissue that can be extracted from the tissue by lipid solvents can be considered as an approximation and, in an empirical sense, the lipid soluble fraction. This soluble fraction varies depending especially on the species from which the pineal tissue is taken, which solvent or mixture of solvents is used, and various conditions of the tissue preparation and extraction process. An early tabulation (Fenger, 1916)[270] gives the fraction of fresh (wet) pineal tissue soluble in petroleum ether as 2.2 percent (cattle in March), 2.8 percent (cattle in December and January), 2.5 percent (sheep in December and January) and 2.5 percent (lambs in December and January). Cattle pineals extracted in a Soxhlet apparatus for 24 or 48 hours were stated by Roux[868] to show an ether-soluble fraction consisting of 2.51 percent of the wet weight (12.35% of dry weight) and an absolute alcohol-ether soluble fraction of 3.47 percent of the wet weight. This is less than the total lipid fraction of whole mammalian brain (10.47% of its gray (5.0–6.2%) or white matters (16.0–22.0%).[281] The lipid-soluble fraction from pig pineals has been reported as 3 percent.[656] Histochemical studies also suggest greater lipid content in pig pineals than in those of sheep or cattle.[40] A recent report on extraction of cattle, sheep and human pineals with chloroform-methanol (2:1 by volume) gave lipid fractions of 5.8, 10.8 and 9.2 percent, respectively.[190] The higher yields from cattle and sheep pineals in this study probably resulted from the particular solvent system and extraction procedure used. Excess lipids extracted by this system and procedure applied to brain, as compared with previous methods of extraction, have been identified as proteolipids and strandin.[280]

Soluble fractions from rodent pineal glands have been measured by Quay,[776,781,790] who used whole pineals dried on aluminum foil pans. A similar reduction in dry weight was obtained by extraction at 60°C with any one of several solvents used alone; these were ethanol, methanol, chloroform and pyridine (Table XV). Ethanol was favored over pyridine since it did not leave a grease-like residue,

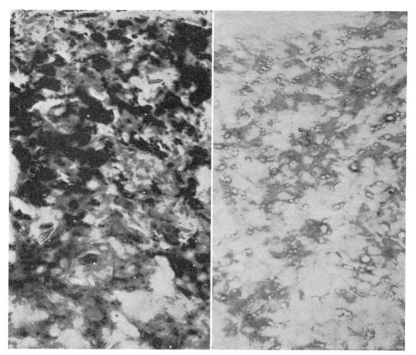

Figure 14. Adjacent frozen tissue sections from a posterior and peripheral part of an adult male rat's pineal gland stained according to the Seligman and Ashbel method for carbonyl lipids. The section on the right was extracted with absolute ethanol at 37°C for twenty-four hours prior to staining simultaneously with the section at the left. (Modified from Quay.[769])

was easier to handle and gave more consistent and somewhat larger soluble fractions (Table XV). Absolute ethanol, however, can be expected to extract some non-lipid tissue constituents and to be relatively ineffective in extracting some lipids. Nevertheless, histochemical studies and several kinds of experiments[768,776] support the belief that most of the rodent's pineal lipids are extracted by hot ethanol (Fig. 14).

Experimental and Daily Changes

The lipid-soluble fraction of the rodent pineal gland can be decreased in amount by various experimental or environmental treatments of the animals prior to removal and analysis of the pineal tissue. The most extensively studied experimen-

TABLE XV

Lipid-soluble fractions (means ± standard errors) of dry rodent pineal glands and the effects of continuous light (LL) as compared with a normal day-night rhythm with fourteen hours of light per day (LD). Also shown are results where LL and LD treatments followed either bilateral surgical transection of the optic nerves intraorbitally (OPTIC X) or bilateral adrenalectomy (ADREN X). Such experimental test groups are compared with appropriate sham-operated control (SC) groups.*

Solvent	Species, sex & age (weeks)	Treatment groups	'Lipid'—soluble fraction			
			μg	†P	% of pineal dry wgt.	†P
Pyridine	Rat, ♀ , 26–39	LL	27.0 ± 4.3		14.8 ± 1.1	
		LD	47.6 ± 3.5	< 0.01	19.5 ± 0.9	< 0.01
Pyridine	Rat,♂ , 25–26	LL	27.6 ± 1.6		15.1 ± 0.8	
		LD	40.0 ± 2.8	< 0.001	17.6 ± 0.5	< 0.02
Ethanol	Rat,♂ , 8.5–9.5	LL	37.9 ± 1.8		29.5 ± 0.7	
		LD	50.8 ± 3.3	< 0.01	31.7 ± 0.1	

				P[†]	
Ethanol	Hamster, ♂, 26–52	LL	9.1 ± 0.8		24.4 ± 2.1
		LD	13.4 ± 0.8	< 0.001	28.3 ± 1.4
Ethanol	Rat, ♀, 9–11	OPTIC X + LL	34.5 ± 1.7	< 0.01	25.3 ± 0.8
		SC + LL	27.8 ± 1.7		24.0 ± 0.6
		OPTIC X + LD	30.1 ± 1.5		23.8 ± 0.6
		SC + LD	31.0 ± 1.8		24.8 ± 0.6
Ethanol	Rat, ♂, 14–17.5	OPTIC X + LL	43.2 ± 2.1	< 0.001	23.9 ± 0.6
		SC + LL	32.2 ± 1.8		23.0 ± 0.5
		OPTIC X + LD	41.3 ± 2.5		24.3 ± 0.5
		SC + LD	41.8 ± 1.5		24.3 ± 0.4
Ethanol	Rat, ♂, 24–26	ADREN X + LL	39.0 ± 2.1	< 0.02	24.7 ± 0.5
		SC + LL	46.8 ± 1.9		25.7 ± 0.6
		ADREN X + LD	40.9 ± 2.0		25.3 ± 0.7
		SC + LD	44.8 ± 2.4		25.1 ± 0.7

* Data of Quay.[776]
† P = probability based on Student-Fisher t

Pineal Chemistry

TABLE XVI

Ethanol-soluble fractions (means ± standard errors) of adult male Long-Evans rat pineal glands in three experiments in which matched animals in individual suspended wire mesh cages were either in or away from the path of a continuous motor-driven blower.[820] Ten animals were present in each group in each experiment.

Experiment Number	Length of Treatment (days)	Ethanol-soluble fraction (= % of dry wgt.)		
		Blown	Controls	*P
1	30	25.21 ± 0.32	26.50 ± 0.43	< 0.05
2	28	27.86 ± 0.26	28.52 ± 0.22	< 0.01
3	31	25.13 ± 0.29	24.90 ± 0.31	n.s.

* P = probability based on pair-wise analysis and Student-Fisher *t*.

tal effect is the decrease produced by continuous light.[775, 776] In hamsters and in rats of different ages continuous illumination of moderate intensity (five to seventy foot candles) and lasting four weeks or less was sufficient to cause marked and significant decrease in the pineal lipid-soluble fraction (Table XV) and in the histochemically demonstrable lipid droplets in the pinealocytes.[775, 776] The effect is blocked by bilateral surgical transection of the optic nerves (Table XV), indicating that this effect of continuous light on the pineal gland is mediated by the lateral eyes and the central nervous system. Since laboratory rats and hamsters are naturally nocturnal animals and are somewhat photophobic, it might be hypothesized that, for them, continuous illumination may elicit stress responses of a possibily non-specific nature. Following this line of thought, it might be supposed that the pineal effect may originate from this circumstance rather than from an indirect but specific pineal response to light. However, bilateral adrenalectomy does not abolish this pineal response (Table XV). Nevertheless, experiments with chronic stimuli other than light suggest that chronic stress or irritation can be expected to produce decreases in the rat pineal's ethanol-soluble fraction. One such experiment that has not been published previously, and which can serve as an example, is summarized in Table XVI. It is seen that pineal glands of adult male rats in the path of a blower generally have a slightly smaller ethanol-soluble fraction than do those of matched control animals in identical cages close by but out of the direct path of the blown air. The variation in the three experiments, and probably the degree of difference between the experimental (blown) and control animals is attributable partly to differences in the time of day at which the animals were killed and analyzed. The reason for this suggestion will be evident from results in a subsequent paragraph showing a daily or twenty-four hour rhythmicity in the pineal's ethanol-soluble fraction.

The effect of continuous light on the rodent pineal gland is probably not due solely to a general physiological response to stress. Continuous light has various effects on the rat's central nervous system, and certain of these possibly are more directly related physiologically to those occurring in the pineal gland. For example, continuous light causes a significant reduction in cerebral sodium and potassium content in rats receiving a sodium-deficient diet.[787,800] It also reduces the amplitude of the circadian rhythm in the neurohypophyseal content of antidiuretic hormone (ADH) in rats.[510]

The rat pineal's ethanol-soluble fraction follows a daily or twenty-four-hour rhythm (Fig. 15).[790] Although the amplitude of the rhythm is slight, representing only about 3 percent of the ethanol-soluble fraction, it is highly consistent. The question as to whether this rhythm does, in fact, represent a rhythm in pineal lipid content can be at least partially supported by circumstantial and another kind of evidence. Counts of pinealocytes in tissue sections stained for lipids reveal a twenty-four hour rhythm in percentage of cells containing microscopically visible lipid droplets (Fig. 16). The approximate times of maximum and minimum values coincide with those shown by the ethanol-soluble fraction. The secondary peak suggested immediately following the onset of darkness is not secure statistically (Fig. 16).

The twenty-four-hour rhythm in the pineal ethanol-soluble fraction is not free-running or *circadian*, according to the restricted use of this term by some investigators. At least in conditions of continuous light, the rhythm is lost or is no longer detected in the data at hand through a period of four days, the first two of which are shown in Figure 17.[790]

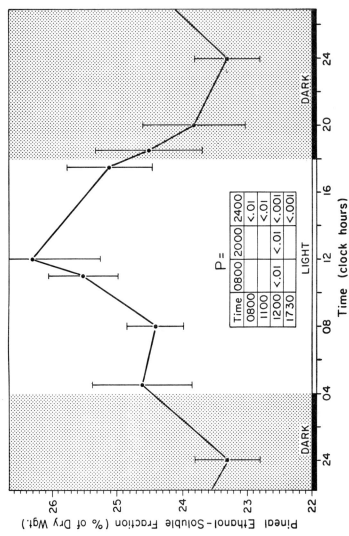

Figure 15. Twenty-four-hour rhythm in pineal ethanol-soluble fraction. Each point represents the mean from 10 male rats twenty-eight to twenty-nine weeks old; the vertical lines through each point extend twice the standard error of the mean on each side. The significances (P) of the differences between means for selected sample times of the cycle are tabulated. (Modified from Quay.[790])

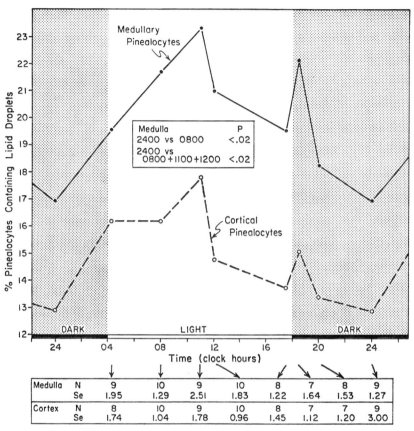

Figure 16. Twenty-four hour rhythm in percentage of pinealocytes containing microscopically detectable lipid droplets in cortical and medullary zones of the pineal glands of adult male rats.[820] N = number of animals: Se = standard error of the mean; P = probability based on Student-Fisher *t*. Fixation in formalin-ammonium bromide was followed by chromation at 60°C for twelve hours, routine histological technique and staining of sections with Sudan black B. Additional technical information is available in Quay and Renzoni.[826]

It is interesting to note, however, that when darkness does not occur at the end of the first light phase, the pineal ethanol-soluble fraction climbs to a new peak whose timing is near in clock hours to the usual time of a nocturnal minimum value (Fig. 17). In identical conditions of continuous light, the twenty-four hour rhythm in rat running activity continues

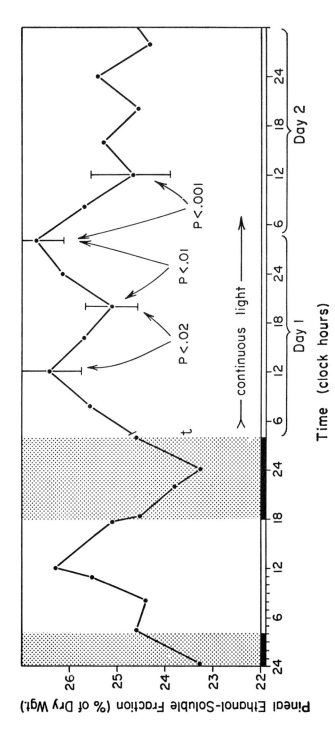

Figure 17. Rhythmicity of the pineal's ethanol-soluble fraction in adult male rats after transfer (t) to a continuously lighted room. Each point represents the mean of ten to twenty-three animals; vertical bars through some of the means extend in each direction for a distance equal to twice the standard error of the mean; P = probability based on Student-Fisher t. (Modified from Quay.[790])

for many days and is, therefore, free-running and circadian in the strict sense of the term.[790] Since the behavior of the pineal ethanol-soluble fraction is so different (Fig. 17), it is unlikely that it is in any way related to the muscular or general body activity of the animal. Furthermore, the pattern shown by the rat pineal's ethanol-soluble fraction during the first forty-eight hours of continuous light (Fig. 17) appears to be unique. It should be recognized, however, that very few metabolites or cellular constituents have been measured at timed intervals after the start of a regime of continuous light. This problem will be considered again in relation to the pineal's content of indoleamines and their changes in response to continuous light and other modified schedules of illumination.

CELLULAR LOCALIZATIONS

Histochemistry

Microscopic localization of lipid within mammalian pineal glands has been known for many years and has been described frequently. Descriptions of pineal lipid localizations started becoming common in the literature about sixty years ago, with Jordan's (1911) work on sheep,[445] Ruggeri's (1914) on laboratory rats[873] and Polvani's (1913) on man.[748] From the beginning, contradictory interpretations and speculations were presented by these and other authors concerning the physiological significance of pineal lipid. This aspect of the subject is treated in a subsequent section. The present section is concerned with lipid localization rather than its quantitative changes and their possible meaning.

The physical disposition of lipids in pineal, as well as other kinds of cells, is subject to artifactual modification, leading to increased number and size of lipid droplets or globules and the formation of myelin figures.[467,752] In varying degrees such changes from the natural *in vivo* appearance are recognizable in the published figures and descriptions of the physical nature and distribution of pineal lipids. These artifactual changes are more prevalent and are more difficult to avoid in pineal specimens having greater amounts of lipid, more labile lipid, more phospholipid, and more exposure to trauma. Thus, the outer or cortical zone of the rat pineal gland is more apt to be affected than the center or medulla, and the rat organ more affected than that of man.

Pineal lipid histochemistry has been studied most frequently and in most detail in laboratory rats. Small lipid droplets are present in pinealocytes of newborn animals. They increase for about a week at least, and then, later gradually decrease.[753,1099] Greater amounts or larger droplets of lipid often are found in the peripheral or cortical zone, especially at the posterior or distal end of the organ (Fig. 18, top).[470,769,1099] Nevertheless, it can be demonstrated that often a greater percentage of the central or medullary pinealocytes contain lipid droplets than do the peripheral or cortical pinealocytes (Fig. 16). Medullary lipid droplets, however, are usually smaller and more diffuse when examined following histochemical procedures (Fig. 18, bottom).

Lipid histochemistry has been employed by Quay[470,778] to attempt to distinguish and classify kinds of parenchymal cells or pinealocytes within adult rat pineal glands. Table XVII presents an outline of the resulting classification. Studies of various kinds are still needed in order to determine the reliability of this classification. Some data now available concerning rat pineal ultrastructure and physiology are relevant to this problem since they suggest correlations between particular of these histochemical cell types and ultrastructural ones and particular physiological and pharmacological effects. These will be considered in subsequent sections. The most generally accepted of the rat pineal cell types containing lipid is the one noted as the *type I cell* (Table XVII). These contain cytoplasmic lipid droplets easily seen with the light microscope, both in normal or untreated animals and others that have been operated upon or given hormones or drugs.

The *type II cells*, on the other hand, are less uniform and are more open to question as to the nature of their lipid content. Furthermore, they are seen more fully or in larger numbers after massive injections of norepinephrine or amphetamine three to six hours before removal and fixation

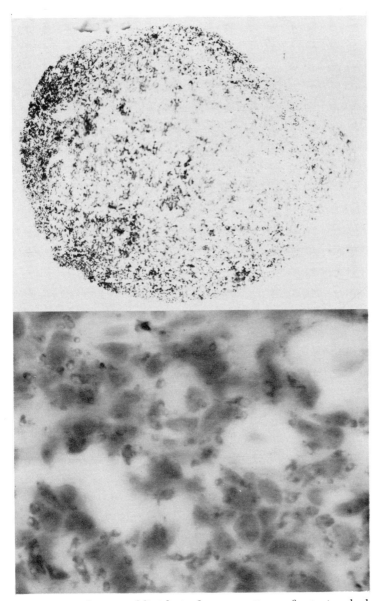

Figure 18. Distribution of lipids in frozen sections of rat pineal glands.

Top: Horizontal section of entire pineal gland of an adult female. Lipid droplets are colored with Sudan black B. The distal or posterior tip (left) shows more lipid than the proximal or anterior end, which is attached to the pineal stalk.

Bottom: Typical central or medullary area in an adult female rat pineal stained with Oil red O and acid alum hematoxylin. Lipid droplets enclosing vacuoles are present in most of the parenchymal cells. (Modified from Quay.[769])

TABLE XVII

Classification of rat pineal parenchymal cell (pinealocyte) types on the basis of lipid cytochemistry, staining reactions and cell structure. (After Quay[769,778]).

Type I Cells:

Numerous ethanol-soluble, cytoplasmic lipid droplets, containing triglycerides[753] and covered with phospholipid; in histological preparations the cytoplasm is vesiculated and weakly stained; widely distributed through the pineal gland and often are closely adjacent individually to type II cells.

Type II Cells:

Cytoplasmic matrix with very few and small lipid droplets, and staining heavily with Baker's acid hematein method, orange G or phloxine.[766]

Subtype 1–Orthocytes:

Cells of medium to large size, resembling fibrous astrocytes, but differing in being relatively few in number, having cell bodies largely restricted to the anterior or proximal quarter of the pineal organ, having a greater amount of cytoplasm in the perikaryon, and possessing long $(80+\mu)$ and smooth cytoplasmic processes.

Subtype 2–Spirocytes:

Cells of medium to large size; relatively few in number, but more numerous than the orthocytes and having more cytoplasm in the perikaryon; numerous, long $(90+\mu)$, spiraling, granular and network-forming cytoplasmic processes, which wrap around and terminate on other cells—usually on type I cells—but also in the vicinity of capillaries; largest examples are usually in the anterior or proximal quarter of the organ, but small ones are scattered throughout.

Subtype 3–Polygonocytes:

Medium-sized, multiangular cells with short $(5–25\mu)$ and irregular cytoplasmic processes; most numerous of the type II cells but probably less numerous than the type I cells; scattered throughout the pineal organ and usually closely adjacent individually to type I cells.

Subtype 4–Contocytes:

Small, angular cells with little cytoplasm and a large nucleolus; distribution scattered but often adjacent to capillaries; not always distinguishable from subtype 3, of which it may represent a physiological phase or developmentally related category.

---

of the pineal tissue.[778] The question of their lipid content centers on the meaning and chemical specificity of Baker's[70] acid hematein method, the histochemical staining technique most clearly revealing the *type II cells.* Originally proposed as a method for phospholipids, it has been restudied and its specificity reargued. Pearse[725] has concisely reviewed this history. The current conclusion, stemming especially from the studies by Adams and co-workers,[6,7] is that the acid hematein reaction depends on the presence of choline (lecithin or sphingomyelin), but that it is enhanced by ethylenic bonds and that possible participation of non-lipid cell contents must be kept in mind. Additional chemical studies on the method have been presented recently by Roozemond.[861-863]

Although some of the *type II cells* resemble astrocytes, evidence is available supporting belief in their individuality and suggesting their participation in particular histophysiological mechanisms. In a previous review, the general distribution through the rat pineal organ and the typical nature of pineal astrocytes were noted.[786] Typical astrocytes, therefore, can be both identified in rat pineals and cytologically distinguished from the *type II cells*. A detailed study by Kroon[523] on hypothalamic cells staining with Baker's acid hematein procedure indicates that it is principally certain populations of neuronal or ganglion cells that are stained and not the astrocytes. In relation to the increased staining and apparent number of pineal *type II cells* after treatment with norepinephrine[771,778] and staining with acid hematein, it is interesting to note the effect of norepinephrine on the incorporation of ^{32}P into brain phospholipids. In protracted (20–120 minutes) incubations of homogeneates of rat brain, norepinephrine (NE) has been shown to cause increased incorporation of ^{32}P into phospholipid of the synaptosomal and mitochondrial fractions.[920] Increased incorporation was noted in the phosphatidylcholine fraction, as well as the three others separated chromatographically. Similarity occurs in the specificity of the response to NE by pineal *type II cells in vivo* and brain ^{32}P incorporation into phospholipids *in vitro*. Neither response occurs after treatment with 5-hydroxytryptamine or histamine.[771,778,920]

Histochemical studies of lipids in human pineal glands have revealed pinealocytes which resemble the *type I cells* of rat pineal glands, but *type II cells* have not been demonstrated. This is not surprising since pharmacological manipulation and more rigorous attention to postmortem events are important for the demonstration of *type II cells*, at least by the acid hematein reaction. Fine and diffusely distributed cytoplasmic lipid droplets can be identified in pinealocytes from human pineals of diverse ages (Fig. 19, Table XVIII).[769] The number, distribution and composition of the lipid-containing

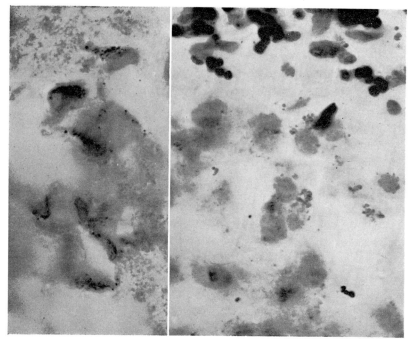

Figure 19. Distribution of lipids in frozen sections of human pineal glands stained with Oil red O and acid alum hematoxylin. (Modified from Quay.[769])

Left: Pinealocytes with numerous lipid droplets and associated vacuoles in four-year-old male (U.M.H.-A577BH).

Right: Interlobular (top) and intralobular (bottom) areas within the pineal gland of a thirty-three old woman (W.R.U.-13924). The large, densely stained (with hematoxylin) bodies in the interlobular zone are corpora arenacea. Adjacent to them are interlobular cells with large masses of lipid; pinealocyte lipids (center and bottom) are in the form of small droplets, mostly in the perikaryon.

parenchymal cells change with age. In youth, they are peripherally distributed in the organ, are few in number and usually do not contain pigment. In adulthood and later life, they are found within lobules throughout most of the organ, and some of them contain yellow to brown pigment granules, some of which are capped with lipid. A second kind of lipid-containing cell becomes more prominent in adulthood and older age. These contain larger lipid droplets and lie primarily within the stromal areas and interlobular septa (Figs. 19 and 20). They are principally neuroglial and phagocytic in nature,

TABLE XVIII

Percent occurrences of lipid- and pigment (lipofuscin)-containing cells in human pineal glands according to age.*

Age and Sex	Without Lipid or Pigment	Pinealocytes			Interlobular Cells	
		Lipid Only	Lipid + Pigment	Pigment Only	Lipid Only	Pigment Only
Series A†:						
2 mos.♂	95.9	2.8	0	0	1.1	?0.2
14 mos.♀	94.8	2.5	0	0.1	4.6	0
1½ years♀	93.3	2.7	0	0	4.0	0
2 years♀	96.5	1.2	0	0	2.3	0
2 years♀	95.5	2.3	0	0	2.2	0
3½ years♂	97.4	1.0	0	0	1.6	0
4 years♂	93.9	3.6	0	0	2.5	0
5 years♀	94.6	1.1	0	0	4.3	0
5 years♀	85.5	7.3	0.1	0	7.1	0
5 years♂	85.6	8.5	0	0	5.9	0
5 years♂	80.6	4.3	0	0	15.1	0
9 years♂	89.6	6.6	0.2	0.1	4.5	0

Age and Sex	Pinealocytes + Interlobular Cells			
	Without	Lipid Only	Lipid + Pigment	Pigment Only
Series B‡:				
5 days premature	97	3	0	0
13 mos. ♂	90	10	0	0
3 years ♂	89	11	0	0
4 years ♂	77	23	0	0
33 years ♀	26	23	35	16
62 years ♀	26	13	16	45
65 years ♀	40	11	11	38

* Blood and endothelial cells omitted from counts.
† Series A specimens from Detroit, Michigan.[820]
‡ Series B specimens from Ann Arbor, Michigan and Cleveland, Ohio.[768]

rather than some type of parenchymal cell. These interlobular or stromal lipid-containing cells increase in number with age and in younger pineals are notable largely around cysts and similar regions of reaction on the part of the stromal tissue constituents. They have irregular cytoplasmic extensions and are structurally distinctive, readily enabling their microscopic differentiation from other kinds of cells, such as granular leucocytes and mast cells. Correlations between increased numbers of human pineal lipid-containing cells and particular premortem physiological or disease states or causes of death have not been successful. Many opinions have been

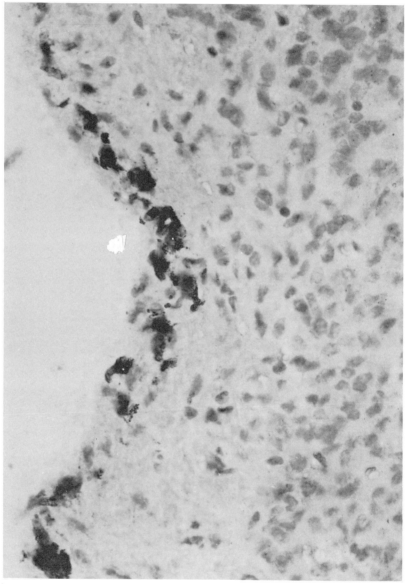

Figure 20. Stromal cells containing lipid droplets around a pineal cyst (left); parenchymal (pinealocyte) nuclei predominate in right third of the figure. Five year old human female (leukemia + pneumonia); Oil red O and acid alum hematoxylin.

expressed concerning the physiological or pathological significance of the human pineal lipid-containing cells, but without the support of quantitative analyses or convincing
evidence.[22,91,134,205,301,478,517,700,748,761]

The reality of age changes in human pineals is beyond
doubt and includes the phenomena observed in both the
intralobular pinealocyte lipid-containing *(type I?)* cell and
the interlobular or stromal lipid-containing cell. Comparable
changes have not been described in the pineal glands of rats
or of other mammalian species. It is probable that the age
changes in the interlobular cells have some histopathological
significance. They are associated with a poorly understood
and age-related increase in thickness of the interlobular septa
which suggests decrease in transport facility between the
pinealocytes within the lobules and the nearest blood vessels.
The histophysiological significance of the increased cytoplasmic lipid and associated pigment in aging human pinealocytes
is not clear. There is no direct evidence suggesting that such
cells are either metabolically or functionally less active.

Electron Microscopy

Information on cellular localization of lipid in pineal cells
is now also available from electron microscopic studies.
However, such information is scattered and has not been the
main topic of any ultrastructural study of the pineal organ.
The laboratory rat's pineal has been studied most frequently
and in the greatest detail. Many electron microscopic investigations of it have figured its lipoidal inclusions, and diverse
opinions have been expressed concerning their localization
and physiological significance.[165,212,345,347,470,482,524,626,627,
638,886,1056] Lipid droplets have been found in pinealocytes
of rats of all ages from newborn[580] to old age.[124] An analysis
and summary of the rat pineal's parenchymal cells or
pinealocytes with particular attention to lipid or lipoidal inclusions is presented in Table XIX. This is largely derived from
the detailed studies and descriptions provided by Arstila and
Hopsu (1964).[38] A lessened adherence to such a scheme of
mutually exclusive parenchymal cell types is suggested by
a later report by this group.[37] Futhermore, many other inves-

TABLE XIX

Tentative classification of rat pineal parenchymal cell (pinealocyte) types on the basis of lipoidal inclusions and other ultrastructural characteristics. (Modified from Arstila and Hopsu,[38]).

Cell Types By Lipid Histochemistry (from Table 17)	Ultrastructural Cellular Correlates and Their Characteristics
Type I Cells:	"Chief" or "light" cells of most authors: the most common and most often described cells; lipid droplets or inclusions with a homogeneous content and lacking a limiting membrane occur in various cytoplasmic regions, but only seldom within the cytoplasmic processes ending in the pericapillary space; Golgi complex smaller than in other cell types; mitochondria numerous and polymorphic.
Type II Cells:	"Dark cells" of most authors: less numerous than type I cells and not always readily distinguished from them; cytoplasm dark and more abundant in the processes than in the perikarya; contains small lipid inclusions, numerous mitochondria, large Golgi complex, abundant granular endoplasmic reticulum with parallel cisternae, lysosomes, and—most characteristically—neurofilaments and *synaptic* structures (= synaptic membrane thickenings, vesicles and intracellular spines). = The most neuron-like pineal cell, and possibly equivalent to the pineal basophil of Constantini[173] and of Hungerford and Pomerat[415,416]
No equivalent in rat described, but probably = subpopulation of neuroglial or interlobular cells, as described in human pineal organs.	"Type III" or "fat-laden" cells: diverse cytoplasmic lipoidal inclusions are most characteristic and include: (1) small lipoidal granules, usually with a single limiting membrane, and found near nucleus, as well as in cell processes; (2) largest lipoidal granules, with limiting membrane and suggestions of a lamellar and granular internal structure—found most often in cell periphery and especially in the endings of the processes; (3) other kinds of lipoidal inclusions and granules; nucleus lacks invaginations, cytoplasm with abundant granular endoplasmic reticulum and a Golgi complex; processes contain "glial" fibrils; cells lie in or near the pericapillary spaces. = Probably the fat-laden cell *in vitro* of Hungerford and Pomerat[415,416], O'Steen and Dill[702] and the type B cells (in part) of Orofino[699] and a subpopulation of interstitial cells.

tigators of mammalian pineal ultrastructure have been reluctant to support the identification of distinctive or mutually exclusive parenchymal cell types.[344] The possibility of light and dark cells, or *type I* and *II*, being merely different metabolic or secretory phases often is either implied or mentioned. However, the radically different morphologies and distributions of at least some of these cells, as shown in rat pineals by light microscopy (Table XVII), suggests that distinctive parenchymal cell types do exist. Obviously, more research is needed before the question of pineal cell types can be treated satisfactorily and convincingly. What information that is now available, is, nonetheless, sufficient to suggest several conclusions in regard to pineal lipid inclusions. (1) Lipid or lipoidal inclusions are detectable in pinealocytes of apparently all mammalian species examined with the electron microscope[24,544,879,903,1027,1028] and in human pinealoma cells.[644] (2) The occurrence of appreciable lipid in two or more different types of pineal cells suggests that comprehensive generalizations concerning the functional significance of pineal lipid may be faulty without attention to particular cellular localizations and particular cellular functions. (3) Since the distribution of lipid inclusions in pinealocytes (*types I* and *II*) is less in the ends of the cytoplasmic processes than near the nucleus, their possible significance as the immediate precursors of secretion is doubtful. (4) Lipid droplets of simple structure in pinealocytes (*types I* and *II*) are most likely to be of basic importance in cell metabolism, while those of complex and variable structure in interlobular cells (neuroglial and stromal) are probably phagocytized and represent variable tissue and/or vascular biproducts.

Quantitative Changes in Tissue Sections

Tissue sections of rat pineal glands have been examined for lipid droplets after various treatments of the animals before autopsy. The results of such studies are summarized in Table XX. It should be emphasized that the analytical methods used in different studies varied considerably and many were not supported with analyses of variance by the original authors.

Many conditions or treatments lead to a reduction in the

TABLE XX

Effects of diverse treatments on estimated lipid contents of rat pineal glands, primarily as visualized in cytoplasmic droplets in *type I cells* by light or electron microscopy. Reference sources are noted in the appropriate columns for increase in amount (↑), no change (≂), change in structure and/or distribution (▲), and decrease in amount (↓).

Treatments	↑	≂	▲	↓
Continuous light				754,776
NaCl added			753	
NaCl deficient				
—*in vivo*				599,714,715
—*in vitro*			417	
Pineal extracts		754		345
Hypophysectomy				715,886,1099,1100
+ ACTH		715		
+ gonadotropin (PMS or HCG)	1099,1100 (= restoration)	(no restoration)		
Gonadotropin (PMS)	1099			
Orchidectomy	873			132
Ovariectomy	703,886,1098-1100			132
+ estradiol				1099,1100
+ progesterone		1099,1100		
Adrenalectomy				599,714,715
Adrenal enucleation	470			
DOCA	715			
Hydrocortisone		715		
Thyroid hormones —*in vivo* & *in vitro*		417,715		
Propylthiouracil				715
Angiotensin II				
—*in vivo*				715
—*in vitro*		417		
Superior cervical ganglionectomy + continuous light		1100		
Norepinephrine	143		345	
Niamid (inhibition of monoamine oxidase)	143			469
Reserpine	469			

rat pineal's content of lipid, as seen microscopically in the form of lipid droplets (Table XX). These treatments range from continuous illumination and sodium deficiency to diverse endocrine extirpations and administrations of particular hormones and drugs. It is impossible to suggest a mechanism that might serve as a common explanation for the results of all of these treatments. Nevertheless, a pair of mechanisms, or really, a pair of general physiological systems can be suggested as tentative correlates of these pineal effects: (1) modification of tissue water and electrolytes, and (2) modification of endocrine and/or metabolic balances. The broad and diffuse relationships suggested by these tentative correlations do not lend themselves easily to critical discussion. If we ignore some of the data in Table XX and focus selectively instead on data from the two most frequently studied systems, some other relationships, and problems, appear. These two systems are the hypophyseal-gonadal endocrine system and the sympathetic division of the autonomic nervous system.

Most intensively and frequently studied are the rat pineal's responses to changes in the hypophyseal-gonadal endocrine system (Table XX). As background for review of this work, the more than 20 percent drop in rat pineal lipid at proestrus in normal, untreated animals should be noted (Fig. 21). Consistent with this change during proestrus in the untreated animal is the depression in pineal lipid in the animal injected with estradiol and the lasting increase in the ovariectomized animal (Fig. 22). On the other hand, hypophysectomy causes a reduction in pineal lipid in female rats (Fig. 23). This effect can be prevented or counteracted by either human chorionic gonadotropin or pregnant mare's serum gonadotropin (Fig. 23). Contrary to what at first might be supposed, the presence of the ovaries is not required for the effect of gonadotropin on pineal lipid in hypophysectomized animals. In fact, the same daily dose of PMS produces the same level of increase in pineal lipid in hypophysectomized + ovariectomized as in hypophysectomized female rats (Fig. 24). ACTH has no clear effect on pineal lipid in the hypophysectomized rat, and progesterone is without effect on pineal lipid in the normal animal (Table XX). This summarization of hypophyseal and gonadal effects on pineal lipid depends most strongly on the careful quantitative analyses by Zweens,[1098,1100] although it must be recognized that contradictory results from gonadectomy have been claimed by Bostelmann.[132]

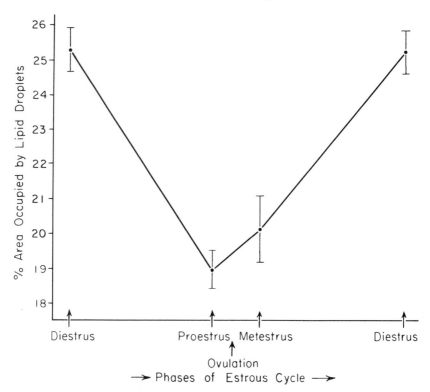

Figure 21. Pineal lipid content at different phases of the estrous cycle in virgin rats ten and one-half weeks old. Percentage of tissue section area occupied by lipid droplets after controlled chromation and staining with Sudan black B in propylene glycol was determined. Means and ranges are plotted for the six animals used at each phase. (Adapted from Zweens.[1098,1099])

The second system to which pineal lipid can be made to respond in rats is the sympathetic and pharmacological sympathomimetic one. Available results (Table XX), however, present more contradictions and problems in interpretation. Possible effects following injection of norepinephrine likely depend closely on dose and time of administration, and on time of sacrifice of the animal. Less labile or longer acting agents, such as Niamid and reserpine, may be expected to be easier to control in their particular effects. But, studies on the effects of sympathomimetic agents on pineal succinic

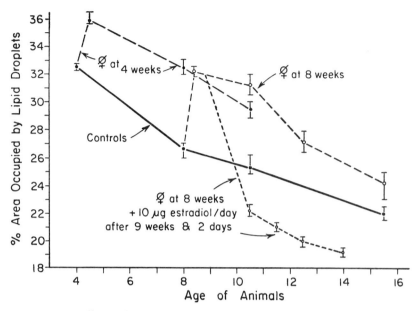

Figure 22. Effects of bilateral ovariectomy (=♀) at two ages and subsequent subcutaneous administration of estradiol benzoate on pineal lipid content in virgin female rats. Means (dots) and ranges (vertical lines) are shown for each sample; six animals present in each sample. (Adapted from Zweens.[1099])

dehydrogenase activity indicate that the particular times of drug administration and of subsequent tissue removal and analysis govern the direction of the resulting metabolic change. This is likely to be based on the twenty-four hour rhythmicity in pineal composition and metabolism, which includes its content of norepinephrine. Thus, to extrapolate from other pineal metabolic systems, it is likely that particular responses of pineal lipid to either norepinephrine or related drugs depend upon critical timing within the twenty-four-hour daily physiological cycle.

There is evidence that responses of the rat pineal's content of lipid in droplets to the two systems, hypophyseal-gonadal and sympathetic, are not mediated by the same external mechanism. An experiment by Zweens shows that pregnant

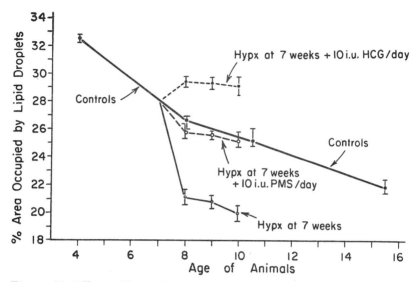

Figure 23. Effects of hypophysectomy (Hypx) and subsequent daily injections of gonadotropins (HCG = human chorionic gonadotropin; PMS = pregnant mare's serum) on pineal lipid content in virgin female rats. Means (dots) and ranges (vertical lines) are shown for each sample; 6 animals in each sample. (Adapted from Zweens.[1099])

mare's serum gonadotropin elicits the same increase in pineal lipid in rats that have had the operation bilateral superior cervical ganglionectomy, as in ones that have not been operated upon (Fig. 25). If the pineal's innervation, stemming from the superior cervical ganglia, were the common pathway for the mediation for such hormonal effects, the response of ganglionectomized animals to PMS would be expected to be different.

All of the above studies, based on microscopic evaluation of quantitative changes in pineal lipid, and summarized in Table XX, concern lipid in droplets in pinealocytes, primarily if not exclusively of the *type I* category. There are results available, also, for experimental changes in the *type II cells*. These relate to changes in lipid content insofar as a positive reaction to Baker's acid hematein test is a reliable quantitative indicator of lipid. The number of *type II cells* strongly positive to the acid hematein technique was determined in rat pineal tissue sections by Quay following selected sets of ex-

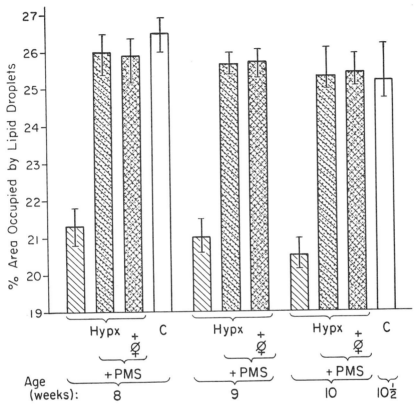

Figure 24. Effects of hypophysectomy (Hypx) and bilateral ovariectomy (♀) at 7 weeks of age and subsequent daily injection of pregnant mare's serum gonadotropin (PMS, 10 i.u. subcutaneously/day) on pineal lipid content in virgin female rats (C = control groups). Means are represented by the upper limit of the bar, ranges by the vertical lines through the means; six animals are present in each sample. (Adapted from Zweens.[1099])

perimental treatments. Statistically significant increases in the number of positive *type II cells* per pineal cross section were obtained following subcutaneous injections of DL-norepinephrine or of DL-amphetamine ($P < 0.01 - < 0.02$), and possibly significant increases were obtained following either a vitamin E-deficient diet for 72 days or a rachitogenic diet supplemented with 10μg calciferol per day for 21 days ($P < 0.05$).[771,778] Many other hormonal, pharmacological and dietary treatments were without detectable or significant effects. The effect of norepinephrine occurred only after rela-

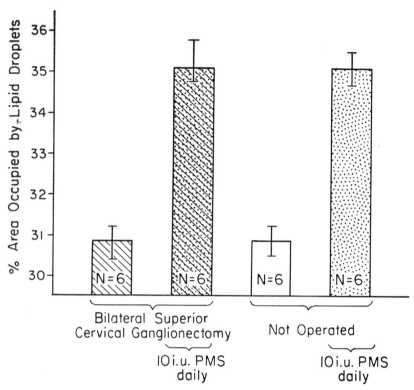

Figure 25. Effects of bilateral superior cervical ganglionectomy (at thirty days of age) and subsequent daily injections of ten i.u. of gonadotropin (= PMS—pregnant mare's serum) on pineal lipid content in virgin female rats sacrificed at thirty-seven days of age. Means are represented by the upper limit of the bars, ranges by the vertical lines through the means. (Adapted from Zweens.[1099])

tively massive doses (0.50 mg/151–386 gm rat) (P < 0.02) and within six hours. Similarly, increased acid hematein reactivity of *type II cells* occurred within three to four hours after large doses of amphetamine (2 mg/18–26 gm young rats; 10 mg/160–360 gm adult rats) and disappeared by 24 hours after injection.

An increase in stainable pineal lipid content has been claimed to occur in rats of both sexes following experimental induction of fibrosarcomas in the hind legs. The mechanism of the effect is not known, but the investigators speculated

that the finding afforded indirect evidence of a pineal relation
to control of malignancy.[421]

STRUCTURAL CLASSES OF LIPIDS

Lipid Classes in Mammalian Pineal Tissue

Chemical analyses of the structural classes or named vari-
eties of lipids comprising pineal tissue lipids have succeeded
in showing similarity between man and other mammalian
species. They have shown, also, significant differences
between pineal lipid composition and that of other organs
or tissues with which the pineal gland might be compared
most naturally on the basis of known or suspected developmental, histological or physiological relationships.

A survey of the classification of lipids which are known
to occur in mammalian pineal tissue, and others which might
logically be expected to occur, is presented in Table XXI.
This tabulation may serve as a programmatic preview for the
following discussion, and as a checklist of pineal lipid classes
and the authorship of their detection and measurement. Some
of the lipids in this table will be scarcely if at all discussed,
due to the circumstance of their low levels in the pineal and
lack of additional significant information concerning them.
It can be suggested that some lipids listed here as present
in pineal tissue in small amounts may owe their inclusion
to technical variables, such as accrue from differences in
anatomical dissection of the pineal away from adjacent tissues,
and differences in chemical fractionation of the lipoidal contents. At the same time, other minor lipid constituents may
remain unrevealed, due to very low levels, inadequate
techniques for separation from other lipid fractions, or otherwise deficient general knowledge concerning them.

Free cholesterol and glycerides comprise the major
ingredients of the neutral lipid fraction of pineals of man
and other mammals (Table XXII). Histochemical evidence
suggests that a major localization of the glycerides is within
the cytoplasmic lipid droplets of the *type I cells*.[467,753] A
discrepancy in results occurs in regard to pineal cholesterol.

TABLE XXI
Annotated classification of pineal lipids

I. Simple Lipids (= esters of fatty acids with alcohols)
   A. Glycerides (= esters with glycerol)—present[467,752,753]
   B. Cholesterol esters—small amount present[90]

II. Compound Lipids (= fatty acids + alcohols + other molecules)

   A. Phospholipids (= phosphatides; a phosphoric acid molecule is a part of
      the structure)—usually comprise > 50% of pineal lipid[90,190,270,448,467,656,752,1098,1100]

      1. Glycerophosphatides (glycerol = the alcohol molecule within the
         structure)
         (a) Phosphatidyl choline (= lecithin)—the major phosphatide present[90,190,448,467,752]
         (b) Lysolecithin (= lecithin—one fatty acid molecule)—present[448]
         (c) Phosphatidyl ethanolamine (= cephalin)—present[90,448,467,752]
         (d) Lysocephalin—present[448]
         (e) Phosphatidyl serine—present[90,190,448,467,752]
         (f) Diphosphatidyl glycerol—small but consistent amount present[90]
         (g) Acetal phosphatide (= plasmalogen)—small amount present[90]
      2. Phosphoinositides (inositol = the alcohol molecule within the structure)
         (a) Monophosphoinositide—present[90,190]
         (b) Polyphosphoinositide—not present[90]
      3. Sphingomyelins (= phosphosphingosides; = sphingosine + a single
         fatty acid + phosphoric acid + choline)—present[90,190,448]
      4. Phosphatidic Acids (including cardiolipin)—present[90,190,448]

   B. Cerebrosides (= galactosphingosides)—lacking[296,336,752,753]
   C. Gangliosides—small amount present[90,336]

III. Derived Lipids (= derivatives of class I and II above obtained by hydrolysis
    and which retain lipid solubility characteristics; contains the major components
    of the so-called non-saponifiable fraction)

   A. Fatty Acids—present[90,467,752]
   B. Alcohols
      1. Sterols
         (a) Cholesterol—a major constituent[90,190]

   C. Hydrocarbons—not yet demonstrated in pineal tissue
      1. Carotenoids and vitamin A

IV. Complex Combinations of Lipids with Other Classes of Compounds

   A. Lipoproteins

      1. Lipofuscin—present in pineals of man and discussed in Chapter Thirteen on pigments; also, see Table XVIII

The Schultz reaction for cholesterol and cholesterides has failed repeatedly to demonstrate these compounds in tissue sections from human[768] and bovine[751] pineal glands. A probable explanation can be derived from considerations of the insensitivity of the histochemical method[6] and the possibily

TABLE XXII
Total lipid composition of pineal glands of different mammalian species*

Species	Total Lipid (% of wet wgt.)	% of Total Lipid					
		Phospholipids	Free Cholesterol	Ester Cholesterol	Glycerides	Other P-free Lipids	Total P- & Cholesterol-free
Man	2.9–9.2	58	13.6	0.4	n.d.†	n.d.	28
Cattle	3.7–5.8	71	15.0	0.8	12	1	13
Sheep	4.0–10.8	60	13.4	0.5	n.d.	n.d.	26
Pig	5.3	59	13.2	1.1	n.d.	n.d.	n.d.

* Data of Czarnocki et al.[190] and Basinska et al.[90]
† n.d. = not determined.

TABLE XXIII

Composition of mammalian pineal phospholipids (percent)

Compounds	Man*	Cattle*	Sheep*	Pig†
Phosphatidyl choline	44.6	46.4	44.6	47
Phosphatidyl ethanolamine	22.0	22.6	21.6	27
Sphingomyelin	13.1	13.8	14.0	11
Phosphatidyl serine	9.6	7.6	8.6	—
Monophosphoinositide	8.3	7.0	8.9	—
Diphosphatidyl glycerol	2.4	2.6	2.4	—
Phosphatidic acids	—	—	—	12
Lysolecithin	—	—	—	3

* Data of Basinska *et al.*[90]
† Data of Jouan *et al.*[448]

diffuse and membrane-associated distribution of pineal cholesterol. The same circumstances can also be offered as an explanation for the lack of positive results with human and rat pineal sections treated according to the Windaus digitonin method for cholesterol.[768] Evidence for pineal contents and biosynthesis or metabolism of sterols and steroids can be expected from studies employing gas chromatography and the uptake and conversion by pineal tissue of radioactive precursors. Young rat pineal glands *in vivo* have a notable uptake and binding of ^{3}H-estradiol,[331] and those from both young and old chickens contain cholesterol, identified by thin-layer and gas-liquid chromatography.[1048]

Phospholipids constitute more than half of the pineal's total lipid content and nearly all of the pineal's compound lipids (Tables XXI and XXII). Comparisons of the results of Jouan *et al.* (1964)[448] and Basinska *et al.* (1969)[90] show that although the exact total percentage of phospholipid within pineal lipids can vary considerably, depending on extraction and fractionation techniques, the proportional representation of the subtypes of phospholipids turns out to be similar after various methods (Table XXIII). The pineal's relatively great content of phospholipids has been known, in fact, for many years. In 1916 Fenger[270] published data on phosphorus contents of petroleum ether extracts of diverse bovine endocrine glands. Recent investigations, although not citing his work, essentially confirm his results. Among pineal phospholipids, phosphatidyl ethanolamine merits particular interest and further study, due to its showing the greatest variation in human pineals from individuals of different ages.[190]

The fatty acid composition of individual phospholipids from bovine pineals has been described by Basinska *et al.* (1969).[90] The chief components are C16:0, C18:0 and C18:1, followed by C16:1 and C14:0 fatty acids (Table XXIV). Also, monophosphoinositide and phosphatidyl ethanolamine contain significant amounts of C20:4. Two-thirds of the total fatty acids are saturated, and one-third unsaturated. Human and sheep phospholipid fatty acid compositions were found by Basinska and co-workers[90] to be about the same as that of bovine pineals and, therefore, were not reported. The fatty acid composition of pineal sphingomyelin is described in Table XXV. Beef pineal sphingomyelin has a base composition consisting mainly of C18 sphingosine with a trace of C18 dihydrosphingosine.

Comparisons with Other Tissues

Comparisons of the pineal gland's lipid composition with that of other organs are of interest for at least two reasons. Similarities in composition between pineal and certain other organs or tissues may suggest similarities in lipid metabolism and some attributes of functional activity. Unique features in pineal lipid composition may serve as clues for detecting which metabolic systems and what related functional activities may be specialized or unique in this organ.

Broad categorical comparisons of pineal lipid contents in man and large domestic mammals are presented in Table XXVI. The pineal's total lipid content is considerably lower than that of whole brain and some glandular tissues. In most of its major categories of lipids it is most similar to such cytologically and functionally dissimilar organs as testes, liver and kidneys.

A more satisfactory comparison with brain tissue is possible when the separate cellular elements of the young brain are analyzed, in contrast to what is obtained in analysis of adult brain when myelin and its lipid content are included. Mam-

TABLE XXIV

Fatty acid composition of phospholipids of bovine pineal glands (percent).*

Fatty Acids†	Phosphatidyl-choline	Phosphatidyl-ethanolamine	Phosphatidyl-serine	Diphosphatidyl-glycerol	Monophospho-inositide
12:0	0.4	0.5	1.6	0.8	0.8
13:0		0.1	0.3	0.2	0.2
14:0	1.6	3.0	8.1	6.6	4.7
14:1	0.2	0.4	1.0	0.9	0.8
15:0	0.9	1.6	3.8	3.6	2.8
15:1	0.2	0.4	0.7	1.0	0.6
16:0	34.2	17.7	24.0	25.5	21.0
16:1	2.5	3.4	5.4	7.8	6.3
17:0	1.0	1.4	1.3	2.0	1.4
18:0	29.3	37.3	29.4	15.4	34.0
18:1	20.9	20.8	16.6	18.6	10.8
18:2	1.9	2.5	2.0	5.2	1.8
19:0	0.3	0.2	0.1	0.5	0.5
20:0	0.6	0.6	1.6	0.8	0.8
20:4	2.0	4.9	1.0	2.2	9.0
21:0	0.4	0.6	0.4	1.8	0.8
22:0	2.0	2.0	1.0	2.5	1.5
24:1				2.2	
Total saturated	70.4	65.0	71.6	59.7	68.5
Total unsaturated	28.9	34.2	28.3	40.5	31.1

* From Basinska et al.[90]

† Fatty acids expressed as number of C atoms : number of double bonds.

TABLE XXV
Fatty acid composition of pineal sphingomyelin (percent).*

Fatty Acids†	Species Method‡	Man A	Man B	Cattle A	Cattle B	Sheep A
12:0		0.8	0.8	0.7	——	1.0
13.0		0.2	0.2	0.1	——	0.3
14:0		3.7	5.6	2.8	0.5	4.1
14:1		0.6	1.1	0.6	0.3	1.6
15:0		2.5	3.4	1.5	0.3	2.4
15:1		0.8	1.3	0.6	——	0.4
16:0		17.6	18.1	14.6	10.3	18.2
16:1		6.6	10.2	3.0	——	6.4
17:0		1.4	1.7	1.2	0.9	1.2
18:0		30.0	20.2	33.0	44.0	34.4
18:1		9.8	10.4	9.2	2.4	11.7
18:2		1.4	1.8	2.0	0.3	1.3
19:0		1.0	1.8	0.6	0.6	0.8
20:0		2.8	2.7	4.2	4.7	2.1
20:4		1.6	1.0	3.4	1.9	1.1
21:0		0.6	0.6	1.1	——	1.1
21:1		——	——	0.3	——	0.8
22:0		3.6	3.9	6.0	9.8	2.8
23:0		0.8	1.8	1.4	1.3	——
24:0		4.7	5.4	8.9	12.7	3.3
24:1		7.0	4.4	3.0	8.7	1.9

* Data from Basinska *et al.*[90]
† Fatty acids expressed as number of C atoms : number of double bonds.
‡ Method A = separation of sphingomyelin by silicic acid paper chromatography; Method B = separation of phospholipids by column chromatography with subsequent mild alkaline hydrolysis of phosphatides and extraction and purification by silicic acid column chromatography of the remaining sphingomyelin.

malian pineals and brains have a closely related embryological origin, and the adult pineal is like young brain in having very little myelin and in having some of the same kinds of cells, particularly astrocytes and others which, at least superficially, have some characteristics of neurons. As demonstrated by Table XXVII, pineal lipid composition is like that of neurons and glia in some of its constituents but different in others. The pineal differs from neurons in its cholesterol and phosphatidyl serine levels, from astrocytes in its phosphoinositide content, and from both cell types in its content of sphingomyelin, acetal phosphatides and galactolipid (Table XXVII). Thus, in its lipid composition the pineal has a distinctive individuality and shows nearly equivalent degrees of differentiation from astrocyte as from neuronal lipid compositions.

TABLE XXVI
Comparisons of lipid contents of pineal and other mammalian tissues*

Tissue	Total Lipid (% of wet wgt.)	% of Total Lipid				
		Phospholipids	Free Cholesterol	Ester Cholesterol	Glycerides	Other P-free Lipids
Pineal	2.9–5.3	58–71	13–15	0.4–1.1	12	1
Brain	10–13	45–76	19–27	n.d.†	n.d.†	28
Pituitary	n.d.†	33	7	0.4	51	8.6
Adrenal	20–27	10	4.5	40.5	45	0
Testes	2.2	80	9.5	0.5	10	0
Pancreas	15	24	10.9	2.1	61.7	1.3
Liver	2.5	55	12.6	3.4	26.9	2.1
Kidney	2.7	78	15.4	0.6	5.5	0.5

* Primarily from Basinska et al.[90] but slightly modified by data from references 281, 690, 936.
† n.d. = not determined.

TABLE XXVII

Comparison of adult mammalian pineal lipid composition with that of neuronal perikarya and astrocytes from young rat brains (percent of total lipid).*

	Neurons†	Astrocytes†		Pineal
Cholesterol	10.6 ± 0.6	14.0 ± 1.9		13–16
Total Phospholipid	72.3 ± 2.9	70.9 ± 2.0		58–71
Phosphatidyl Choline	39.9 ± 2.5	36.3 ± 2.1		26–33
Phosphatidyl Ethanolamine	18.2 ± 0.6	20.1 ± 1.8		13–16
Phosphatidyl Serine	3.9 ± 0.3	5.2 ± 0.4		5.2–5.6
Phosphoinositides	4.9 ± 0.4	3.5 ± 0.5		4.8–5.3
Sphingomyelin	3.2 ± 0.3	3.7 ± 0.6	<	6.5–9.8
Acetal Phosphatides	7.0 ± 0.7	7.6 ± 0.9	>	low
Galactolipid	2.1 ± 0.4	1.8 ± 0.4	>	very low

* Data derived from references 90, 448, 690.
† Means ± standard deviations from six samples.

The appreciable pineal sphingomyelin content, like that of whole brain, is higher than that of isolated neurons and astrocytes, but it is distinctive in its low concentration of C24:1 fatty acid (Table XXV). Two methods of separation give yields of C24:1 fatty acids lower than those reported for nervous tissue, blood, spleen, placenta, liver and kidney, but similar to that of fetal whole brain.[90]

A comparatively low pineal content of acetal phosphatides (plasmalogens) is characteristic. While rat brain contains 11.8 μ moles/g wet wgt., human, bovine and sheep pineals contain 2.3, 2.6 and 3.0 μ moles plasmalogen, respectively.[90]

In their apparent lack of cerebrosides[296] and very low content of gangliosides, pineal glands show additional differences with respect to brain tissue. Ganglioside preparations from pineals of man, cattle and sheep show, by analysis of their neuraminic acid content, less than 0.2 μ moles/g wet wgt. for all three species.[90] A higher value (5.85 μ moles/g tissue) for bovine pineal total neuraminic acid was obtained by Green *et al.* (1962),[336] who, however, did not isolate the fraction derived from gangliosides. Ganglioside preparations from bovine brain gave 1.28 μ moles neuraminic acid/g tissue wet wgt.,[90] which is at least six times greater than that of bovine pineal. A greater ganglioside content occurs, also, in bovine retina, with total lipid equaling 2.82 percent of the wet weight, and ganglioside comprising about 0.6 percent of the total lipid, or 0.58_μ moles neuraminic acid/g wet wgt. of whole retina.[367]

Quantitative analyses of pineal lipid classes, reviewed above, have not revealed any lipid fraction or specific compound unique to this organ. The possibility still remains that further studies will succeed in demonstrating such compounds. However, at the present time, the pineal's known lipid composition is consistent with the interpretation that pineal lipids are primarily concerned in general metabolism and in membrane structure and function rather than as having roles as hormones or precursors to hormones.

LIPID METABOLISM

No studies concerned specifically with pineal lipid metabolism have been reported. Only few and small bits of evidence can be pulled together at this time to provide a preliminary view of this subject. Such fragmentary evidence has two origins: (1) studies of uptake of inorganic phosphate and its incorporation in phospholipids, and (2) histochemical and chemical demonstrations of enzyme activities involved or potentially involved in pineal lipid metabolism or mobilization.

The classic studies by Borell and Örström[128,129] showed that the rapid uptake and turnover of ^{32}P in the rat pineal gland *in vivo* proceed in two ways. About 90 percent of the bound radioactivity is quickly found in a fraction soluble in trichloroacetic acid, and representing, at least largely, phosphorylated metabolic intermediates most often associated with carbohydrate and energy metabolism. The remaining smaller fraction of bound radioactivity is slower in its rise and turnover, and is insoluble in trichloroacetic acid. It is presumed to include phospholipid and protein. A more extensive and detailed metabolic analysis of pineal phosphate incorporation by newer methods would be timely. Many studies of this kind have been performed recently using sympathetic ganglia and other nervous tissues and have shown profound effects of ions, neurotransmitters and other chemical agents.[297,406,537,538,920,1092]

Acetone-fixed frozen sections of adult rat pineals were found by Leduc and Wislocki[541] to be capable of hydrolyzing long-chain fatty acid esters (Tweens 40 and 60), but to be relatively weak in this activity as compared with choroid plexuses and some other brain structures. Prop[753] succeeded subsequently in using Tween 80 as a substrate and in showing a relatively high enzyme activity on, or associated with, the rat pineal's cytoplasmic lipid droplets. Most recently, Markina,[599] in combined application of lipid staining and the "Tween method," has shown an increase in enzyme activity and decrease in lipid in rat pineals after adrenalectomy or after a salt free diet. These histochemical results based on Tween substrates do not succeed, however, in distinguishing between the activities of true lipase and so-called nonspecific esterases.[142,724]

A peptide having weak lipolytic activity when tested on rabbit adipose tissue has been purified from bovine and ovine pineals and has been found to have a molecular weight between 1000 and 3500.[871] It is not known whether this compound has any physiological significance as a lipolytic agent, either within the pineal or systemically.

CONCLUSIONS

1. Lipids occur in the pineal glands of man and other mammals, but the amounts vary according to species and age, and, at least in the laboratory rat, a great variety of other conditions and treatments.

2. Human intralobular pinealocytes containing cytoplasmic lipid droplets increase in apparent number with age, and they increase, also, in their content of a lipofuscin-like pigment. Interlobular or stromal cells containing lipid droplets of larger size also increase in apparent number with age, especially in relation to formation of pineal cysts and increases in thickness of interlobular septa.

3. No correlations have been made between relative numbers or other characteristics of human pineal lipid-containing cells and particular premortem physiological or disease states or causes of death.

4. Lipid-containing cells in rat pineals can be subdivided into two categories: *type I* (light) *cells,* consisting of pinealocytes containing ethanol-soluble cytoplasmic droplets with a high content of neutral lipids; and *type II* (dark) *cells,* consisting of more glioid pinealocytes, demonstrable primarily by the acid hematein technique for staining structures having a composition with choline-containing phospholipids.

5. Rat pineal lipid, particularly that in *type I cells,* has a twenty-four hour rhythm. The maximum lipid content is near midday, and the minimum is near midnight, in relation to the timing of the daily photoperiod. This rhythm is not free-running and is rapidly depressed, and probably lost, in continuous light.

6. During phases of the rat's estrous cycle, pineal lipid content is lowest during proestrus and highest during diestrus. Ovariectomy or gonadotropin administration raises pineal lipid content, and hypophysectomy or administration of estradiol lowers it.

7. Structural classes of lipids and their relative amounts are similar in man and large domestic species of mammals. From 3 to over 10 percent of the organ's wet weight is lipid, and more than half of this is phospholipid. Most of the remaining lipid is free cholesterol and glycerides.

8. Pineal phospholipids in man and other investigated large mammals are primarily phosphatidyl choline (45–47%), phosphatidyl ethanolamine (22–27%) and sphingomyelin (11–14%). In comparisons with isolated neuron cell body and astrocyte fractions from young rat brains, pineal phospholipid composition differs from both most greatly in having a greater relative (to total lipid) content of sphingomyelin and lesser contents of acetal phosphatides and galactolipids.

9. No lipid compounds have been isolated or identified which are peculiar to pineal tissue. As currently known, pineal lipids can be interpreted as probably being involved primarily in general metabolism and in membrane structure and function within the organ. Little is known about pineal lipid metabolism.

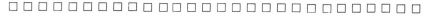

Chapter Five

CARBOHYDRATES

METABOLITES

CARBOHYDRATES FORM A large group of compounds with an empirical formula close to $C_x H_{2x} O_x$, and consisting of polyhydroxyaldehydes or polyhydroxyketones and their derivatives. The primary members of this group are saccharides. They are classified according to the number of unit saccharide or sugar molecules which form their structure. Monosaccharides comprise the simplest members. They are soluble in most aqueous solutions and are metabolically very labile in animal tissues. Mammalian pineal tissue can be expected to contain such monosaccharides as glucose and related nearly ubiquitous derivatives and metabolites. But, measurements of most of these are not available. This is due largely to the technical difficulties of measuring such labile compounds. Even for larger compounds, the polysaccharides such as glycogen, lability and solubility are causes of controversy concerning accurate tissue analyses. At the presently primitive state of knowledge about pineal carbohydrates, we can lump the demonstrated members together under the heading of metabolites. Nevertheless, it is to be recognized that while a larger proportion of these are taken up in energy metabolism, a significant proportion can be expected to be involved in pineal structural composition, especially within stromal regions and within the intercellular substances.

Ascorbic Acid

Ascorbic acid (L-xyloascorbic acid) or vitamin C has been measured by many methods, most of which are based on

TABLE XXVIII

Concentration of ascorbic acid in bovine pineal glands from animals of different ages.*

	Number of Individuals	mg Ascorbic Acid g Tissue Wet Wgt.
Fetal		
5.2 months	1	0.15
7.2 months	1	0.24
8 months	1	0.27
Postnatal		
Calves	5	0.12–0.16
Adult Cows	4	0.07–0.12

* Data of Glick and Biskind.[322]

its strong reducing power. The only data discovered on human pineal ascorbic acid content are based on microtitration with methylene blue and necropsy tissue samples taken long after death.[145] The specificity of the latter determinations (range 0.025–0.400 mg/g) and their significance remain doubtful. The usual and preferred method for measuring tissue ascorbic acid is microtitration with dichlorophenol indophenol. This method has been used by Glick and Biskind[322] to measure the ascorbic acid contents of bovine pineal glands from animals of different ages (Table XXVIII). Higher concentrations in adult cattle and horse pineals were obtained by Giroud and co-workers (means and ranges, respectively: 0.277, 0.208–0.245; 0.367, 0.207–0.520 mg/g).[320] Bovine pineal ascorbic acid has a developmental pattern (Table XXVIII) similar to that of some other tissues, including brain.[489] Thus, in a recent study rat brain ascorbic acid was found to rise from 0.43 mg/g six days before birth to 0.66 mg/g by five days after birth and to subsequently decline to 0.28 mg/g in adults.[18] About 40 percent of this decline occurred during the first three weeks after birth. Similar results are available from older investigations of age changes in human brain ascorbic acid.[489] The similarity between pineal and brain developmental and age changes in ascorbic acid concentration suggests that the decrease in the adult pineal cannot be automatically construed as evidence for reduction in general functional activity. Ascorbic acid normally is present in brain, pituitary gland and adrenal medulla in relatively high concentrations, and is also present in cerebrospinal fluid.[607] Among brain regions of adult larger mammals, its concentration ranges from 0.10 to about 0.18 mg/g.[299,607] This is close to concentrations in adult bovine pineal glands (Table XXVIII). It is interesting to note that histochemical studies of ascorbic acid distribution within the brain show major localizations within autonomic centers and regions having a very active metabolism of monoamines.[299] This is another parallel with the pineal gland.

Only one histochemical method is recognized for the demonstration of ascorbic acid in tissues, and it depends on a relatively non-specific reduction of silver nitrate. The serious limitations of the method have been reviewed by Pearse.[724] It, nevertheless, remains capable of providing results of value in carefully controlled studies. Early applications to human pineal tissue sections by Leopold[545] and Clara[162] revealed some scant reduced silver grains partly in the cytoplasm of pinealocytes and especially in glial and connective tissue cells. Since it was not possible to rule out cell pigment granules, and perhaps certain other inclusions, as the reactive centers, these findings are of doubtful validity as demonstrations of pineal localizations of ascorbic acid. The same method was applied by Collier[170] to pineal tissue sections from untreated rats and mice, as well as those that had been injected subcutaneously with ascorbic acid. In pineals of neither group could he detect a positive reaction microscopically. Bacchus' variant of this method was applied by Prop and Kappers[755] to pineal glands of adult untreated rats. A small number of irregularly distributed granules was found in pinealocytes, as well as in other cells. The same variant of the technique has been combined with electron microscopic examination of normal rat pineal glands.[345] Fresh tissue was treated first with alcoholic silver nitrate in the dark (Bacchus' variant)[723] and then fixed in OsO_4 for fifteen minutes. In almost all of the pineal cells an intensively electron-dense and finely granular precipitate was found. The granules ranged from 150 to 250 mμ in diameter and were, thus, partly within and partly below the limits of resolution by light microscopy. The rather general distribution and frequent binding of these granules to organelles such as mitochondria were noted. These characteristics and the lack of any control specimens or supporting experiments lead to doubts concerning the identification of the reduced silver granules as sites of pineal ascorbic acid.

Neuraminic Acid

Neuraminic acid is a 9-carbon, 3-deoxy-5-amino sugar. Various *N*- and *O*-acyl derivatives of it form the group known as sialic acids. These are ubiquitously distributed in animal tissues and have been identified as constituents of lipids, polysaccharides and mucoproteins. Green and co-workers[336] have found a relatively high concentration of neuraminic acid in bovine pineal glands, 5.85 μmoles/g tissue as compared with 3.92 μmoles/g bovine brain gray matter. Brain sialic acids are found in both glycoprotein and glycolipid components of cell membranes and have been studied recently by intracerebral injection of radioactive precursors (L-fucose-^{3}H and *N*-acetyl-^{3}H-D-mannose).[759] Similar studies with pineal tissue may provide results of especial interest, in view of the high concentration of neuraminic acid, and the relatively low concentrations of known glycolipids (Table XXI) in the pineal gland.

Glycogen

Glycogen is a polysaccharide composed of branched chains of glucose molecules and is the nutrient storage form of carbohydrate in animal tissues. Reported molecular weights range from 270,000 to 100,000,000. It has been studied in pineal glands by both biochemical and histochemical techniques. However, two circumstances give the available findings only a severely limited significance. The first of these is the rapidity of the loss of tissue glycogen after the killing of the animal. A five minute delay before freezing of mouse brain for glycogen analysis has been reported to lead to an 82 percent loss.[418] Although it is possible that postmortem loss of glycogen from pineal glands may not be as rapid as that from brain or other investigated organs, there are no data available to support such a possibility. The second circumstance providing difficulties is the still controversial relative demonstrability of protein-bound glycogen (desmoglycogen) in comparison with easily extractable or *free* glycogen (lyo- or lysoglycogen).[87,526,553] No reliable information of either direct or indirect sorts is available on what fraction of bound glycogen is likely to have been revealed in pineal glands so far by either biochemical or histochemical methods. The small size of the organ in laboratory mammals has been a handicap until recently for discriminating chemical studies of pineal glycogen fractions. Now, enzymatic and microchemical methods provide the technical advances necessary for such studies on pineal composition.

The only chemical measurements of pineal glycogen are apparently those of Quay,[781] who was interested primarily in determining the effect of continuous light on relative levels of pineal metabolites and metabolic activities. Krisman's modification of the colorimetric iodine method for glycogen was used.[522] The pineal concentrations found by this method fall within the range of glycogen concentrations (0.4–2.0 μg/mg) reported recently in adult rat brain by other investigators, using other methods. Of probably greater significance is the much lower pineal glycogen concentration revealed in rats that had been subjected to continuous environmental illumination (Table XXIX).

A circadian (twenty-four hour) rhythm has been found recently in mouse pineal glycogen content, based on a semiquantitative histochemical method. Glycogen in pinealocytes was least at the end of the daily dark period, and was greatest in amount at the end of the light period. A rhythm in pinealocyte glycogen could not be detected in blinded mice.[456]

Histochemical studies on distribution of glycogen within mammalian pineal glands have been made for over sixty years on a wide variety of species and with a diversity in results. In adult human pineals Quast[761] found glycogen granules only in cells of the interlobular connective tissue. Bayerová and Bayer[91] studied human pineal sections stained by Bauer,

Pineal Chemistry

TABLE XXIX
Effect of continuous light for twelve weeks on pineal glycogen content of adult female rats.*

Group	Number of Samples†	Pineal Wet Wgt. (mg)‡	Pineal Glycogen Content	
			μg/pineal‡	μg/mg‡
Continuously Lighted	5	0.876 ± 0.14	0.48 ± 0.03	0.55 ± 0.04
Controls (14 hr. light/day)	5	1.084 ± 0.026	1.40 ± 0.10	1.30 ± 0.11

* Data of Quay.[781]
† Each sample contained the pineal glands from nine to ten animals.
‡ All results are mean ± standard error of the mean; P < 0.001 for differences between means of the experimental and control groups.

Best's carmine and periodic acid-Schiff (PAS) techniques and compared them with control sections previously treated with saliva. Only traces of glycogen were found and only in a few cells. Wislocki and Dempsey[1053] studied glycogen distribution in pineal sections of rhesus monkeys (*Macaca mulatta*) stained by Bauer and PAS methods and compared with saliva-treated controls. The Bauer technique for glycogen was completely negative, but the more sensitive PAS technique differentiated two kinds of parenchymal cells in the monkey pineal on the basis of presence or absence of glycogen. This was suggested to be indicative of either two different types of parenchymal cells or parenchymal cells in different stages of functional activity. Pineal localization of glycogen has been investigated in several kinds of domesticated ungulates. Jordan,[445] using an insensitive iodine reaction, was unable to detect glycogen in sheep pineal glands. But Toryu,[980] with Best's carmine stain, found it to be abundant in the interstitial tissue of horse pineals. He found it was easily removed by prior treatment with either saliva or diastase. In a study using similar methods for glycogen, and employing pig and goat pineals as well as those of horses, Mikami[622] concluded that cytoplasmic glycogen characterized one of the two observed kinds of pineal parenchymal cells. Within this cell, glycogen was found in close association with alkaline phosphatase activity in the cytoplasmic extensions or processes. Mikami's other stated structural and cytochemical characteristics for the two parenchymal cell types suggest that the glycogen-containing cells may have been either *type II* pinealocytes or astrocytic glial cells. It is also likely that his interpretation of the cytological distribution of pineal glycogen was influenced significantly by that of Wislocki and Dempsey[1053] based on monkey pineals and noted above.

Cytoplasmic glycogen granules have a characteristic appearance in electron micrographs of animal cells. On this basis glycogen often can be identified, or its presence surmised, in pinealocyte cytoplasm in published reports on pineal ultrastructure. However, the texts of these same reports seldom mention glycogen, probably because its presence is frequently taken for granted. Wartenberg,[1026] nevertheless, did note the occurrence of glycogen granules within what he identified as glial cell processes in mammalian pineal organs. A systematic study on the intrapineal distribution and abundance of these granules at the ultrastructural level is still needed.

Other Polysaccharides and Derivatives

With the aid of various staining reactions, many investigators have noted the probable presence within mammalian pineals of more complex and relatively insoluble materials containing polysaccharide or related or derivative compounds such as mucopolysaccharides and glycoproteins.[91,152,824,983] Some of these materials are in, or associated with, interlobular cells and structures, including fibroblasts, mast cells, phagocytic cells and corpora arenacea. Much more problematical are other stained materials which possibly lie within lobules or their parenchymal cells. Separation of peptides from beef pineals has yielded one fraction that has the staining reactions of glycoprotein.[966] It remains to be determined whether this product has biological or humoral activity.

METABOLISM

Characteristics of pineal carbohydrate metabolism are revealed by both direct and indirect means. The direct means consists of tracing metabolic products from radioactively labeled carbohydrate substrate. In the case of studies of pineal metabolism, this has meant brief incubations of pineal tissue with glucose, either uniformly labeled with ^{14}C or with particular ones of its C atoms so labeled in order to differentiate metabolites formed through modifications or ruptures of the glucose molecule at different ones of its C-C bonds. Indirect avenues of viewing pineal carbohydrate metabolism consist of data on the presence and levels of particular enzymes and metabolites within pineal tissue. However, these data have greater qualitative rather than quantitative significance, since the level of a particular enzyme activity demonstrated by a homogenate, mince or tissue fragment may differ considerably from that possible *in vivo,* where membrane systems are intact, critical concentrations of cofactors maintained, and supporting metabolic activities are allowed to continue. Tissue levels of carbohydrate metabolites are often exceedingly labile postmortem, and distorted relative levels of some of them can be expected in specimens taken even a few minutes after death.

Hellman and Larsson[380] studied metabolism of uniformly labeled ^{14}C-glucose by pineal glands from goats of four different age groups. Consumption of O_2 and conversion of ^{14}C-glucose into $^{14}CO_2$ and ^{14}C-lactic acid by pineal tissue decreased with age (Table XXX). Bidimensional chromatography of extracts of the homogenized pineal tissue after incubation revealed the highest levels of radioactive amino acid products in the samples from the youngest animals (Table XXXI). This is most distinct in the cases of alanine and glutamic acid. Pineal tissue from the youngest animals also had the greatest incorporation of glucose into the insoluble residue, while only traces of such incorporation were detectable in that from the oldest ones. In incubations of tissue from the one- to three-month-old group, 1.3 ± 0.2 μg glucose was found in the insoluble fraction per 25 mg of tissue, and in that from the groups of intermediate age, 0.6 ± 0.1. The moderate conversion of glucose to GABA (γ-aminobutyric acid) is a characteristic shared by pineal and neuro-

TABLE XXX

Respiratory exchange and lactic acid production by goat pineal tissue according to age of donor animals.*

Age	N†	O_2 Uptake† (μl O_2/25mg tissue)	Glucose (μg) Converted to:†		Free Glucose† (in tissue extract after incubation)
			CO_2	Lactic Acid	
1–3 months	5	30.2 ± 2.2	9.9 ± 0.6	149.5 ± 9.2	5.0 ± 0.3
4–6 months	4	27.8 ± 2.1	4.3 ± 1.0	58.3 ± 6.3	1.7 ± 0.3
2–3 years	7	22.1 ± 1.5	4.4 ± 0.3	72.0 ± 5.5	5.7 ± 0.4
> 6 years	4	13.5 ± 0.6	2.7 ± 0.2	27.0 ± 4.5	trace

* From Hellman and Larsson.[380]
Incubation for 1 hour at 37°C in 0.1% glucose (20 μc/mg) in a phosphate buffer.
† N = number of animals (and incubations).
‡ Means ± standard errors.

hypophyseal tissue, but is lacking in hypophyseal anterior lobe and pancreatic islets. It is interesting, also, that at least in terms of absolute values, the pineal's formation of alanine from glucose seems especially high (Table XXXI).

Parallel tissue incubations with $[1-^{14}C]$-glucose and $[6-^{14}C]$-glucose have been employed to reveal the relative activities of two routes of glucose oxidation. These are, respectively, the pentose phosphate pathway, or "shunt" and the Embden-Meyerhof pathway leading through pyruvate. The pentose phosphate pathway is known sometimes, also, as the hexose monophosphate (HMP) or phosphogluconate pathway. Its primary purpose in most cells is the generation of chemical reducing capacity in the extramitochondrial cytoplasm in the form of reduced nicotinamide adenine dinucleotide phosphate (= $NADPH_2$ or TPNH). A second common function of this pathway is the generation of pentoses, particularly D-ribose, used in the synthesis of nucleic acids. The ratio of the fractional recoveries of radioactive CO_2 from $1-^{14}C$- and $6-^{14}C$-labeled glucose substrates provides a measure of the relative activities of the two metabolic pathways, so long as certain assumptions are accepted. However, as pointed out by B. Axelrod[44] and others, the quantitative interpretation of the resulting data can have uncertainties due to possible occurrences of alternative metabolic mechanisms.

TABLE XXXI

Metabolic conversion of glucose into amino acids by incubated goat pineal tissue according to age of donor animals.*

Age	N†	Glucose (μg) converted (per 25 mg tissue) to:‡					
		Alanine	Aspartic acid	Glutamic acid	Glutamine	Arginine	GABA
1–3 months	5	3.4 ± 0.1	0.5 ± 0.1	3.8 ± 0.2	1.2 ± 0.1	1.2 ± 0.3	0.6 ± 0.1
4–6 months	4	1.1 ± 0.2	0.3 ± 0.1	1.5 ± 0.1	0.3 ± 0.1	0.5 ± 0.2	0.3 ± 0.1
2–3 years	7	1.3 ± 0.2	0.3 ± 0.1	1.5 ± 0.3	1.8 ± 0.2	0.6 ± 0.1	0.2 ± 0.1
> 6 years	4	trace	—	trace	trace	—	—

* From Hellman and Larsson.[380]
Incubations for one hour at 37°C in 0.1% glucose (20 μc/mg) in a phosphate buffer.
† N = number of animals (and incubations).
‡ Means ± standard errors.

Nevertheless, results from such studies remain strongly suggestive of the relative activity of the pentose phosphate pathway, especially when related tissues are compared or when samples of the same kind of tissue from animals of different ages or physiological states are compared.

Krass and LaBella have studied bovine pineal, brain and lobes of the pituitary gland by this method.[520,521,530] A C-1/C-6 ratio greater than 1.0 was considered indicative of an active pentose phosphate pathway. The pineal gland was found to share with the pituitary and other studied endocrine tissues the distinction of having a high C-1/C6 ratio (Table XXXII). In this characteristic, pineal tissue differs greatly from all regions of the brain which have been examined, including that region lying immediately adjacent to it. Krass and LaBella calculated that in anterior pituitary, posterior pituitary and pineal gland, 5 percent, 4 percent, and 3 percent of the utilized glucose, respectively, is metabolized via the pentose phosphate pathway, while in brain the activity of this pathway is negligible. Although activity by this pathway is correlated with tissues having endocrine capacity, its precise role or roles within specific adult cells or tissues remains unclear. A higher activity in young or rapidly proliferating cells can be associated with synthesis of nucleic acids. In order to accommodate the circumstance of a low C-1/C-6 ratio in hypothalamic neurosecretory nuclei where synthesis of neurohypophyseal hormones occurs, and a high ratio in the posterior pituitary where storage and secretion of these hormones occurs, Krass and LaBella proposed that the pentose phosphate pathway may be more involved in either the storage and/or secretion of hormones rather than in their synthesis.[521] This distinction in regard to relative involvement in hormone synthesis probably depends also on the chemistry of the hormone, as for example, oligopeptide as compared with steroid hormones.

Additional insights concerning the possible significance of the pineal's and pituitary's relatively high C-1/C-6 ratio can be obtained by considering the relative incorporation of ^{14}C from $[1-^{14}C]-$ and $[6-^{14}C]$-glucose into other prod-

TABLE XXXII

Comparison of oxidation *in vitro* of [1-^{14}C]- and [6-^{14}C]glucose by bovine pineal, anterior pituitary, posterior pituitary and cerebral cortex according to age.*

Organ Age	$^{14}CO_2$ counts x 10^{-3}/min/g†			% Difference Young > Adults		
	1-^{14}C	6-^{14}C	C-1/C-6	1-^{14}C	6-^{14}C	Ratio C-1/C-6
Pineal						
5–10 months	72.7 ± 10.2	7.0 ± 0.8	10.6 ± 1.0	+89	+ 56	+18
3–8 years	38.5 ± 3.9	4.5 ± 0.1	8.6 ± 0.7			
Anterior Pituitary						
5–10 months	15.5 ± 1.7	1.6	12.7	+42	+100	−24
3–8 years	10.9 ± 1.9	0.8	16.7			
Posterior Pituitary						
5–10 months	271.5 ± 36.9	37.0 ± 6.8	7.3 ± 1.2	+47	+107	−24
3–8 years	185.3 ± 24.4	17.9 ± 2.6	9.7 ± 1.4			
Cerebral Cortex						
5–10 months	117.8 ± 22.3	70.5	1.4	−31	− 49	+27
3–8 years	184.0 ± 31.0	139.0	1.1			

* Calculated from data of Krass and LaBella.[520]

† Means ± standard errors, from tissue minces incubated for 30 minutes.

ucts, as well as CO_2 (Table XXXIII). Thus, in comparison with cerebral cortex, pineal and pituitary parts have relatively greater incorporation of ^{14}C into lactate and fatty acids, from [6-^{14}C]-glucose, in comparison with that from [1-^{14}C]-glucose. In its distribution of specific yield, the pineal is seen to be remarkably similar to the posterior pituitary. Anterior pituitary differs from both of these neuroectodermal derivatives, as well as from cerebral cortex, in having greater incorporation of ^{14}C into fatty acids and glycerol, and especially from [6-^{14}C]-glucose (Table XXXIII). Therefore, it can be suggested that greater diversion of C-6 glucose metabolites into synthetic pathways and into other metabolic systems, such as those for lipids, can enhance a relatively high C-1/C-6 ratio based on incorporation into CO_2.

Nevertheless, studies on specific enzyme activities of pineal tissue lend support to belief in a relatively more active pentose phosphate pathway in pineal than in brain. Two enzymes are especially interesting in this connection, glucose-6-phosphate dehydrogenase and aldolase. Glucose-6-phosphate dehydrogenase catalyzes the first distinctive step in the pentose phosphate pathway, that from glucose-6-phosphate to 6-phosphogluconate. Histochemical studies have shown this enzyme to have relatively strong activity in human pinealomas,[479] as well as in normal rat pineal glands. The latter study comprehensively compared activities throughout the rat brain, and found those of the greatest magnitude in the paraventricular and supraoptic nuclei of the hypothalamus and the pineal body or gland of the epithalamus. Other parts of the epithalamus had lower activities; medial habenular nuclei had moderate activity, lateral habenular nuclei faint activity and the stria medullaris was negative. In guinea pig pineals, glucose-6-phosphate dehydrogenase has an uneven distribution among the pinealocytes,[1029] suggesting that differences in the activity of this pathway occur in relation to parenchymal cell type or to phase in a synthetic and secretory metabolic cycle. Aldolase catalyzes in the Embden-Meyerhof path the critical step from fructose-1,6-diphosphate to glyceraldehyde-

TABLE XXXIII

Relative incorporation of ^{14}C of labeled $[1-^{14}C]-$ and $[6-^{14}C]$glucose into CO_2, lactate, fatty acids and glycerol by bovine pineal, anterior pituitary, posterior pituitary and cerebral cortex *in vitro*.*

	Specific yield†							
	CO_2		Lactate		Fatty acids		Glycerol	
Tissue	1-C	6-C	1-C	6-C	1-C	6-C	1-C	6-C
Pineal	0.087	0.019	0.850	0.920	0.004	0.005	0.058	0.055
Anterior pituitary	0.130	0.019	0.605	0.535	0.010	0.125	0.260	0.435
Posterior pituitary	0.130	0.026	0.770	0.915	0.003	0.005	0.096	0.058
Cerebral cortex	0.094	0.081	0.885	0.880	0.004	0.003	0.021	0.037

* Calculated from data of Krass and LaBella[521]; 200 mg tissue in 3 ml pH 7.4 phosphate buffer containing 50 mg glucose including $2\mu c$ of either $[1-^{14}C]$glucose or $[6-^{14}C]$glucose, at 37°C, under 95% $O_2-5\%$ CO_2 for two hours.
† Specific yield = fraction of the total glucose utilized; means of results of two experiments, each of which was based on triplicate incubations.

TABLE XXXIV

Effect of epinephrine on oxidation *in vitro* of [1–^{14}C]- and [6–^{14}C]glucose by bovine pineal glands from 'young' (5–10 months) and 'adult' (three to eight years) animals.*

Age Treatment	$^{14}CO_2$ counts x 10^{-3}/min/g†		% Increase by epinephrine		Ratio C-1/C-6	
	1–^{14}C	6–^{14}C	1–^{14}C	6–^{14}C	Control	Epineph-rine
Young Control	55.3	7.65				
			171	41	7.2	13.9
Epinephrine	150.0	10.86				
Adult Control	32.2	5.16				
			157	33	6.2	12.0
Epinephrine	82.6	6.87				
Control	144.0	24.60				
			183	63	5.9	10.1
Epinephrine	408.0	40.20				

* Data of Krass and LaBella.[520]

† Each value is the mean of triplicate thirty-minute incubations of tissue minces.

3-phosphate. Its activity in pineal homogenates has been found to be lower than that obtained in parallel incubations of brain tissue from cerebral cortex and from the epithalamus.[967] Other enzymes relevant to carbohydrate metabolism and known to occur in the pineal gland are reviewed in a later chapter devoted specifically to enzymes.

Another area of interest concerning pineal carbohydrate metabolism is that of control mechanisms. Epinephrine has been shown to stimulate *in vitro* the oxidation of [1-^{14}C]- and [6^{14}C]-glucose by bovine pineal tissue, although the metabolism of the latter label to $^{14}CO_2$ was affected to a lesser degree (Table XXXIV). Oxidation of [6-^{14}C]-glucose to $^{14}CO_2$ by brain, anterior and posterior pituitary *in vitro* is not affected by epinephrine, but oxidation of [1-^{14}C]-glucose to $^{14}CO_2$ is stimulated by epinephrine in these tissues.[520,530] It may be recalled from the chapter on pineal lipids that massive injections of norepinephrine or amphetamine caused *in vivo* an increase in numbers of cells reacting to the acid hematein technique. Catecholamines have other metabolic effects, as well, on the pineal organ.

Some more general metabolic aspects of control mechanisms are suggested from studies on pineal respiration and activity of enzymes of the citric acid cycle. In comparison with tela chorioideal or choroid plexus samples, consisting in large part of ependymal cells, rat pineal tissue has the greatest increase in O_2 uptake when succinate or glutamate are added substrates.[780] Pineal succinic dehydrogenase activity *in vitro* is modified by previous treatments of the animals. All of the effective stimulatory treatments fall within the category of sympathetic and sympathomimetic agents, but the direction of their effect depends upon timing of treatment and autopsy.[770,773]

CONCLUSIONS

1. Carbohydrates in pineal tissue are known primarily from a few nearly ubiquitous compounds that are somewhat less labile postmortem than glucose. These are ascorbic acid, neuraminic acid and glycogen.

2. Ascorbic acid concentrations in bovine pineal glands show a decline from young to adult animals similar to that described in rat brain. Also similar are adult concentrations of ascorbic acid in bovine pineal and brain tissue from large mammals.

3. Neuraminic acid occurs in greater concentrations in bovine pineal glands than in brain of the same species. Pineal derivatives of neuraminic acid, especially those of glycoprotein composition, merit study as possibly distinctive and functionally significant products of pinealocytes.

4. Although demonstrated within pineal cells by diverse methods, glycogen measurements are few and localizations varible according to species and author. Reduction in rat pineal glycogen content occurs under continuous illumination; under normal day-night conditions there is a circadian rhythm.

5. Metabolism of ^{14}C-labeled glucose *in vitro* by ungulate pineals leads to labeled CO_2, lactic acid, amino acids (alanine, aspartic acid, glutamic acid, glutamine, arginine,

GABA), fatty acids, glycerol and insoluble residue. Reduction in level of pineal glucose metabolism occurs with age (cattle and goats), but there is no evidence that this decline is significantly greater than that occurring in other tissues which are known to be functionally active throughout life.

6. Studies with parallel incubations of tissue with [1-^{14}C]- and [6-^{14}C]-glucose suggest that the pineal differs from brain and resembles other endocrine glands in having a relatively active pentose phosphate pathway, as compared with the Embden-Meyerhof pathway in the production of CO_2 from glucose. Consistent with this is the finding of relatively strong glucose-6-phosphate dehydrogenase and weak aldolase activities in pinealocytes, as compared with most brain cells or regions.

7. *In vitro* oxidation of both [1-^{14}C]- and [6-^{14}C]-glucose to $^{14}CO_2$ by bovine pineal tissue is stimulated by epinephrine. The oxidation of the latter label to $^{14}CO_2$ by brain, anterior and posterior parts of the pituitary gland is not stimulated by epinephrine. Distinctive pineal responses to sympathetic and sympathomimetic agents include other metabolic systems as well.

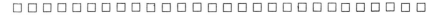

Chapter Six

AMINO ACIDS

FREE AMINO ACIDS

Tissue amino acids are found in two states, *free* and *bound*, most of the latter consisting of the unit molecules within peptides and related macromolecules. Free amino acids have been separated and measured from the pineal glands of three kinds of mammals (Table XXXV). Similarities, but also very great differences, are observed. Probably these differences can be ascribed to one or more of the following variables: postmortem time before tissue freezing or stabilization, particular techniques of amino acid separation, variable freeing of weakly bound amino acids, species and age of the source animals. Probable significance and possible origins of these differences can be considered most intelligibly in terms of the major structural or metabolic groups of amino acids. Likewise, discussion of tissue comparisons, and of origins and fates, of the pineal amino acids can be considered most coherently according to major groups and their constituent member amino acids and metabolites. The more important and interesting of the free amino acids known to occur in pineal tissue each can be allocated to one of three groups: aliphatic, sulfur-containing, and cyclic amino acids. Within each of these groups are some amino acids which are known often to be constituents of protein molecules and others which are known only in the free and sometimes weakly bound state.

Aliphatic Amino Acids

Pineal contents of aliphatic amino acids lacking sulfur can be compared with those of brain and astrocytomas (Table

TABLE XXXV

Free amino acids in mammalian pineal glands according to three studies.*

Amino acid	Man † Amount	%	Cattle ‡ Amount	%	Sheep %
Taurine	3.01 ± 0.50	15.7	5.19	18.2	—
Glutamic acid	2.98 ± 0.37	15.5	5.10	21.0	3.5
Alanine	1.74 ± 0.10	9.1	0.89	2.2	37.2
Glycine	1.67 ± 0.16	8.7	1.60	3.4	20.0
Serine	1.29 ± 0.29	6.7	§0.55	§1.6	—
Leucine	0.85 ± 0.07	4.4	0.30	1.1	4.6
Aspartic acid	0.83 ± 0.14	4.3	0.40	1.5	—
Valine	0.72 ± 0.04	3.8	0.46	1.5	8.9
Threonine	0.60 ± 0.10	3.1	0.26	0.9	—
Lysine	0.57 ± 0.08	3.0	0.18	0.7	—
Proline	0.39 ± 0.07	2.0	0.14	0.4	6.4
Arginine	0.38 ± 0.04	2.0	0.14	0.7	—
Phenylalanine	0.34 ± 0.03	1.8	0.09	0.4	3.2
Isoleucine	0.34 ± 0.03	1.8	0.17	0.6	3.2
Tyrosine	0.33 ± 0.02	1.7	0.11	0.6	3.2
Methionine	0.29 ± 0.07	1.5	≏0	≏0	
γ-Aminobutyric acid	0.23 ± 0.03	1.2	0.10	0.3	—
Citrulline	0.23 ± 0.04	1.2	0.08	0.4	—
Histidine	0.21 ± 0.02	1.1	0.17	0.8	—
Cystathionine	0.20 ± 0.02	1.0	5.76	35.9	—
Cystine	0.15 ± 0.04	0.8	0.04	0.3	—
Ornithine	0.12 ± 0.05	0.6	0.08	0.3	—
Methionine sulphoxide	0.03 ± 0.01	0.2	0.08	0.4	—
α-Aminobutyric acid	0.03 ± 0.01	0.2	—	—	—
β-Aminobutyric acid	—	—	0.21	0.6	—
Hydroxyproline	—	—	0.04	0.1	—
Glutamine	—	—	0.82	3.4	—
Tryptophan	—	—	≏0	≏0	—
3-Methylhistidine	—	—	0.01	0.1	—
Others of above in groups	—	—	—	—	4.1
Totals	19.17	100%	22.97	100%	94.3(?)%

* Data from references 447, 532 and 1006 respectively.
† Mean ± standard error, μmoles/g pineal tissue from fifteen patients forty-five to eighty-nine years old and obtained 13–96 hours postmortem.
‡ Original data converted to μmoles/g tissue
§ Includes asparagine.

XXXVI). In most instances in which the human pineal concentration of a particular amino acid falls significantly outside of the range of concentrations known for brain, it is within the range for astrocytoma, or at least closer to it. Thus, brain concentrations of leucine, valine, lysine, arginine and isoleucine are less than those for pineal and astrocytoma, and brain concentrations of glutamic acid and γ-aminobutyric acid are greater (Table XXXVI). The first group

TABLE XXXVI

Tissue comparisons of contents of aliphatic, non-sulfur-containing, free amino acids.*

Amino acid	Man		Other Mammals	
	Pineal	Brain (frontal lobe)	Brain (whole)	Astrocytomas
Glutamic acid	2.98	10.50—19.90	7.44—12.80	3.02—5.06
Alanine	1.74	—	0.42— 1.25	2.69—4.07
Glycine	1.67	—	0.86— 2.70	3.81—5.50
Serine	1.29	1.21	0.66— 5.80	2.34—5.49
Leucine	0.85	0.56	0.06— 0.10	0.07—0.48
Aspartic acid	0.83	—	0.44— 3.38	0.60—2.16
Valine	0.72	—	0.07— 0.12	0.52—0.64
Threonine	0.60	0.53	0.14— 1.60	—
Lysine	0.57	—	0.04— 0.41	0.49—0.74
Arginine	0.38	—	0.08— 0.16	0.16—0.88
Isoleucine	0.34	0.18	0.02— 0.09	0.18—0.33
γ-Aminobutyric acid	0.23	2.00—5.50	1.35— 7.10	trace—0.14
Citrulline	0.23	—	⁼0.04	—
Ornithine	0.12	—	trace—0.02	trace—0.02
α-Aminobutyric acid	0.03	—	0.01	—

* All values are μ mole/g fresh tissue; data from references 12, 13, 647, 958, 959, 1006.

is primarily proteinagenous, and the second has special functional significance in nervous tissue. γ-Aminobutyric acid (= GABA) is formed specifically from glutamic acid through the action of glutamic acid decarboxylase, and in nervous tissue has been considered to function like an *inhibitory neuron transmitter*.[985] Transamination of GABA with α-ketoglutarate forms glutamate and succinic acid semialdehyde, thereby providing a pathway for the oxidation of the carbon chain of GABA via the citric acid cycle. Within the brain, glutamic decarboxylase and GABA-transaminase activities have a somewhat similar but not identical distribution.[299,616] In general, the distribution of enzyme activities suggests that pathways for glutamate metabolism are present in both gray and white matter of the brain and in the pineal gland, but that pathways for GABA metabolism are partially restricted to gray matter of the brain. Glutamate is second only to succinate as a substrate increasing oxygen uptake by pineal tissue *in vitro*.[780] As noted earlier (Table XXXI), glutamic acid (glutamate) and glutamine are major amino acid products from glucose incubated with pineal tissue. Other aliphatic amino acids produced from glucose by pineal incubations are alanine, aspartic acid, arginine and GABA.[380] The pineal thus appears to have an active metabolism of glutamic acid although it has been thought to lack glutamic acid decarboxylase,[14] and to have very low GABA-α-ketoglutarate transaminase activity.[900] In summary, and extrapolating from known metabolic pathways in brain, at least four routes for metabolism of glutamic acid (glutamate) can be suggested as probably occurring in the pineal gland.

(1) glutamic acid + NH_3 $\overset{ATP,\ Mg^{++}}{\underset{phosphate}{\rightleftarrows}}$ glutamine

(2) glutamic acid $\overset{DPN}{\rightarrow}$ α-iminoglutaric acid $\rightarrow$ α-ketoglutaric acid + NH_3 (to TCA cycle)

(3) glutamic acid $\rightarrow$ GABA; with α-ketoglutarate $\rightarrow$ succinic + CO_2 semialdehyde (& to TCA cycle)

(4) glutamic acid $\rightarrow$ peptides, including glutathione

Glycine and alanine are aliphatic amino acids which, in the pineal, are similar in concentration and probable metabolic significance to glutamic acid. Some of the amino acids found in smaller and more variable quantities in pineal tissue might be considered problematical as measurable *in vivo* constituents. For example, ornithine and citrulline (Tables XXXV and XXXVI) can be obtained through the hydrolysis of arginine.[985] However, it is probable that metabolically these compounds occur in the pineal along with an active urea cycle. Urea has been measured in bovine pineal tissue at 13 mg/100 g fresh tissue, a concentration close to and intermediate in relation to those of pituitary and cerebral cortex.[532]

Sulfur-containing Amino Acids

Amino acids containing sulfur hold special interest in pineal biochemistry at this time for three reasons: (1) they occur

in high but variable concentrations within the pineal (Tables
XXXV and XXXVII);[348] (2) they are involved in the provision
of the methyl donor, S-adenosylmethionine, required in the
biosynthesis of melatonin; and (3) they constitute a large fraction of the amino acids within certain pineal peptides and
proteins. Metabolic pathways of primary interest in relation
to these compounds are summarized in Figure 26.

Available data on tissue levels of these compounds suggest
that significant species differences exist. Thus, in brain, cystathionine has been found at levels of 0.02—0.10 μmoles/g
tissue in man, mouse and rat; but at 0.11–0.59 μmoles/g in
the rhesus monkey.[946] It is not known to what extent the
very high cystathionine content recorded for cattle pineal
tissue (Table XXXVII) is a species characteristic. It is higher
in the pineal than in the pituitary and brain of the same
species, but the difference is much greater in cattle pineals.
Vellan and co-workers suggested that this could be due conceivably to the difference in postmortem time before removal
of the glands, about 30 minutes in the studies on cattle pineals
and thirteen to ninety-six hours in the human pineal
studies.[1006] However, they cite other work showing no significant change in brain occipital lobe cystathionine content in
biopsies at room temperature for ten hours, nor in human
necropsy pineals in their own studies taken at different times
from thirteen to ninety-six hours postmortem. The data in
Table XXXVII support belief in species differences between
man and cattle in tissue contents of cystathionine, as well
as related sulfur-containing amino acids. Thus, in both pineal
and pituitary greater concentrations of methionine and cystine
and a lesser concentration of cystathione occur in man than
in cattle (Table XXXVII).

Preliminary hypotheses to explain this pattern of differences can be formulated from a consideration of the pathways
shown in Figure 26. Results from studies on brain cystathionine levels and metabolism indicate that regional or
tissue accumulations of cystathionine are not simply reflec-
tions of excessive production by cystathionine synthase nor
diminished breakdown by cystathionase. Studies comparing

TABLE XXXVII

Concentrations of sulfur-containing, free amino acids in mammalian pineal, pituitary and brain.*

Organ & part →	Pineal		Pituitary			Brain	
			Whole	Ant. Lobe	Post. Lobe	Various Regions	Cerebral Cortex
Species	Man	Cattle	Man	Cattle	Cattle	Various	Cattle
† Methionine	0.32	0.08	0.39	0.16	0.18	0.01—0.09	0.11
Cystathionine	0.20	5.76	0.03	0.18	0.16	0.02—0.59	0.11
Cystine	0.15	0.04	0.19	0.09	0.07	0.05	0.05
Cysteic acid	—	0.70	—	—	—	trace	—
Taurine	3.01	2.10—5.19	3.10	2.88	3.92	0.09—9.13	0.29

* Means or ranges, μ moles/g fresh tissue; data from references 12, 13, 336, 441, 532, 647, 672, 849, 850, 946, 958, 959, 1006.

† Includes 'methionine sulfoxide.'

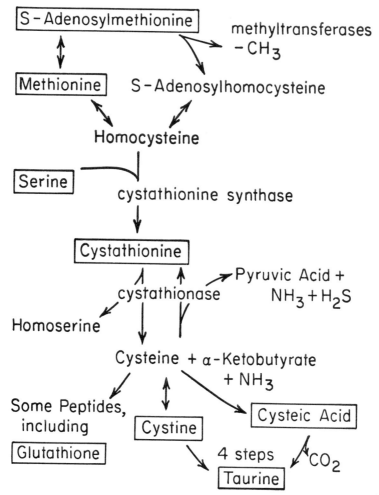

Figure 26. Metabolic pathways of primary interest in relation to pineal sulfur-containing amino acids and related compounds (in boxes).

different regions of the primate brain in the activity of cystathionine synthase, as compared with that of the methionine-activating enzyme (ATP-L-methionine S-adenosyl-transferase), suggest that in some regions the methylation pathway predominates, whereas in others transulfuration predominates (S of methionine transferred to serine to form cystathionine).[1013] A similar situation may exist in the pineal of different species and perhaps in the same species in different physiological situations. Such possibilities, not yet studied in the pineal however, have great potential interest in experimental analyses of the biochemical control of pineal methyltransferase activities.

Present knowledge allows very little to be said directly about the functional significance in the pineal of relatively high levels of products of transsulfuration from methionine. About the best that can be done at this time is to draw on information derived from studies on other tissues, especially brain. There is no strong evidence reported so far supporting a physiological role for cystathionine in the brain. However, preliminary suggestions based on circumstantial evidence have been made for its association with myelination,[1013] pathogenesis of certain inborn errors of metabolism[483] and with energy metabolism.[473] Brain cystathionine synthase requires pyridoxal phosphate[137,473] as a cofactor and increases rapidly in activity in the postnatal rat brain. A large part of the activity is particulate bound, and the developmental changes in the brain activity resemble closely those of respiratory enzymes, particularly of succinic dehydrogenase.[473] In comparisons with cystathionine, taurine in the brain shows a number of interesting characteristics. Brain levels decrease with maturation and age. Outside of its conjugation with bile acids in the liver, taurine often has been considered a metabolic end product. However, current reviewers believe this assumption is almost certainly erroneous.[434] Although taurine has remarkably few pharmacological effects, it inhibits the transmission of nerve impulses in a number of mammalian and non-mammalian test systems. This effect is considerably less than that obtained with GABA, of which it is a structural analogue. A physiological role for taurine as an inhibitor of nerve impulse transmission is attractive but is not sufficiently supported by experiments directed to test this possibility.[434]

Biochemical constituents of the pineal gland receiving the greatest attention in recent years are the methylated indole derivatives, of which melatonin (5-methoxy-*N*-acetyltryptamine) has been favored with the greatest

TABLE XXXVIII
Specificity of methyl donor for pineal hydroxyindole-*O*-methyltransferase (HIOMT).*

Methyl donor	† Relative Amount of Product
None (blank)	24
S-Adenosylmethionine	2150
Methionine	23
Choline	35
Betaine	24
N-Dimethylglycine	17
Sarcosine	21
Creatine	25
Dimethylpropriothetin	21

* Data from Baldessarini and Kopin[77].

† [^{3}H] melatonin formed (= counts/min. of chloroform-extractable product) by incubations of 0.02 units of partially purified ox pineal HIOMT (= hydroxyindole-*O*-methyltransferase), 200 μ moles phosphate buffer, 1.0 μ mole potential methyl donor and 0.1 μc (m μmoles) N-[^{3}H]-acetylserotonin in total volume of 2.0 ml.

attention. The last step in the pineal's synthesis of these compounds requires an enzyme catalyzing methylation and a methyl donor.

All evidence points to S-adenosylmethionine (SAMe) being that donor (Table XXXVIII). This compound is practically ubiquitous in mammalian tissues, but its concentrations are greatest in adrenal and pineal glands (Table XXXIX), tissues which are engaged in the methylation of catechol- and indoleamines, respectively. Therefore, among pineal derivatives of sulfur-containing amino acids, SAMe is of the greatest interest. Its concentration in the bovine pineal, 0.096 μmoles/g (from 48.0 μg/g, Table XXXIX), is similar to that of methionine (Table XXXVII). Pineal synthesis of SAMe from methionine through the activity of a "methionine-activating enzyme" or methionine adenosyltransferase (EC 2.5.1.6) is presumed, but has not received detailed study in this tissue. The reaction is, ATP + L-methionine + H_2O → S-adenosylmethionine + orthophosphate + pyrophosphate. Increased levels of SAMe have been produced in liver and brain by the administration of large doses of methionine, and decreased tissue levels by pyrogallol, a compound which is rapidly methylated.[76] No information is available, however,

TABLE XXXIX
Tissue levels of S-adenosylmethionine (SAMe).*

† Tissue	‡ SAMe
Adrenal	48.0 ± 10.0
Pineal	38.4 ± 2.7
Liver	28.8 ± 1.5
Heart	25.7 ± 6.2
Spleen	24.0 ± 4.2
Kidney	20.4 ± 5.4
Lung	11.1 ± 2.2
Brain	10.6 ± 1.0
Serum	0.47 ± 0.02

* Data from Baldessarini and Kopin.[77]
† Pineal from ox; other tissues from adult Sprague-Dawley rats.
‡ Mean μg/g ± standard error of the mean.

on experimental modification of pineal levels of SAMe *in vivo*.

S-Adenosylhomocysteine (Fig. 26) has been shown to be a potent inhibitor *in vitro* of the activity of hydroxyindole-*O*-methyltransferase and related methyltransferases. A factor stimulating these enzyme activities, and found in the supernatant fraction from brain homogenates, has been identified as an enzyme which enhances transmethylations by hydrolyzing S-adenosylhomocysteine.[199] The interesting possibility is raised that this compound and related metabolic activities might control transmethylations of biogenic amines.

Cyclic Amino Acids

Cyclic amino acids occurring in pineal tissue can be subdivided into four groups on the basis of their ring structures. These are illustrated in Figure 27.

Proline and 4-hydroxyproline are the pineal representatives (Table XXXV) of the amino acids containing the pyrrolidine ring. Proline in mammals occurs in various proportions in a large number of proteins; whereas, hydroxyproline is limited, being found in relatively few. It is quantitatively most significant in mammalian tissues as a major component of elastin and collagen, proteins of connective tissue fibers.[985] Chemical analyses of collagen show a composition of proline and hydroxyproline of 1.32 and 1.07 mmoles/g, respectively.

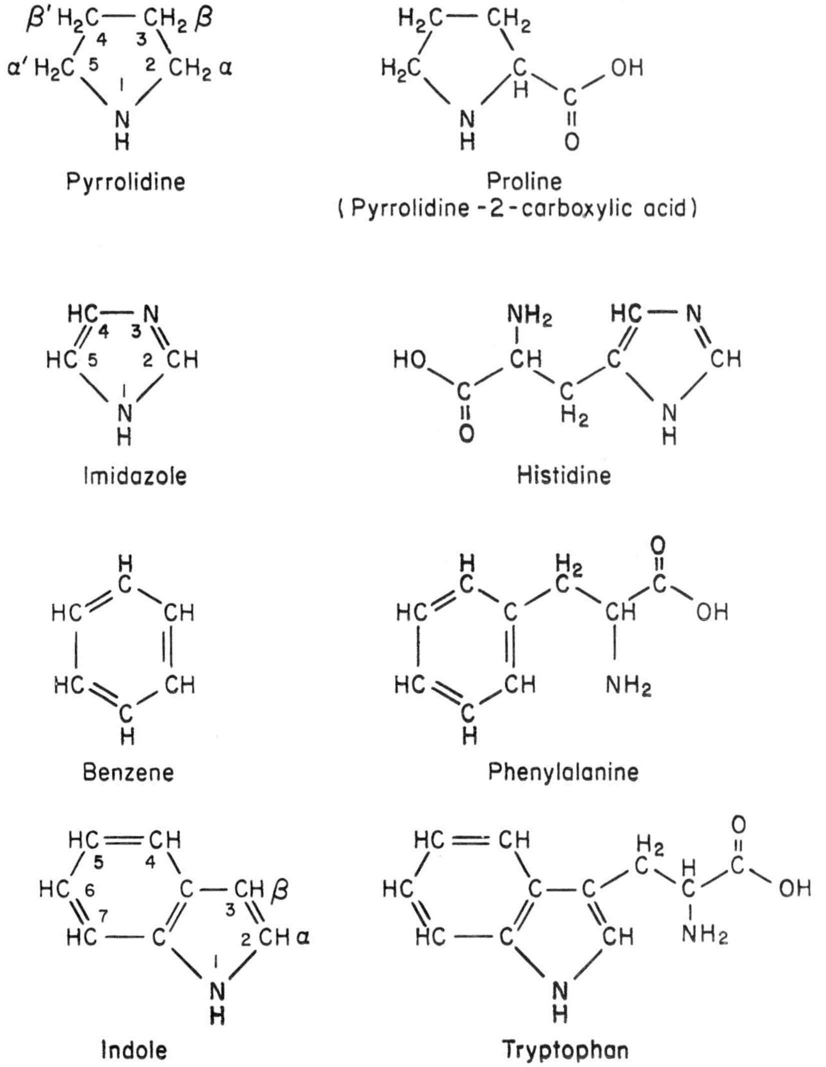

Figure 27. Ring structures (left) and example, derivative, cyclic amino acids (right) illustrating major categories found in pineal tissue.

Their contribution to collagen is exceeded only by that of glycine (3.50 mmoles/g).[348] Although proline has been isolated from a pineal peptide ('pinéaline'),[624] it is likely that appreciable fractions of both proline and hydroxyproline are associated with pineal connective tissue or stroma rather

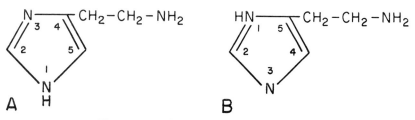

Figure 28. The tautomers of histamine.

than only with some possibly pineal-specific pathways or products. Both free and bound hydroxyproline arise from proline. Ascorbic acid (vitamin C) aids in this process, in bringing about a rapid hydroxylation of proline in ribosomal-bound protocollagen, thus leading to the formation of free collagen.

Histidine is the primary imidazole amino acid known in pineal glands (Table XXXV).[965] Nevertheless, a low content (2.0 μg/g) of 3-methylhistidine has been extracted, also, and identified from bovine pineal.[532] Although histidine is a component in many proteins, in the pineal gland its only derivative about which much is known is histamine. As one of the so-called biogenic amines, histamine is found prominently in nervous tissue, mast cells and certain other sites.[965] It can exist in two tautomeric forms (Fig. 28), which have not been separated. Current evidence suggests, however, that the dominant one is A, but that the presence of B can be inferred from studies demonstrating metabolites of 1-methyl-5 (β-aminoethyl) imidazole in urine.[335] The earliest measurements of pineal contents of histamine gave values of 10 μg/g and 0.5 μg/g fresh tissue, in cattle and dog, respectively.[5,314] A more comprehensive study by Machado and co-workers[582] has shown variability in pineal histamine content both between and within species (Table XL). Among the human specimens examined no correlations could be found between pineal histamine content and either age or cause of death. A significant correlation was found, nevertheless, between the histamine content of one half of each gland and the mast cell content of the other half. For the human pineals, r (the correlation coefficient) = 0.94 (P < 0.001) and for the cattle pineals r = 0.71 (P < 0.001). Experiments *in vitro* with cattle

TABLE XL
Pineal histamine contents in different mammals*

Group Species	† N	Histamine content ($\mu g/g$) Mean ± standard error	Range
Primates			
Man (2—89 years)	11	6.30 ± 0.9	3.3— 14.6
Ungulates			
Cattle	12	76.4 ± 10.1	33.6—145.3
Goat	4	18.9	
Sheep	2	2.6	
Pig	4	0.0	
Horse	1	0.0	
Lagomorphs			
Rabbit	7	0.0	
Rodents			
Rat	54	0.0	

* Data from Machado, Faleiro and DaSilva.[582]
† Number of individuals, glands or gland halves analyzed.

pineal tissue showed release of histamine after treatment with octylamine, but not after compound 48/80 (a mixture of polymers of *p*-methoxy-*n*-methyl-phenylethylamine nuclei).[582] Tissue cultures of rat pineals revealed to Bernád and Csaba[110] basophilic cells containing histamine according to results with the fluorescence histochemical method using *o*-phthalaldehyde on frozen, dried cultures. These same cells showed by other techniques: cytoplasmic contents of 5-hydroxytryptamine, Alcian blue-positive granules, circumnuclear granules staining dark blue with May-Grünwald-Giemsa stain, weakly with PAS (periodic acid-Schiff) and strongly with aldehyde fuchsin. Inspite of the obvious similarity in characteristics with mast cells, these pineal cells were believed not to be mast cells but rather the pineal basophils, a separate cell type described earlier in rat pineal cultures by Hungerford and Pomerat.[415] It can be noted parenthetically that true mast cells are extremely rare in rat pineals *in vivo*. In conclusion, therefore, it is not entirely clear what kind or kinds of cells contain histamine in the mammalian pineal gland.

Histamine is synthesized in tissue by decarboxylation of histidine (Fig. 29). At least two decarboxylases may be involved, a specific histidine decarboxylase, and a non-

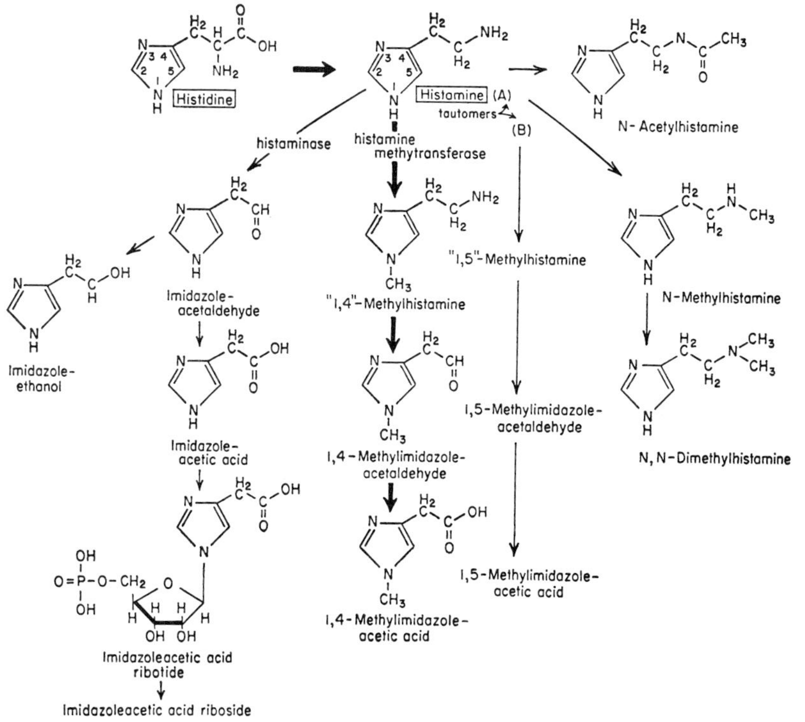

Figure 29. Biosynthesis and main pathways of catabolism of histamine.

specific L-amino acid decarboxylase. Although early work claimed the absence of both histidine decarboxylase and histaminase from the bovine pineal,[314] the possible pineal occurrences and characteristics of these and other enzymes involved in histamine synthesis and metabolism should be re-examined. Direct oxidative deamination of histamine to imidazole acetaldehyde is an important pathway in most species, including man. This reaction is catalyzed by histaminase (= diamine oxidase?). On the other hand, methylation of histamine is probably the more important catabolic route. The enzyme involved, histamine-methyltransferase (= imidazole-N-methyltransferase, E.C. 2.1.1.8) is highly specific for histamine as its substrate and is widely distributed among mammalian tissues. Its concentration or activity is very high in the pineal gland, being exceeded only by the neurohypophysis among a host of monkey tissues and brain regions sampled.[50] In a series of human pineal glands this enzyme's activity was high, and essentially without significant differences from age groups of three to twelve years to fifty-five to seventy years.[1075]

The remaining two major groups of pineal cyclic amino acids contain benzene and indole rings, and give rise, respectively, to catecholamines and indoleamines. Since so much interesting information has been obtained about these compounds in the pineal, and since they probably play major roles in the control and expression of the gland's functional activity, separate chapters will be devoted to them. It will suffice at the moment to point out that the pineal's major neurotransmitter, norepinephrine, is synthesized from phenylalanine and tyrosine, and its series of neurohumoral indoleamines are derived endogenously from tryptophan. It is to be noted that although these products are important in the pineal, the precursor free amino acids are found at rather low levels in the tissue (Table XXXV). This observation may serve to reinforce the idea that the tissue concentration of a particular free amino acid, or other precursor molecule, may have little relation to the importance or tissue levels of its products.

AMINO ACID DERIVATIVES

Some of the structurally simpler amino acid derivatives found in pineal tissue have been discussed above in relation to their amino acids of origin. The subjects of the next chapters, indole- and catecholamines, are likewise amino acid derivatives of simpler structure. The structurally most complex derivatives are the pineal polypeptides, proteins and related compounds. These will be reviewed in a later chapter, also. A third group of derivatives of mostly small to intermediate molecular size is the subject of the present section. They form a miscellaneous and artificial assemblage (Table XLI), brought together as constituents frequently revealed by chromatography along with the free amino acids discussed earlier. Carnosine and glutathione are small peptides which have been isolated from brain as well as many other tissues.

TABLE XLI
Miscellaneous pineal amino acid derivatives.*

Species Compound	Pineal	Pituitary		Cerebral Cortex
Man		whole		
Carnosine	0.15 ± 0.03	0.07 ± 0.05		—
Ethanolamine	1.18 ± 0.20	3.28 ± 0.61		—
Phosphoethanolamine	0.31 ± 0.07	1.77 ± 0.24		—
Cattle		anterior	posterior	
Phosphoethanolamine	0.61	7.09	3.97	1.98
Glycerophosphoethanolamine	0.26	0.24	0.47	0.51
Phosphoserine	0.03	0.07	0.09	0.04
Glutathione	0.65	1.04	0.49	0.98
Creatinine	2.21	——	1.06	6.63
Urea	2.16	3.00	2.50	1.33
Ammonia (NH)	2.11	2.17	3.41	1.64

* μmoles/g tissue wet weight; data from references 532, 1006.

Carnosine, a dipeptide, is β-alanyl-L-histidine. Glutathione (γ-L-glutamyl-L-cysteinylglycine) is a cofactor for several enzymes.[616]

Of particular interest in the tissue comparisons in Table XLI are the lower concentrations of ethanolamine and its phospho- derivatives in pineal, as compared with pituitary and brain tissues. Furthermore, a sexual difference was found in the concentrations in human pineal glands. Ethanolamine in female pineals was 1.83 ± 0.24, and in males 0.98 ± 0.19 μmoles/g. Phosphoethanolamine in female pineals was 0.50 ± 0.16, and in males 0.15 ± 0.04 μmoles/g. An opposite sexual difference occurred in the concentrations of these two compounds in the pituitary glands of some of the same individuals.[1006] The significance of, and mechanisms behind, these differences are not known. However, on the basis of demonstrated effects of particular sex hormones on amino acid transport and metabolism in other tissue systems, various preliminary hypotheses could be projected for explaining the sexual differences in the pineal.

CONCLUSIONS

1. Pineal contents of free amino acids of the aliphatic group resemble more closely those of astrocytoma than those of whole brain. Thus, pineal and astrocytoma concentrations of

leucine, valine, lysine, arginine and isoleucine are greater, and those of glutamic acid and γ-aminobutyric acid are less than in brain. An active pineal metabolism of glutamate, nevertheless, occurs over several pathways which are discussed.

2. Remarkably high concentrations of sulfur-containing amino acids, especially of cystathionine and taurine, are found in pineal tissue. These amino acids are of great interest in this organ as precursors and possibly regulators of transmethylations of biogenic amines and other compounds, and as constituents of particular peptides and proteins.

3. Cyclic amino acids in the pineal gland are representatives of four groups on the basis of molecular ring structure. Three of these give rise to biogenic amines of probably humoral and neurotransmitter activity within the gland. Thus, histidine gives rise to histamine, tryptophan to the indoleamines and phenylalanine and tyrosine to the catecholamines.

4. Pineal histamine contents are variable and, at least in some species, show a positive correlation with the number of mast cells. However, the very high level of the enzyme histamine-methyltransferase in pineal tissue and the deficiency in other information concerning pineal histamine metabolism, indicate needs for caution in conclusions at this time and for more investigations in the future.

5. Among various pineal amino acid derivatives considered here, ethanolamine and phosphoethanolamine are interesting on two counts. They are present in lower concentrations in pineal as compared with pituitary tissue, and they occur in higher concentrations in pineals of females than in those of males.

Chapter Seven

INDOLEAMINES

INTRODUCTION

MORE ATTENTION HAS been given to indoleamines dur- ing the recent decade than to any other group of pineal compounds. This is due in large measure to the follow- ing circumstances, listed approximately in their chronological order of discovery or most active espousal, from 1957 to 1965: (1) Melatonin, 5-methoxy-N-acetyltryptamine, was isolated and identified by Lerner and co-workers[548,550,551] following studies to isolate the pineal constituent responsible for blanching amphibian skin. (2) Pineal concentrations of 5-hydroxytryptamine (5-HT) were found to be higher than those of other mammalian tissues.[314,316,637,823] (3) The enzyme responsible for the O-methylation of 5-hydroxy-N-acetyltryptamine in the biosynthesis of melatonin and some other 5-methoxyindoles was discovered, isolated and characterized from pineal tissue by Axelrod and Weiss-bach.[56,57] (4) Derivatives of tryptamine and 5-HT, and espe-cially N-methylated derivatives and structural analogues with psychoactive or hallucinogenic activity, were presented as possible abnormal metabolites responsible for some kinds or symptoms of mental disease.[608,612,696,937,1064] (5) Melatonin, and related 5-methoxyindoles, were brought into prominence as possible antigonadotropic pineal hormones, especially by Wurtman and colleagues.[613,1071,1076] (6) Twenty-four hour rhythms of great amplitude and sensitivity to environmental illumination were demonstrated in pineal 5-HT and related compounds.[782,784,785] Although these findings suggest the pos-sibility of future therapeutic or clinical uses for pineal indole

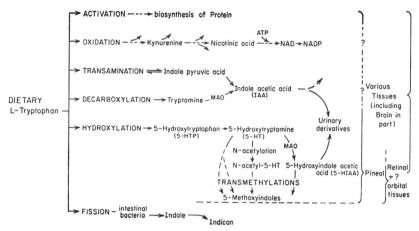

Figure 30. Major pathways of tryptophan metabolism in pineal as compared with other tissues according to current knowledge.

compounds, hopes for such uses are still unfulfilled. Thus melatonin has not been found to be effective as a drug for the control of mammalian melanocytes or melanoma, and there is no general agreement on the consistency and specificity of effects of melatonin or related compounds on the reproductive or nervous systems. This situation should not obscure the fact, however, that basic research on pineal indoleamines has provided us with new insights concerning control mechanisms in brain and neuroendocrine systems.

PINEAL INDOLE DERIVATIVES AND THEIR METABOLIC RELATIONS

The common precursor of pineal as well as brain indoleamines is L-tryptophan, the only indole amino acid and one of the *essential amino acids,* required in the diets of man and other mammals. Major pathways in the body's metabolism of tryptophan are outlined in Figure 30, with particular reference to comparative localizations in pineal and other tissues. The best known pineal pathways are those from 5-HT to 5-HIAA, 5-methoxyindoles and conjugated urinary derivatives. The only known features in these pathways thought to be unusual in the pineal gland are the overall level of activity of certain of the enzymatic steps and the pineal-specificity of the O-methylation of 5-hydroxyindoles. The latter enzymatic activity, however, has been revealed more recently as well in mammalian retina and Harderian gland and in yet other tissues of submammalian vertebrates. Other possible avenues of pineal tryptophan metabolism, such as via oxidation and transamination (Fig. 30) have not been studied. But pineal incorporation of tryptophan into protein has been demonstrated.[915],[1090]

The pineal indoleamine derivative of tryptophan having the highest tissue concentration is 5-hydroxytryptamine (= serotonin, or 5-HT). Its pathways of synthesis and metabolism within the pineal are summarized in Figure 31. Organ cultures of rat pineal glands readily synthesize 5-HT from tryptophan in the culture medium[899] and there is good reason to believe that circulating tryptophan is similarly utilized by the pineal gland *in vivo*. The initial step is catalyzed by tryptophan hydroxylase, which has high activity in pineal tissue of all examined species,[572] and is found in a particulate fraction sedimenting at 10,000 g. The resulting 5-hydroxytryptophan (5-HTP) is relatively unstable, at least in mammalian tissues, and is rapidly decarboxylated to 5-HT. The responsible enzyme, aromatic L-amino acid decarboxylase, is thought by some to similarly catalyze decarboxylation of dopa, histidine, tyrosine and 5-HTP.[574] In at least several kinds of mammals (rat, rabbit, cattle and pig) it has higher activity in the pineal gland than in any other tissue.[356],[357],[924] While there is but a single path for the biosynthesis of 5-HT in pineal and other mammalian tissues, there are several routes for its metabolism, especially in the pineal (Fig. 31). The major route quantitatively remains the same in pineal as in other tissues, namely that to 5-hydroxyindole acetic acid. The unstable intermediate, 5-hydroxyindole acetaldehyde, is not recovered from tissues analyses. The product, 5-HIAA, is biologically inactive and is, for the most part, excreted.

Pineal indole products which have received the greatest attention are the O-methylated derivatives of 5-HT (Fig. 31). These are believed by some investigators to include com-

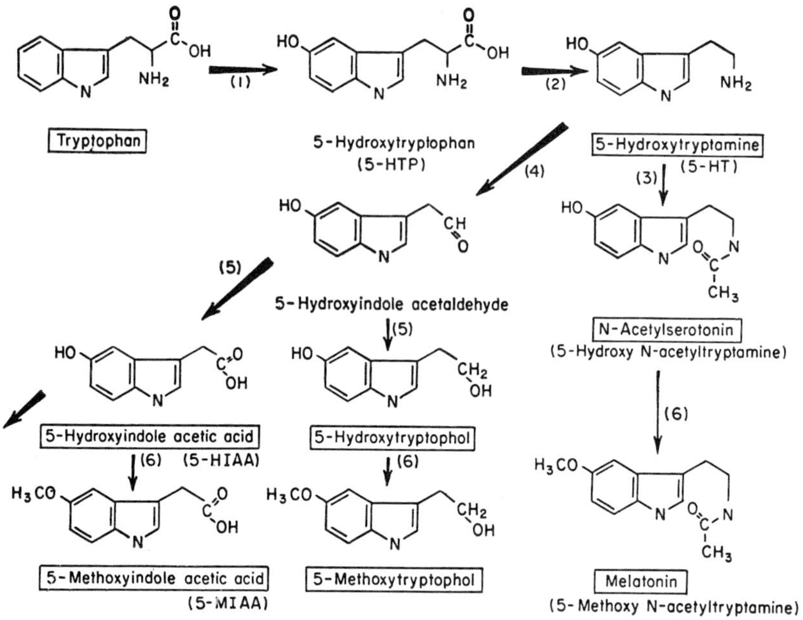

Figure 31. Pathways of synthesis and metabolism of 5-hydroxytryptamine within mammalian pineal glands. Heavier arrows indicate the major pathways; compounds in rectangles are measurable within pineal tissue. Enzymatic steps: (1) tryptophan hydroxylase, (2) aromatic L-amino acid decarboxylase, (3) N-acetyltransferase, (4) monoamine oxidase, (5) aldehyde dehydrogenase, (6) hydroxyindole-O-methyltransferase.

pounds, such as melatonin, which satisfy at least many of the criteria for being hormones. Due to the interest these compounds are receiving this chapter will place a major emphasis upon them.

Methods of separation and measurement of tissue indoleamines and their derivatives have seen important improvements during the past fifteen years. These have enabled reliable chemical determinations to be made from individual pineal glands weighing 1 mg. or less, such as those of laboratory rats. Separation techniques applied to pineal homogenates have most often been differential extractions or various kinds of chromatography. The most important chemical techniques for measurement of individual indoleamines have employed fluorometry. Either the native fluorescence of the separated indole, or that of its product

TABLE XLII
Mean percent recoveries of indole compounds by six
differential extraction methods.*

Compounds	† Methods					
	I	II	III	IV	V	VI
5-Hydroxytryptamine	92	3	3	0–1	0–1	0–1
N-Acetylserotonin	0–1	69	2	0–1	1	2
5-Hydroxytryptophan	30	3	59	0–1	0–1	0–1
5-Hydroxyindole-3-acetic acid	0–1	2	12	84	2	0–1
5-Methoxyindole-3-acetic acid	0–1	2	0–1	13	27	0–1
Melatonin	0–1	6	3	0–1	2	73
5-Methoxytryptamine	3	2	3	0–1	0–1	5
Bufotenine	0–1	3	3	0–1	0–1	0–1

* From Quay.[779]
† Methods (in brief):
  I. washed with diethyl ether while at acidic then basic pH's, then extracted with n-butanol (high pH).
  II. washed with p-cymene (low pH), then extracted with diethyl ether.
  III. washed with tert-amyl alcohol (high pH), then extracted with tert-amyl alcohol (low pH).
  IV. washed with diethyl ether (high pH), then extracted with diethyl ether (low pH).
  V. washed with diethyl ether (high pH), then extracted with p-cymene (low pH).
  VI. extracted with p-cymene (high pH).

with ninhydrin or o-phthaldialdehyde is utilized. Different laboratories often have their own preferences in separation and fluorometric procedures. Technical reviews and evaluations can be consulted for the details about these.[78,221,230,447,453,454,499,641,779,791,798,802,997] To be kept in mind is the variation in the specificity of these techniques and in the extent to which their chemical specificity has been critically evaluated by laboratory tests. Since fluorometry by itself is rarely absolutely specific for any one pineal indole compound, preliminary separation procedures remain useful. Examples of the relative degrees of success of these are provided in Tables XLII, XLIII and XLIV.

Tryptophan

Amino acid surveys (Chapter 6) have shown relatively little tryptophan in mammalian pineal tissue. However, recent microchemical studies devoted to measuring this compound in rabbit pineal glands suggest appreciable levels (0.5–6 μ

Pineal Chemistry

TABLE XLIII

Rf values (x100) from thin-layer chromatography (silica gel G sprayed with ascorbic acid) of pineal indoles and related compounds in six solvents.[*]

Compounds	† Solvents					
	I	II	III	IV	V	VI
Tryptophan	0	0	0	26	—	0
5-Hydroxytryptophan	0	0	0	39	85	0
5-Methyltryptophan	0	0	0	28	—	0
Tryptamine	0	0	0	46	—	0
5-Hydroxytryptamine	0	0	0	25	24	0
5-Hydroxy, 6-methoxytryptamine	0	—	0	—	40	—
5-Methoxy, 6-hydroxytryptamine	0	—	0	—	30	—
5-Methoxytryptamine	2	0	3	5	38	0
N-Acetylserotonin	5	0	29	62	83	74
N-Acetyl, 5-hydroxy, 6-methoxytryptamine	3	—	24	—	85	—
Melatonin	8	0	35	52	77	77
6-Hydroxymelatonin	5	—	24	—	81	—
5-Hydroxytryptophol	46	—	71	—	84	—
5-Methoxytryptophol	59	—	77	—	84	—
Indole-3-acetic acid	55	30	54	85	—	89
Indole-3-butyric acid	55	39	56	85	—	92
Indole-3-proprionic acid	55	39	56	85	—	92
5-Hydroxyindole-3-acetic acid	63	0	75	78	86	94
5-Methoxyindole-3-acetic acid	60	0	76	87	84	96
Bufotenine	0	0	0	0–1	23	2
5-Hydroxyindole	89	0	88	85	87	95
5-Methoxyindole	92	0	89	82	87	94
Gramine	4	0	—	—	—	—
5-Methoxygramine	8	—	83	—	30	—

* From Quay.[820]
† I. diethyl ether; II. dichloromethane; III. ethyl acetate; IV. n-butanol; V. - methanol; VI. acetone.

moles/g).[915] A modification of the method of Folbergrová *et al.* (1969)[279] was used for extracting the tryptophan from this tissue. This was followed by a procedure involving (1) the cleavage of the tryptophan by tryptophanase, (2) the conversion of the resulting pyruvate to lactate by lactate dehydrogenase while NADH is transformed to NAD^+, and (3) the measurement of decrease in NADH fluorescence.

5-Hydroxytryptophan (5-HTP)

This intermediate in the biosynthesis of 5-HT is believed to occur in mammalian pineal tissue but its levels are low

TABLE XLIV

Rf values (x100) from thin-layer chromatography (silica gel G) of
pineal indoles and related compounds in five solvent systems.*

Compounds	† Solvent Systems				
	I	II	III	IV	V
Tryptophan	0	0	30	51	13
5-Hydroxytryptophan	0	0	22	43	10
5-Methyltryptophan	0	0	33	54	20
Tryptamine	0	2	78	65	63
5-Hydroxytryptamine	0	0	62	58	40
N-Acetyltryptamine	14	49	84	76	85
N-Acetylserotonin	4	24	80	66	71
5-Methoxytryptamine	0	1	72	59	63
Melatonin	11	50	88	70	88
Tryptophol	24	53	91	80	85
5-Methoxytryptophol	25	53	86	78	83
5-Hydroxyindole-3- acetic acid	6	2	24	64	17
5-Methoxyindole-3- acetic acid	40	7	33	74	24

* From Ebels *et al.*[230]
† I. chloroform-glacial acetic acid; 95:5 (v/v)
 II. chloroform-methanol; 90:10 (v/v)
III. ethyl acetate-propanol-2-25% ammonia; 45:35:20 (v/v/v)
IV. n-butanol-pyridine-glacial acetic acid-distilled water; 15:2:3:5 (v/v/v/v)
 V. chloroform-methanol-25% ammonia; 12:7:1 (v/v/v)

due to its rapid decarboxylation to 5-HT.[791] To be kept in
mind, however, is the probability of the levels being increased
after certain dietary or drug treatments and the variable and
incomplete capacity of some of the chemical and histochemical methods for 5-HT to distinguish 5-HT from 5-HTP.

5-Hydroxytryptamine (5-HT, serotonin)

The indoleamine that attains the greatest concentration
within pineal tissue is 5-HT. The concentrations, however,
vary, even in normal or untreated animals, according to
species and time of day (Table XLV). The latter point will
be examined in a later section within this chapter. Species
differences in pineal contents of 5-HT are confirmed by histochemical studies, which show in addition some species variability in 5-HT localization.[708,709] Usually, however, the
pinealocyte cytoplasm is the chief site of the pineal's 5-HT
localization and the probable site of its synthesis within the
organ. Secondary uptake by pineal sympathetic nerve termi-

Pineal Chemistry

TABLE XLV

Pineal content of 5-hydroxytryptamine (μg/g tissue) in some mammalian species.

Group Species	* (N)	Time of Death Day	?	Night	† Assay Method	References
Primates						
Man (*Homo sapiens*)	(11 adults)	—	0.4–22.8	—	I	316
Rhesus monkey (*Macaca mulatta*)	(17)	—	1.2–10.0	—	I	316
Rhesus monkey (*Macaca mulatta*)	(56)	40–80	—	10–30	II	792
Ungulates (domestic)						
Goat (*Capra hircus*)	(5)	—	1.2–7.0	—	I	743
Cattle (*Bos taurus*)	(13)	—	0.2–0.6	—	I	314–316
Cattle (*Bos taurus*)	—	—	2.7	—	II	453
Swine (*Sus scrofa*)	—	—	20–56	—	II	453,709
Sheep (*Ovis aries*)	(8)	—	1.1–6.6	—	II	820
Rodents (laboratory)						
Rat (*Rattus norvegicus*)	(40+)	—	10–17	—	I	739
Rat (*Rattus norvegicus*)	(400+)	60–120	—	10–60	II	113,258,641, 782,823,925
Guinea pig (*Cavia cobaya*)	—	—	6	—	II	709
Carnivores						
Dog (*Canis familiaris*)	(3–4)	—	7.4	—	II	641
Pinnipeds (feral)						
Fur seal (*Callorhinus ursinus*)	(6)	—	39–138	—	II	239
Marsupials (feral)						
Red kangaroo (*Megaleia rufa*)	(6)	—	—	0–4.1	II	822
Grey kangaroo (*Macropus canguru*)	(3)	—	—	1.3–1.9	II	822

* (N) = number of specimens or samples.
† I = bioassay, II = chemical assay.

nals has been found in some circumstances.[707] Analyses of adult human pineals taken at necropsies within twenty-four hours postmortem showed great variation but correlations with age (thirty-seven to ninety years), sex or specific chronic diseases were not apparent.[316]

Consistently lower values for pineal contents of 5-HT were obtained by the earlier investigations which employed bioassay methods using the heart of *Venus mercenaria*[316] or the rat fundic stomach strip (of Vane). It is now generally agreed that the chemical methods are superior. The diverse separation or extraction methods coupled with three different

TABLE XLVI

Radioactive indole metabolites separated after twenty-four-hour organ culture of rat pineal glands with 5-HT-C[14].*

† Compounds (by TLC)	‡ counts/minute
5-Hydroxyindole-3-acetic acid	2000 ± 350
5-Hydroxytryptophol	630 ± 13
5-Methoxytryptophol	100 ± 20
Melatonin	50 ± 4
5-Methoxyindole-3-acetic acid	30 ± 5

   * Adapted from Klein and Notides.[499]
   † Remaining at the origin of the thin-layer chromatograms would be 5-HT, 5-HTP, tryptophan and 5-methoxytryptamine, having a combined counts/min of 40000 ± 2000.
   ‡ Mean ± standard error from 4 organ cultures.

fluorometric methods produce equivalent values for rat pineal 5-HT and have confirmed in many laboratories the early chemical results.

5-Hydroxyindole-3-acetic acid (5-HIAA)

The chief pathway of metabolism of 5-HT is by oxidative deamination (Fig. 31) to 5-HIAA in the pineal gland as well as in other mammalian tissues. The order of magnitude of this path's activity can be seen in the results of pineal organ cultures incubated with labeled 5-HT (Table XLVI). The enzyme primarily involved in the pineal formation of 5-HIAA is monoamine oxidase, an enzyme category having a high activity and wide distribution through pineal tissues. Although 5-HIAA is believed to lack biological activity within the animal body and to be merely excreted, its concentrations within pineal glands are of some interest in relation to physiological and daily changes in pineal indoleamine metabolism. Published measurements (Table XLVII) are based on various kinds of extraction techniques followed by fluorometry.

N-Acetylserotonin

The pineal concentrations of this biosynthetic precursor to melatonin are normally very low. Appropriate differential extraction of pineal homogenates followed by reaction with o-phthaldialdehyde and fluorometry have given values of

TABLE XLVII
Pineal content of 5-hydroxyindole-3-acetic acid (μg/g tissue)
in mammalian species.

Group Species	* (N)	Day	?	Night	References
		Time of Death			
Primates					
Rhesus monkey (*Macaca mulatta*)	(31)	†10.2 ± 0.8	—	—	820
Langur (*Presbytis cristatus*?)	(1)	5.2	—	—	820
Ungulates					
Cattle (*Bos taurus*)	—	—	2.0	—	550
Rodents					
Rat (*Rattus norvegicus*)	(122)	8–18	—	4–6	784
Marsupials					
Red kangaroo (*Megaleia rufa*)	(6)	—	—	0.9–8.8	822
Grey kangaroo (*Macropus canguru*)	(3)	—	—	1.5–2.0	822

* (N) = number of specimens or samples.
† Mean ± standard error.

7.80 ± 0.09 and 0.92 ± 0.11 μg/g for rat and dog pineal glands respectively.[641] A very sensitive and specific assay for pineal N-acetylserotonin has been described by Klein and Weller.[505] It employs the conversion by purified hydroxyindole-O-methyl transferase of N-acetylserotonin to melatonin (-O-methyl-^{14}C) in the presence of S-adenosylmethionine (methyl-^{14}C). The radiolabeled melatonin is isolated by two-dimensional thin-layer chromatography and is proportional to the available substrate. Male rat pineals *in vivo* were found by this method to contain approximately 0–0.8 μg/g during the day and 12 μg/g at night.[505]

5-Hydroxytryptophol

This indole derivative of 5-HT has been found in cattle pineal tissue by McIsaac *et al.*[611] Its formation from 5-HT by cattle and rat pineals has been demonstrated *in vitro*.[499,704] The unstable 5-hydroxyindole acetaldehyde produced from 5-HT in the presence of monoamine oxidase is then either oxidized to 5-HIAA or reduced to 5-hydroxytryptophol (Figure 31).

5-Methoxyindole-3-acetic acid (5-MIAA)

This metabolite from 5-HT and 5-HIAA was identified in bovine pineal glands by Lerner *et al.* (1960)[550] at a concentration of about 2.0 μg/g tissue. It has been identified recently in sheep pineals also.[230] An early differential extraction and fluorometry of 5-MIAA in rat pineal tissue gave an average value of about 1.0 μg/g,[784] which is at least five times greater than recent results based on different extraction and fluorometric procedures.[641]

Although almost all of the 5-methoxytryptophol administered to rats is converted *in vivo* to 5-MIAA,[202] incubations of pineal tissue with 5-hydroxytryptophol and labelled S-adenosylmethionine give 5-methoxytryptophol and no detectable 5-MIAA.[827] Other data as well (Table XLVI) suggest that at least most of the pineal's content of 5-MIAA is derived through O-methylation of 5-HIAA. Another possible pathway for the pineal synthesis of 5-MIAA is that from 5-HT via 5-methoxytryptamine.[528] However, there is no direct evidence that this path is active in pineal tissue and the possible pineal occurrence of 5-methoxytryptamine is questionable and controversial.

5-Methoxytryptamine (5-MT)

Although claims have been advanced for the presence of 5-methoxytryptamine in pineal tissue the supporting evidence is incomplete.[269,592,641] There is no question that the hydroxyindole-O-methyltransferase in the pineal tissue of some species can methylate *in vitro* 5-HT to form 5-methoxytryptamine.[57] This is true for cattle, sheep and raccoon pineals, but not those of rat, cat and rhesus monkeys.[827] In some gallinaceous birds a pineal hydroxyindole-O-methyltransferase brings about a more active methylation of 5-HT to form 5-methoxytryptamine.[17,49]

5-Methoxytryptophol

5-Methoxytryptophol was identified in cattle pineal glands by McIsaac *et al.* (1965)[611] and the ability of pineal tissue to methylate 5-hydroxytryptophol to form 5-

methoxytryptophol has been demonstrated by several laboratories.[499,611,827] In addition, it has been suggested that methylation could occur at the stage of the intermediate aldehyde, 5-hydroxyindole acetaldehyde (Fig. 31), followed by the reduction of 5-methoxyindole acetaldehyde to 5-methoxytryptophol. *In vitro* studies with cattle pineal tissue by Otani *et al.* (1969)[704] provide support for this possibility and show that the latter step depends on the presence of NADPH.

Melatonin (5-methoxy-N-acetyltryptamine)

It has been known for over fifty years that mammalian pineal tissue contains something having the ability to blanch amphibian melanophores.[313,419,602] The chemical search for the compound primarily responsible for this activity led Lerner and his coworkers to the discovery of melatonin, which they not only isolated and identified, but also named and characterized.[546,548,550,551] Although melatonin has an exceptional potency in affecting melanophores of many lower vertebrates, attempts to use it to modify human or mammalian pigmentation and pigment cells have been predominantly unsuccessful.[167,411,493,605,837,845,921] Most of the physiological interest in melatonin in recent years has centered on its possibly hormonal nature and endocrine effects on hypophyseal-gonadal and related endocrine and metabolic systems. This interest is extending to the central nervous system for localization of the primary target in the effects of melatonin and other hormonal candidates among pineal constituents.[29,787,805,807,809,840]

Remarkable variety characterizes the methods for measuring melatonin in pineal and other tissues. All of the bioassay procedures are based on the response of amphibian melanophores to melatonin. However, the occurrence and potency of melatonin's action on melanophores varies according to species of amphibian, animal age and body region.[62,141,219,693] Whenever a response occurs it consists of a migration of the pigment granules (melanosomes) centripetally within the melanophore's cytoplasm, leading to a punctate appearance for each responding cell. The melanosomes become clustered around the nucleus instead of being dispersed from the perikaryon to the radial cytoplasmic extensions which give the melanophores in darkened skin a stellate appearance. Older methods utilized frog skin samples *in vitro*.[540,552,659] These were usually from a common North American species, *Rana pipiens*, but a toad, *Bufo arenarum*, has been used also as a source of skin samples.[977] Variation in specificity and sensitivity of response and other problems have led to the development of bioassays employing whole larvae or tadpoles, usually of either *Rana pipiens*[475,833] or *Xenopus laevis*.[63,821,997,999] The assay using *Xenopus* larvae is especially sensitive and chemically specific.[578,797,821] The minimum effective concentration of melatonin in aquarium water to cause blanching of the cheek region of *Xenopus* larvae is 0.1 nanogram (10^{-10} g) per ml.[821] Of the very few other compounds capable of provoking this response, 5-methoxytryptamine and N-acetylserotonin have minimum effective concentrations 10^5 times greater (e.g. = 10 μ g/ml). As is true with bioassay systems in general, however, careful control of the development and preparation of the assay organism is important. Thus the lightness or darkness of the background upon which the larvae are reared affects both the number of melanophores which develop and the endogenous levels of melatonin.[72]

Bioassay of tissue contents of melatonin has been applied successfully with both crude homogenates and extracted or partially purified fractions. The latter type of procedure has the disadvantage, however, of frequently adding minute traces of organic solvents or other compounds which may be toxic to the larvae and prevent normal melanophore behavior. Such separation techniques for melatonin as thin-layer chromatography and differential solvent extraction have been noted earlier in this chapter. Others that have been used include paper chromatography,[755] silicic acid column chromatography,[550] gas chromatography,[136,169,197,259,339,742] countercurrent distribution,[81,550] and gel filtration on Sephadex G-10[230] and G-25[454,997] columns. Some of the most

TABLE XLVIII
Pineal content of melatonin (μg/g tissue) in mammalian species.

Group Species	* (N)	Time of Death Day	?	Night	References
Primates					
Man—pinealoma metastasis	(1)	—	0.3	—	168,1085
Rhesus monkey (*Macaca mulatta*)	(30)	†11.5 ± 1.1	—	—	820
Langur (*Presbytis cristatus*?)	(1)	6.4	—	—	820
Ungulates					
Cattle (*Bos taurus*)	—	—	0.2	—	81,550
Rodents					
Rats (*Rattus norvegicus*)	(100 +)	0.4–4.0	—	2.0–7.0	197,576, 755,784
Carnivores					
Dog (*Canis familiaris*)	(3–4)	—	0.2	—	641
Marsupials					
Red kangaroo (*Megaleia rufa*)	(6)	—	—	0.5–7.5	822
Grey kangaroo (*Macropus canguru*)	(3)	—	—	0.0–6.9	822

* (N) = number of specimens or samples.
† Mean ± standard error.

sensitive and discriminating detections and measurements of melatonin have been by means of gas chromatography and mass spectroscopy of melatonin and selected synthetic derivatives.[197, 729]

Melatonin has been detected in human pineal glands[546] and has been measured in a metastasis from a human pinealoma (Table XLVIII). It has been detected or measured in pineal tissue from diverse species, including representative fish,[271] amphibians[71,999] and birds[576,577,793,832,997,999] as well as mammals (Table XLVIII). Its presence in the pineal organs of yet other vertebrate groups including cyclostomes and reptiles is considered likely on the basis of the occurrence in these of the melatonin-forming enzyme, hydroxyindole-O-methyltransferase.[788,820] Melatonin has been measured most frequently in rat pineal glands. Here, considering the great variety of methods used, it is perhaps surprising that the results from most laboratories agree so well. Noteworthy is the fact that in all species where measured, pineal melatonin content is low according to what one might expect for a hormone within its gland of origin. For example, the 0.2–11.5 μg/g concentration of pineal melatonin seems meager indeed in comparison with the 1500–8000 μg/g concentration of adrenal medullary catecholamines.[1050] Combining all *biogenic amines* the pineal concentration is 1/100–1/10 that of the adrenal medulla.[791] Nevertheless, evidence has been presented to support the belief that the pineal releases or secretes melatonin into the blood stream. Melatonin has been identified in chicken blood by mass spectrometry and is not detectable there by bioassay following removal of the pineal gland.[729] The serum of sham-operated (normal control) chickens contained 0.071 ± 0.007 ng melatonin/ml near the middle of the night and less than 0.01 ng/ml near the middle of the day.[728,729] Early reports of melatonin occurrence in human peripheral nerves (0.02 ng/g) and urine[81,549] should be supported and extended by additional studies employing new and improved methods now available. It is probably safe to assume that melatonin occurring in these and other mammalian tissues and fluids is derived from the pineal gland, because of the pineal localization of the enzyme responsible for the last step in melatonin's biosynthesis, and because of the above cited loss of melatonin from chicken serum after pinealectomy. There is no evidence as yet that the low levels of this enzyme, hydroxyindole-O-methyltransferase, detectable in retina[147,148,788] and Harderian gland [1009] can contribute to a release of melatonin from these other tissues.

Melatonin's chemical properties have been studied by Lerner and coworkers[548,550] and by Szmuskovicz *et al.*[955] who synthesized the compound. In crystalline form melatonin is pale yellow and has a melting point of 116–118° C. It is difficult to dissolve directly in water but can first be dissolved in a small drop of ethanol before dilution with aqueous solutions for injection or other uses. In 95 percent ethanol and ultraviolet light it has a distinctive spectrum, with an absorption maximum at 223 mμ. In water it shows a fluorescence similar to that of many other indoles, with excitation maximum at 295–300 mμ and emission maximum at 337 mμ. In strong acid (3N HCl) it shows a fluorescence characteristic of 5-hydroxy- and 5-methoxyindoles, with excitation maximum at 295–300 mμ and emission maximum at 540–550 mμ.[990]

The molecular structure of melatonin has been studied with x-ray diffraction methods and compared with that of 5-methoxytryptamine (5-MT) and 5-hydroxytryptamine (5-HT).[760] Such studies are fundamental in the approach to understanding the basic differences between these compounds in their interactions with enzymes and with receptor sites. Although the benzene ring in melatonin is planar, the indole structure is not; carbons 2 and 10 of the pyrrole ring are out of the plane by 1.8°. In the crystalline state melatonin, unlike 5-MT and 5-HT, assumes a conformation close to that expected from quantum mechanical calculations. Acetylation of the primary amine group (Fig. 31) of 5-MT destroys the ability of the molecule to form a strong N-H-N bond between the nitrogen of the aliphatic side chain and that of the indole ring. The N-H-O hydrogen bonds formed by crystalline melatonin are very weak; the taking on of the calculated minimum energy conformation for the isolated molecule is possible without intermolecular interactions. Partial conjugation of the acetyl group with the indole ring may help stabilize this preferred conformation. Therefore, in comparison with 5-HT and 5-MT, melatonin is not likely to assume a higher energy conformation in a biological environment conducive to the formation of hydrogen bonds.

Beta-Carbolines

Indirect and circumstantial evidence supports the possibility that the pineal gland may synthesize and contain small amounts of *beta*-carbolines. This is a most interesting possibility in view of the neuropharmacological properties of many of these compounds (see last section, this chapter). The proposed pineal *beta*-carbolines would all arise as cyclodehydrogenation products of 5-HT, 5-MT or melatonin (Fig. 32). The first suggestion of pineal *beta*-carbolines was by Farrell and McIsaac (1961)[263] who tentatively identified a cattle pineal constituent that stimulated adrenal aldosterone secretion as 1-methyl-6-methoxy-1,2,3,4-tetrahydro-2-carboline (= 6-methoxy, tetrahydroharman, Figure 32). This chemical identification was later retracted[262,265,377] and subsequent

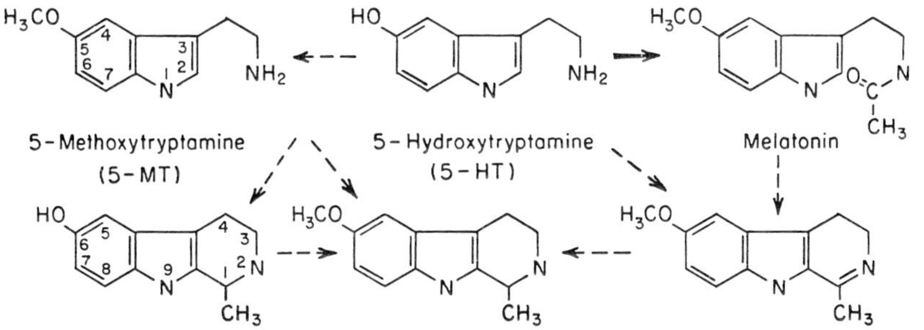

Figure 32. Structures and possible metabolic origins of suggested pineal *beta*-carboline derivatives.

investigations have weakened the case for a pineal hormone stimulating aldosterone secretion.[1069] Nevertheless, McIsaac demonstrated that 6-methoxytetrahydroharman can be formed *in vivo* from 5-MT and acetaldehyde by rats given drugs to block the normally rapid degradation of these precursors. Iproniazid was used to prevent the breakdown of 5-MT by monoamine oxidase, and disulfiram (tetraethylthiuram disulfide) was used to reduce the rate of oxidation of acetaldehyde. Furthermore, it was found that at least *in vitro* 10-methoxyharmalan can be formed from 5-HT.[612] Another route for the pineal synthesis of 6-methoxytetrahydroharman is suggested by the capacity of cattle and sheep pineal tissue to O-methylate 6-hydroxytetrahydroharman (Figure 32).[827] This activity was not found in homogenates of pineal tissue from monkeys, rats, cats or raccoons.

PHYSIOLOGICAL CHANGES AND CONTROLS

Physiological changes in pineal indoleamine levels and metabolism are important as clues to the functional relations of the pineal gland and to roles played by its indoleamine contents. Most of the available information on this subject pertains to either one or both of two broad areas: (1) circadian rhythms and the effects of light and darkness, and (2) correlations with stages of reproductive cycles and the effects of hormones. Especially in the first of these two areas phar-

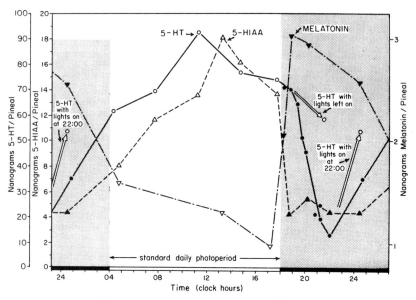

Figure 33. Circadian rhythms in rat pineal 5-hydroxytryptamine (5-HT), 5-hydroxyindole-3-acetic acid (5-HIAA) and melatonin. Arrows point to the different mean values obtained when the onset of light is earlier, or the offset is later than usual. (Data from references 782, 784 and 785; figure adapted from Quay.[806])

macological methods have served to reveal some of the control factors in the changes in pineal indoleamines.

Circadian Rhythms

Circadian rhythms are those rhythms having a cycle length of about (*circa*) twenty-four hours or one solar day (*dies*).[361] However, some authors have restricted the use of the term to those rhythms of this cycle length which are also demonstrably *free-running* or endogenous in the sense of continuing in the absence of timing cues from the environment. For practical reasons alone, we will conform to Halberg's original and broader definition.[361]

A circadian rhythm in the pineal gland was first detected and demonstrated in the rat pineal's content of 5-HT (Fig. 33).[782,785] This finding has since been confirmed in many laboratories.[113,218,618,932,1094] The features that make the pineal rhythm in 5-HT so interesting are the great amplitude

(10–20 to 60–90 ng/pineal from trough to peak) and the correlations of the major changes in the pineal with those in environmental illumination. Experiments modifying the times either of onset of light or of darkness succeeded in significantly modifying the timing of the rise and fall in pineal 5-HT within the same 24-hour period (Fig. 33).[427,782,785] Rat pineal contents of 5-HIAA and melatonin were found also to follow circadian rhythms.[576,784] The patterns of these (Fig. 33) were consistent with the idea that during the daily period of light the 5-HT's metabolism to 5-HIAA was most active and at night that to melatonin was most active.[784] Thus a kind of day-night switching of pineal indoleamine metabolism was suggested.

Pineal 5-HT in a primate, the rhesus monkey, similarly was found to rise during the day and to fall promptly after the start of darkness. Unlike rat pineal 5-HT, however, that of the monkey continues to rise if the lights are left on (Fig. 34). Merely the prolongation of the monkey's daily exposure to artificial light causes within a few hours a pineal 5-HT concentration approximately double the normal daily maximum. Data for daily changes in the other pineal indoleamines of monkey pineal glands are not available, but the melatonin-forming enzyme was shown to be maximum at night just as had been shown earlier in the rat pineal. The pineal glands of birds also have high amplitude circadian rhythms in their indoleamines (Fig. 35).[373,576,793,832,945] In this case, however, the most rapid changes occur following the onset of light rather than the onset of darkness. This may be a significant difference between the indoleamine rhythms in birds and mammals. There is no indication as yet of any correlation of characteristics of these pineal indoleamine rhythms with diurnal versus nocturnal behavior. The pineal 5-HT rhythms of rat and rhesus monkey are not widely divergent in the timing of their daily peaks, but they are nocturnal and diurnal species respectively.

Components in the mechanism of the circadian rhythms in pineal indoleamine contents and metabolism have been studied intensively through recent years, particularly in the laboratory rat. A synthesis of the best evidence for the interrelations among these is summarized in Figure 36. However,

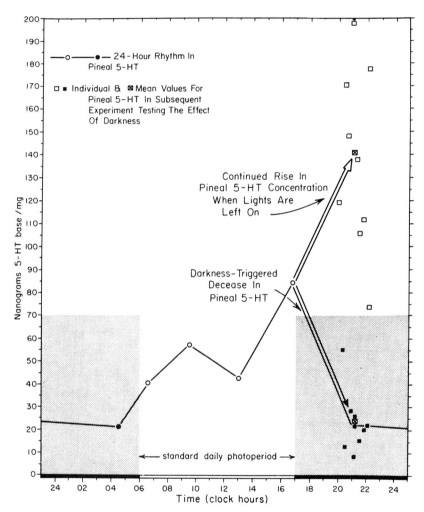

Figure 34. Circadian rhythm in monkey (*Macaca mulatta*) pineal 5-hydroxytryptamine (5-HT) (dots = means) and individual values obtained in an experiment in which the artificial illumination was turned off at the usual time (■) or left on (□). (Data from references 792 and 794; figure adapted from Quay.[806])

it is important to keep in mind several limitations in this scheme and in the evidence upon which it is based:

(1) The components and relations shown here pertain to the adult animal. The adult pineal rhythm, in probable contrast with that

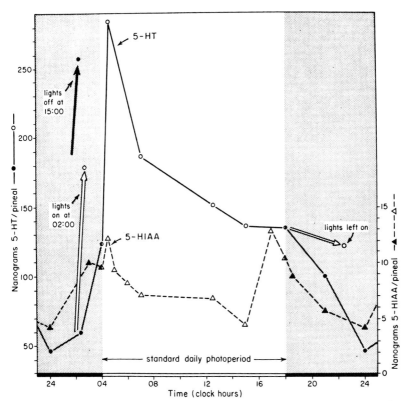

Figure 35. Circadian rhythms in pigeon (*Columba livia*) pineal 5-hydroxytryptamine (5-HT) and 5-hydroxyindole-3-acetic acid (5-HIAA). Arrows point to the different mean values obtained when the onset of light is earlier, or the offset is earlier or later than usual. (Data from reference 793; figure adapted from Quay.[806])

of the infant, has an exogenous drive mechanism imposed upon it by means of its sympathetic innervation.

(2) Pineal components and their daily changes and mechanisms consist of some that are known to be like those in parts of the nervous system, some that are either qualitatively or quantitatively different, and others that are provisionally extrapolated from what is known from the nervous system. These similarities and differences, once they are better known, may be guides to the basis for judging degrees of independency and dependency among aminergic systems within the nervous system and its derivatives, including the pineal gland.

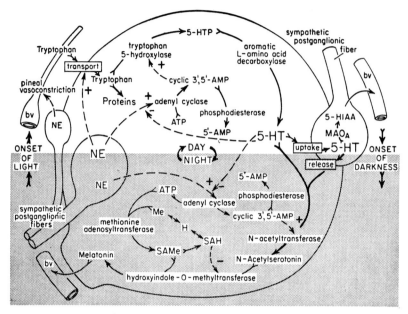

Figure 36. Components and mechanisms in the adult pineal's circadian rhythm in indoleamine contents and metabolism. Abbreviations: 5'-AMP = 5'-adenosine monophosphate, ATP = adenosine triphosphate, bv = pineal blood vessel, H = homocysteine, 5-HIAA = 5-hydroxy-indole-3-acetic acid, 5-HT = 5-hydroxytryptamine, 5-HTP = 5-hydroxy-tryptophan, MAO_A = monoamine oxidase Type A, Me = methionine, NE = norepinephrine, SAH = S-adenosylhomocysteine, SAMe = S-adenosylmethionine.

(3) A great many conditions, drugs and other agents have been shown to affect steps or components in the pineal indoleamine rhythm. But it is still not possible to judge in the case of many of these whether their action is directly on or within the pinealocyte, or whether it is indirect. The latter could involve multiple neuronal links between sensory (photic) input and the pineal cells by way of the nervous system, and possibly other pineal-destined neural or humoral paths.

(4) Effects of continuous light or continuous darkness are frequently not indicative of processes or events during the normal day-night cycle of light and darkness. Continuous light for the normally nocturnal and photophobic rat is a stressing agent with profound and widespread effects on the animal's metabolism, including that of the pineal gland.[276,775,776,781] Furthermore, in either continuous light or continuous darkness, some of the animal's circa-

dian rhythms in physiological functions and behaviors continue and *free-run*. During the latter process the cycles of different animals gradually pass out of phase with each other, so that within a few weeks animals exposed to the same constant environment may be in different phases of their daily cycle at any one selected time.

The events and mechanisms in the adult rat's circadian rhythm in indoleamine metabolism can be described in a sequential manner from the uptake of tryptophan to the secretion of melatonin and other derivatives (Fig. 36):

(1) At the onset of light the daily maximum in pineal norepinephrine (NE) falls, presumably because of release. This release causes constriction of many of the small blood vessels within the pineal[818, 819] and has stimulatory effects on two receptor sites or processes within the plasma membrane of the pinealocyte. One of these, uptake or transport of tryptophan (T), does not require cyclic 3′,5′-adenosine monophosphate (c-AMP); the other one does. NE does not stimulate protein synthesis by pineal organs which in culture contain a previously fixed amount of labeled tryptophan. Nor does it stimulate in culture pineal protein synthesis from labeled methionine or leucine.[1090] The pineal synthesis *in vitro* of ^{14}C-protein from ^{14}C-tryptophan is accelerated by NE or related catecholamines added to the medium, but is not affected by 5-HT, 5-HIAA or melatonin.[1090]

(2) The second process accelerated by NE is the synthesis of 5-HT through stimulation of tryptophan-5-hydroxylase, the rate-limiting step. This requires the mediation by c-AMP.[897] The rat pineal's concentration of c-AMP increases during the daily light phase to a value nearly six times that found at the end of the dark phase.[226] Both NE and c-AMP accelerate synthesis of ^{14}C-5-HT from ^{14}C-T by cultured pineal glands, but neither influence the rate of ^{14}C-5-HT synthesis when pineals are incubated with ^{14}C-5-HTP.[898] It may be noted that in cell-free systems, equally low concentrations of NE and other catechols inhibit pineal tryptophan hydroxylase, presumably because of their capacity for chelation of iron.[438] This enzyme requires a pteridine cofactor and ferrous iron for full activity.[424,573]

Other evidence for the importance of the tryptophan hydroxylase step is available from injections (ip) of either T (200 mg/kg) or 5-HTP (25 mg/kg) at different times of the day and night. Both treatments increase pineal 5-HT, but only T suppresses the rhythm in 5-HT. Moreover, neither the decarboxylation of 5-HTP nor monoamine oxidase activity are believed to show 24-hour rhythms in the pineal.[929]

(3) The next critical step in the cycle is the one dependent on the beginning of darkness. This is also the one having in mammals

the most rapid changes in pineal indoleamine contents. These changes can be explained most easily by shifts in the pineal compartmentalization of 5-HT. Histochemical,[110,112,113,702,708,709,916] autoradiographic[67,309,571] and denervation[739] studies have shown that pineal 5-HT has two localizations, the cytoplasm of pinealocytes where it is synthesized and the terminations of pineal sympathetic nerve fibers where it is taken up secondarily. Approximately 30 percent of the rat pineal's 5-HT has been found within the sympathetic endings.The turnover rate of 5-HT in the pinealocytes has been estimated as about 100 ng/pineal/hours. After inhibition of 5-HT synthesis with *p*-chlorophenylalanine the half-life of decline of pineal sympathetic 5-HT is about ten times faster than that of pinealocyte 5-HT.[680] 5-HT accumulates in the nerve terminals during the day and here is metabolized to 5-HIAA. This is brought about by monamine oxidase$_A$ which is localized within the sympathetic fibers and endings and which can act on 5-HT. Monoamine oxidase$_B$, constituting 85 percent of the rat pineal's total monoamine oxidase, is found within the pinealocytes and can not act on 5-HT.[332,1096] The most rapid chemical event in rat pineals at the start of darkness is the fall in 5-HIAA (Fig. 33).[784,806] This event must signify the release of 5-HT (and 5-HIAA) from the nerve terminals, if monoamine oxidase is not subject to change. From this time in the cycle, the NE content of the pineal (nerves) gradually rises during the dark phase. Much of the released 5-HT probably is reacquired by the pinealocytes, where during the nocturnal phase it is *N*-acetylated and *O*-methylated in the sequence leading to melatonin.

(4) The enzymatic steps prominent during the nocturnal phase are facilitated or stimulated by several mechanisms. First to be noted is *N*-acetyltransferase, which has a circadian rhythm in the rat pineal gland with night-time values more than fifteen times as great as those found during the day-light phase.[502] The activity of this enzyme in pineal cultures is stimulated by NE through c-AMP as an intermediary. 5-HT does not stimulate *N*-acetyltransferase *in vitro*. In practice dibutyryl adenosine 3'.5'-monophosphate is more successful than cyclic-AMP itself in stimulating pineal *N*-acetyltransferase *in vitro*. This is due to the much more rapid degradation of c-AMP by cyclic nucleotide phosphodiesterase. When this enzyme is inhibited in pineal cultures with theophylline the activity of the *N*-acetyltransferase pathway leading to melatonin is increased.[495,1040] Pineal *N*-acetyltransferase *in vitro* can be stimulated also by harmine,[504] which long has been known to have another action, inhibition of monamine oxidase. All of these compounds stimulate melatonin production *in vitro* by a mass action effect; *N*-acetylserotonin is rapidly *O*-methylated in all of these cir-

cumstances.[497] NE's natural role is supported further by the fact that when the preganglionic fibers of the superior cervical ganglia are stimulated electrically, pineal N-acetyltransferase activity is elevated. Return to a basal level of enzyme activity occurs later whether or not nerve stimulation is continued.[1011] This may possibly represent the manner by which pineal melatonin-forming activity is gradually diminished toward the end of the dark phase.

There are differences of opinion about the relative importance of N-acetyltransferase and hydroxyindole-O-methyltransferase (HIOMT) in the regulation of melatonin production during the normal daily cycle. The strongest evidence currently favors N-acetyltransferase, as outlined in the preceding paragraph. However, in some circumstances a higher activity in pineal HIOMT is found at night than during the day. This was once thought to be the basis for the increased melatonin production at night. Proponents of N-acetyltransferase as the limiting and more important enzymatic step have suggested that in some of the studies on pineal rhythms in HIOMT the concentrations of methyl donor, S-adenosylmethionine (SAMe) or the substrate (N-acetylserotonin) may possibly have been too low to saturate the system. Thus, one or more of the other participants in the reaction may have been limiting and have been responsible for the circadian rhythm or for its absence.[1034] SAMe is known to follow a twenty-four hour rhythm in the brain, with lowest values at the middle of the light phase and a maximum 50 percent higher at the middle of the dark phase.[1089] Study of its twenty-four-hour changes and controls in the pineal gland is needed. It has been shown that S-adenosylhomocysteine, (SAH), the product of SAMe in tissues after transmethylations, is a potent inhibitor (25% inhibition at 5×10^{-8} M or 96.7% at 5×10^{-6} M) of HIOMT as well as of some other methyltransferases having monoamine substrates.[199,468] Melatonin, adenosine, homocysteine and some other tested thio compounds have little or no effect on HIOMT.[468] The enzyme is activated by its substrates and certain anions, including those derived from citric acid cycle intermediates.[468] The latter probably contributed to the high

TABLE XLIX

Effects of continuous light (LL) and continuous darkness (DD) on adult mammalian pineal indoleamine contents and metabolism. Symbols: ↑ = increase in level, ↓ = decrease in level, → = no change in level, ⌒↓ = decrease in daily peak, ⌄↑ = increase in daily trough, ⌒ = circadian rhythm continues, X = circadian rhythm suppressed or not detected.

Pineal constituents	LL	DD	References
Tryptophan	?	⌒→	915
Aromatic-L-amino acid decarboxylase	↑	→	383,926,928
5-HT	X ⌒↓ ⌄↑	⌒→	427,823,915,932
Monoamine oxidase	→	→	1081
5-HIAA	→	?	781
N-acetyltransferase	X ⌒↓ ⌄↑	⌒→	502
Hydroxyindole-O-methyltransferase	X ↓	X↑→	32,58,498,672a,795, 799,844,1079,1081
Melatonin	X ⌒↓ ⌄ →	⌒↑→	576,577,835,977

and variable rates of melatonin formation early noted by Quay with incubations of pineal tissue in complex media.[781] Other mechanisms possibly contributing to cyclic and other variations in pineal HIOMT activity can be postulated on the basis of an extensive and detailed study by Karahasanoğlu and Özand.[468]

Continuous Light and Darkness

The effects of continuous light and continuous darkness on pineal indoleamines and enzyme activities involved in their metabolism are summarized in Table XLIX. No data are available for tryptophan-5-hydroxylase, 5-HTP, and N-acetylserotonin. This is probably because of the greater technical difficulty of measuring these pineal constituents. The available data on the measured constituents are nonetheless sufficient to suggest several conclusions: (1) Continuous light and continuous darkness are not opposite in their effects. The particular results of these treatments depend upon which pineal constituent one measures. (2) Continuous light suppresses all of the pineal's circadian rhythms in indoleamines. It is likely that this represents a complex and widespread modification of pineal metabolism, rather than a metabolically sharply localized effect.[781] Continuous light leads to an increased pineal content of c-AMP,[226] along with suppression of rhythms and depression of peak values in pineal 5-HT and *N*-acetyltransferase. These circumstances raise doubts concerning the primacy of cyclic-AMP and c-AMP-mediated activities for the daily stimulation of pineal synthesis of 5-HT during the light period and *N*-acetylserotonin and melatonin during the dark period. (3) Continuous darkness on the other hand has very little effect on pineal indoleamine rhythms or levels, apparently including those of hydroxyindole-*O*-methyltransferase activity and melatonin.[672a] It can be concluded that light is not required for these rhythms, which are thus truly endogenous. The effect of light, superimposed by the pineal's sympathetic innervation, is to synchronize on a daily basis the pineal's indoleamine rhythms with that of the daily light-dark cycle.

Developmental Changes in Pineal Indoleamines and Their Rhythms

Pineal tryptophan-5-hydroxylase, monoamine oxidase (tryptamine as substrate) and *N*-acetyltransferase are present by the time of birth of the laboratory rat (Table L). Significant levels of these enzyme activities precede by several days the first appearance of twenty-four-hour rhythmicity in pineal 5-HT and *N*-acetyltransferase. They are, therefore, not limiting factors in the developmental timing of these rhythms. It appears likely that 5-hydroxytryptophan decarboxylase activity has a critical role in the developmental sequence. Its times of appearance and early augmentation in the rat pineal closely approximate those of 5-HT (Table L). Its postnatal rise can be increased by continuous light, while postnatal continuous darkness has no effect.[383] Continuous light postnatally also suppresses appearance of the infant rat's twenty-four-hour 5-HT rhythm, but the rhythm appears subsequently after the animal is exposed to a twenty-four-hour day-night cycle. Light or an environmental light-dark cycle is not required, however, for the induction of the pineal 5-HT rhythm, since the rhythm is found in twenty day old rats that have been in continuous darkness from the time of birth.[426]

TABLE L

Developmental changes in rat pineal indoleamines and related enzyme activities. Figures are days before (−) or after (+) birth at which first detection or a stated level of a constituent has been recorded. Pineal levels of all constituents are compared in terms of amounts or activities/pineal tissue weight.

Constituent	Absent	First Detected	Rhythm Appears	% of Adult Value 50%	% of Adult Value 100%	References
Tryptophan-5-hydroxylase	0			2 +	30 +	355
Aromatic amino acid decarboxylase(s):						
5-HTP decarboxylase	0.5 +	0→6 +	—	10 +	18→20 +	383,425,1102
DOPA decarboxylase	1 +	12 +	—	30→35 +	60 +	355
5-HT	0–1 +	1→3 +	6 +	7 +	10 +	355,383,426, 588,823
Monoamine oxidase substrates: 5-HT	1 +	12 +	—	20→24 +	?	355
Tryptamine		←0	—	0	10 +	1102
N-Acetyltransferase		←4 −	4 +	5→8 +	10→20 +	245
Hydroxyindole-O-methyltransferase	0→6 +	6→10 +	24→39 +	17→25 +	34→45 +	498,1102

In adult pineal tissue, tryptophan-5-hydroxylase and not 5-HTP decarboxylase has a rate-limiting effect on synthesis of 5-HT. This has been demonstrated with adult female rat pineal organ cultures by Shein *et al.*[899] who found that 5-HT synthesis was progressively increased by additions (10^{-5} to 10^{-3} M) of 5-HTP but additions of tryptophan (10^{-4} to 10^{-3} M) did not cause any such progressive change in 5-HT synthesis.

If 5-HTP decarboxylase has a critical role in the development of pineal 5-HT and its circadian rhythmicity, it is important to look more closely at its properties and behavior in pineal tissue. There are significant differences in these if one compares developing pineal and brain[73,99] in the same species (rat):

    (1) Although the major developmental increase in 5-HT occurs in both tissues after birth, brain 5-HTP decarboxylase activity approaches adult levels by the time of birth, while the pineal's activity does not appear until after birth (Table L).

    (2) Synthesis of brain 5-HT *in vivo* from blood-borne or administered 5-HTP is equally successful in newborn and adult animals. Synthesis *in vivo* of pineal 5-HT on the other hand is not increased by administered (ip) 5-HTP six days after birth but is at twenty days.[383] The activity of pineal 5-HTP decarboxylase is not increased by twenty-four hours after administration (ip) of 5-HTP to newborn, six or twenty day old rats. Thus in the infant rat before twenty days of age, levels of 5-HTP and the metabolic steps preceding that of 5-HTP decarboxylase seem not to be limiting factors in the developmental appearance of the pineal's rhythm in 5-HT. In the brain on the other hand, tryptophan hydroxylase on the basis of good evidence has been credited with being the rate-limiting step in 5-HT synthesis in infants as well as adults.[43,99,334,890]

    (3) Decarboxylation of 5-HTP and DOPA in mammalian tissues has been thought until recently to be catalyzed by a single enzyme, aromatic-L-amino acid decarboxylase. The grossly different rates of development of pineal capacity to decarboxylate 5-HTP and DOPA (Table L) suggest that here more than one enzyme is involved and that they warrant more careful study.

Published data on the development of monoamine oxidase and HIOMT in rat pineal glands are difficult to evaluate at this time. The different results obtained by two laboratories studying pineal monoamine oxidase (Table L) are not readily attributed to the two substrates used since these differ by one hydroxyl group that would seem to be uncritical in location. Variations in the rate of developmental advance of pineal HIOMT activity denoted by the ranges in Table L may be related to the factors discussed in the previous section. Nevertheless, in comparison with most of the other pineal enzymes acting in indoleamine metabolism, HIOMT develops relatively late and could be a limiting factor in the first appearance of melatonin and other 5-methoxy derivatives of 5-HT. Reports are not yet available on the developmental patterns of these compounds.

Sensory Mechanisms

The pineal's circadian rhythm in 5-HT continues in both infant and adult rats that have been either blinded or placed in continuous darkness. In the adult the lateral eyes are required for effects to occur on pineal 5-HT through either continuous illumination or changes in timing of illumination within a particular day-night cycle. Without the lateral eyes and a daily photoperiod or light cue (Zeitgeber) the adult pineal rhythm *free-runs* or continues on an endogenous basis.[932]

However, rat infants do not require the presence of the lateral eyes for the cyclic nocturnal fall in pineal 5-HT to be inhibited by extended environmental illumination.[922,931,1103] The circadian rhythm in six and twelve day old rat pineal 5-HT has a nocturnal decline which can be inhibited by an added four hours of light beyond the usual time of the start of darkness. This occurs in spite of the fact that developmentally the eyelids are still sealed shut. It is likely that significant photoreception by the retinas of infant rat lateral eyes occurs even with the eyelids closed. This was suggested early by Crozier's and Pincus' studies on phototropisms, which began in their rats eight to nine days after birth.[183,184] This is supported also by the fact that when infants are blinded by bilateral orbital enucleation at nine days of age, at twelve days of age four hours of light beyond the usual start of darkness still causes a reduction of the decline in pineal 5-HT. But the blockade of the light-induced inhibition is not complete unless the heads of the animals are completely covered with a black cloth hood (Fig. 37). In these experiments, the hooded animals were said to be able to breathe and move about freely; and they were, like the other groups, presumably similarly separated from the mother at the same time earlier on the last day of the experiment. The investigators concluded that non-retinal photoreception occurred in the infant rats and that photic information from this unknown sensory site was sufficient to cause partial blockade of the light inhibition of nocturnal pineal 5-HT decline in blinded infants.[922,931,1103] This extraretinal photoreception was found to be absent or ineffective by twenty-seven days after birth, since the nocturnal decline of pineal 5-HT in blinded rats of this age could not be blocked by an extended photo-period. The anatomical location of the postulated infantile extraretinal photoreception is not known, but pineal organ and brain are both possibilities. Both have physiologically demonstrated photoreceptive activity in lower vertebrates.[809] In mammals, transient concentric lamellar formations in the cytoplasm of newborn rat pinealocytes form the only, and certainly tenuous, suggested evidence for a possibly photo-receptor organelle.[922] Possibly similar lamellar bodies have been seen in developing chromaffin tissue.[178]

The ontogeny of various physiological and nutritional characteristics[11] in laboratory rats suggests that factors other than light should be looked at in relation to induction and regulation of the pineal's indoleamine rhythms. One may wonder whether the timing of temperature changes, physical stimulation, and nourishment may be significant factors. Experiments testing the importance of such factors on infant pineal indoleamine rhythms remain to be performed.

It also remains desirable to investigate the possibility of natural photochemical responses in infant pineal organs. Although mammalian pineal organ cultures and transplants have been studied chemically in several laboratories, direct photochemical responses have not been demonstrated. Immature pineal glands transplanted to the anterior chamber of the eye in adult rats failed to show any effect of continuous

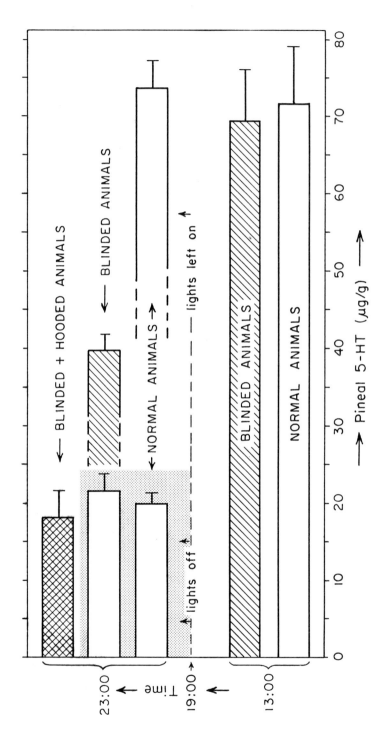

Figure 37. Effects of blinding and blinding + hooding (at 9 days of age) on pineal 5-HT, and on the light-induced blockade of the usual nocturnal depression in pineal 5-HT. Each group contained 16 animals; horizontal bars end at mean; horizontal lines beyond means show the magnitude of the standard errors. (Data of Snyder.[922])

light or darkness ten or fifty-six days later on the fluorescence intensity (level) of the 5-HT in histochemical analyses, or on the HIOMT activity in biochemical incubations.[1068]

Mediation by Sympathetic and Central Nervous Systems

Circadian rhythms and effects of light and darkness involving pineal 5-HT and enzyme activities significant for its pineal synthesis and metabolism have been shown to be mediated in the adult rat by sympathetic and central nervous systems. Techniques of surgical as well as chemical sympathectomy have been used in these studies. Three kinds of surgical pineal sympathectomy have been employed: (1) excision of the superior cervical sympathetic ganglia, (2) *decentralization* of the superior cervical ganglia by cutting the anterior segmental connections between the sympathetic trunk and the spinal cord, and (3) bilateral transection of the nervi conarii within the tentorium cerebelli or close to the pineal organ.[814] Only the first of these procedures has been used extensively in testing the importance of the pineal's sympathetic innervation. It may be important that the superior cervical sympathetic ganglia are responsible for the passage of nerve fibers to diverse intracranial innervations in addition to that of the pineal gland. Innervations of meningeal and cerebral vessels and of choroid plexuses are among these. Modifications in intracranial pressure and in carbonic anhydrase activity of choroid plexuses can follow removal of the superior cervical sympathetic ganglia.[235,236,711] Two kinds of chemical sympathectomy are available at this time: (1) Immunosympathectomy is the selective and permanent destruction of immature sympathetic nerve cells by the injection of newborn mammals for a few consecutive days with an antiserum to the nerve growth factor (NGF).[556,557] (2) 6-Hydroxydopamine injected repeatedly in newborn animals also causes a lasting destruction of sympathetic neurons.[25,26] Only the first of these procedures, immunosympathectomy, has been used in studies on sympathetic regulation of pineal rhythms and responses to light. The relative effectiveness of administration of nerve growth factor antiserum prenatally (*in utero*) and postnatally has been examined in terms of monoamine fluorescence histochemistry and tissue uptake of radioactive NE.[892] Prenatal administration caused a greater reduction in both measures.

Sympathectomized immature rats, unlike adults, still show a circadian rhythm in pineal 5-HT when the animal is in a daily light-dark cycle (Table LI). The pineal glands of such immature animals also respond to light and darkness in the absence or reduction of the sympathetic innervation. This is shown by the blockade by light of the usual nocturnal decline in pineal 5-HT (Fig. 38) and by the abolishing of the circadian rhythm in pineal 5-HT in either continuous light (LL) or continuous darkness (DD) (Table LI). Thus in contrast with those of adults, immature rat pineals are independent of sympathetic control and are dependent on changes in environmental illumination for the circadian rhythm and daily changes in content of 5-HT. The dependence on an external cycle in illumination for the immature's pineal cycle in 5-HT is shown by the effect of continuous darkness. Although the immature's cycle in pineal 5-HT is apparently lost in continuous darkness (Table LI) that of adults continues (Table XLIX).

Machado *et al.*[587] have offered an ontogenetic interpretation of these results. A pineal 5-HT rhythm independent of sympathetic innervation appears shortly after the first appearance of 5-HT in the pinealocytes as visualized by fluorescence histochemistry (Table L). When the pinealocytes become innervated by the ingrowing sympathetic fibers, the regulation of the rhythm within each is taken over by these fibers. This is a non-reversible process in that independence is not restored when the sympathetic innervation is experimentally removed. This implies that the arrival of sympathetic innervation at each pinealocyte causes a fundamental and permanent change in the cell's control mechanism for regulation of its content of 5-HT. Electron microscopy and fluorescence histochemistry show that two to three weeks are required for the development of sympathetic fibers to all members of the population of pinealocytes. During this ontogenetic interval

TABLE LI

Effects of sympathectomy on rat pineal 5-HT and related enzyme activities, in normal daily light-dark cycles (LD), in continuous light (LL) and in continuous darkness (DD). Adults were used in all experiments except as indicated. Symbols: ISX = immunosympathectomized, SGX = bilateral surgical superior cervical ganglionectomy, ↑ = increase in level, ↓ = decrease in level, → = no change in level, ∧↓ = decrease in daily peak, ∨↓ = decrease in daily trough, ∨→ = trough level not changed, ∧∨ = circadian rhythm continues, X = circadian rhythm suppressed or not detected, (X) = situation similar to that in normal animals in LL or DD, ⚡ = blockade of rise during LL or DD.

Pineal Constituent	Procedure	Lighting Conditions			References
		LD	LL	DD	
Adenyl cyclase	SGX	↑			1039
5-HTP Decarboxylase	SGX	↑	⚡		730a,923,926,928
5-HT immatures (8–20 days old)	IGX, SGX	∧∨	X ∧↓ ∨↓	X ∧ ∨ →	587,589,1067
adults (60 + days old)	SGX	X ∧↓ ∨→			275
N-Acetyltransferase	SGX	X ∧↓ ∨→			506
Hydroxyindole-O-methyltransferase	SGX	X ∧ ∨→	(X)	(X) ⚡*	58,844,1077a,1079

*DD = blinded in this experiment.[844]

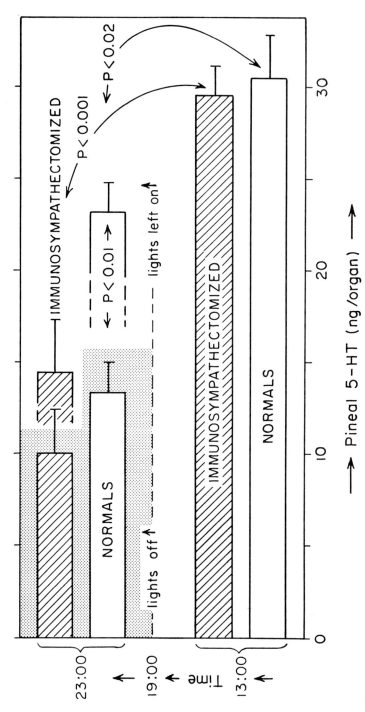

Figure 38. Effects of immunosympathectomy on infant (eight-day-old) rat pineal 5-HT and on the light-induced blockade of its usual nocturnal depression. Bovine nerve growth factor antiserum (1100 units/g) was given within six hours of birth and again twenty-four hours later.[589]

from a few days to three weeks after birth the gland may contain both innervated and non-innervated pinealocytes, responsible respectively for nerve-dependent and nerve-independent rhythms and responses in 5-HT.

Adult rats with the superior cervical sympathetic ganglia either removed or decentralized, no longer show circadian rhythmicity in pineal 5-HT, N-acetyltransferase or hydroxyindole-O-methyltransferase (Table LI). In the case of all three characteristics the loss of apparent rhythmicity involves a depression or blockade of the increased level or activity that occurs in control animals during the daily period of light. The possibility that 5-HTP decarboxylase may be implicated in this effect would seem to gain circumstantial support from the fact that the usual rise in this pineal enzyme activity in continuous light (LL) does not occur after superior cervical ganglionectomy (Table LI). On the other hand, in normal day-night lighting conditions, its pineal activity level is increased after this operation and, as in normal animals, shows no circadian rhythm. It is also not possible to infer for pineal adenyl cyclase a critical role in the denervated animals on the basis of available evidence. Superior cervical ganglionectomy does not cause any change in this enzyme activity in the rat pineal gland but it does enhance its sensitivity to the stimulatory effects of NE.[1039]

The best evidence for sympathetic regulation of a step in adult pineal monoamine metabolism concerns N-acetyltransferase activity. Not only is the daily rhythm in this pineal enzyme activity abolished by blinding, superior cervical ganglionectomy or decentralization, it is increased *in vitro* by norepinephrine (NE) and *in vivo* by stimulation of preganglionic fibers to the superior cervical ganglia.[500,506,1011]

The inferior accessory optic tract has been shown by Moore and co-workers to be the first link in the central mediation of photic effects on adult pineal monoamines and enzyme activity,[54,651,652,653,1078] This demonstration was possible through ingenious use of the different anatomical path taken by the nerve fibers of this system (Fig. 39).[372] Bilateral stereotaxically placed lesions in the lateral hypothalamus to

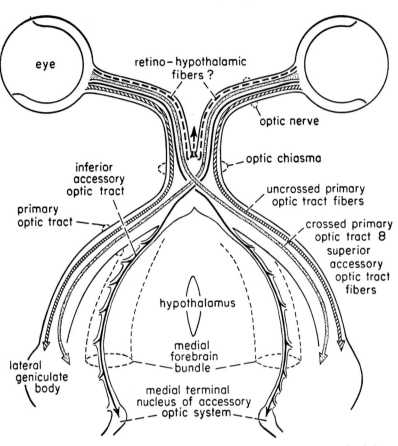

Figure 39. Diagrammatic ventral view of optic fiber systems in the laboratory rat, illustrating the anatomical basis for selective lesions of the inferior accessory optic tract (based on Hayhow *et al.*[372] and Moore *et al*[652]).

interrupt the inferior accessory optic fibers during their course through the medial forebrain bundle (MFB) spare other optic fiber systems. Such bilateral lesions of the MFB or unilateral MFB lesions combined with contralateral orbital enucleation (blinding) block the depressing effect of continuous light on adult rat pineal HIOMT. Bilateral lesions of the primary optic tract or a unilateral lesion of the MFB failed to block the difference in the pineal's HIOMT activity in animals in continuous light as compared with those in continuous darkness.[652] Similar results were obtained in young adult rhesus

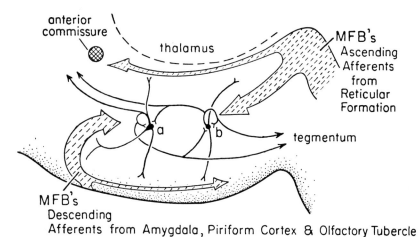

Figure 40. Diagrammatic lateral view of the anatomical relations of the medial forebrain bundle (MFB), its primary afferents and two examples (a and b) of its path neurons in the rat (modified from Millhouse[642]).

monkeys (*Macaca mulatta*) in which the optic chiasma was lesioned in such a way as to destroy all crossing fibers.[651] Those fibers of the primary optic tract which were not crossed were spared and had been shown to be sufficient in such animals for visually guided behavior. Besides blocking the effect of continuous light on adult pineal HIOMT, bilateral MFB lesions also lead to the loss of the circadian rhythm in adult rat pineal norepinephrine (NE).[652] These and related experiments have led to the generalization that behavioral and neuroendocrine responses to light are mediated by separate optic pathways or systems.[154] It is easy to lose sight of the fact, however, that the MFB is a large, complex and heterogeneous system of both nerve cell bodies and fibers. The descending components of this system have been mapped in detail in the rat by Millhouse.[642] The MFB, although clearly a longitudinal fiber system, contains also path neurons (a and b in Fig. 40) that have a quantitative polarity of input along the bundle although the primary sources are the same (Fig. 40). It will be important to determine to what extent, if any, the MFB input from the ascending reticular formation affects the central mediation of photic effects and day-night changes in pineal monoamines and their metabolism. Appreciation of the complexity and the many connections of the MFB system can be readily obtained by making use of Morgane's recent review.[657]

Hormonal Effects on Pineal Indoleamines

Demonstrated hormonal effects on pineal indoleamines and their related enzyme activities are few in number and relatively modest in magnitude. Although the evidence is fragmentary and still weak, the hormonal effects that have been reported can possibly be explained through an intermediate action of norepinephrine or the sympathetic nervous system on the pineal organ. This hypothesis and available direct evidence of hormonal effects on pineal indoleamines will be considered first in relation to observations from human pathology and then in connection with experiments on laboratory rats.

Marked individual variation and relatively little correlation with age was found by Wurtman *et al.*[1075] in human pineal HIOMT and MAO from twenty-five subjects three to seventy years old. Otani *et al.*[750] measured 5-HTP decarboxylase, MAO, and HIOMT in thirty-three adult human male pineal glands obtained at necropsies. Again great individual variation was observed. This did not appear to be due to differences in postmortem time. Furthermore, the investigators saw no correlations between pineal enzyme activities and subject age or extent of pineal calcification. No comment was made concerning other possible correlations.

Nevertheless, examination of their tabulated data suggests to this reviewer the occurrence of relatively low pineal 5-HTP decarboxylase, HIOMT and MAO activities in specimens from subjects with hypertensive and arteriosclerotic disease. This relationship is supportable statistically when the Mann-Whitney U test[908] is applied to the data, and appears similarly valid when the enzyme activities are given in terms either of activity per pineal gland or of activity per unit tissue weight. The case for the suggested relationship is strongest for 5-HTP decarboxylase and weakest for MAO.

Observations on norepinephrine synthesis, storage, retention and turnover in sympathetic nerve endings in experimentally hypertensive rats suggest a means by which hypertensive disease could affect pineal indoleamine metabolism through norepinephrine. In experimental hypertension there is increased turnover of NE in various organs, with a defect in the storage and retention of NE but without a change in its rate of synthesis.[194,195,519] If pineal sympathetic endings are sites of similar changes in NE, a chronically lower level of sympathetic stimulation of pineal indoleamine metabolism would seem to be a likely result.

The circadian rhythm in rat pineal 5-HT is unaffected by hypophysectomy, thyroidectomy, adrenalectomy or oöphorectomy.[932] Adrenalectomy or daily administration of cortisol are both without effect on pineal content of 5-HT measured six days later at the usual time of the peak value.[615] However, pineal levels of metabolic products from 5-HT and content of HIOMT show changes associated with hormone administration and phases of the estrous cycle (Fig. 41). Small but statistically significant differences occur in adult female rat pineal 5-HT and 5-HIAA in relation to day of the estrous cycle as well as in relation to the time of day.[782,784] Rats selected for consistent four-day cycles show higher early morning levels of 5-HT during the last two days and the highest nighttime level during the first (proestrus) day of the cycle. Midday and early evening levels of 5-HT show less evidence of change associated with the days of the estrous cycle. Pineal nighttime melatonin content was found to decrease progressively during the estrous cycle,[784] but its morning HIOMT activity increased during the course of the cycle.[1084] Interpretation of these findings is aided by consideration of three other series of results or experimentally determined relationships: (1) Pineal melatonin content is not always related to relative level of HIOMT activity.[577] (2) Pineal melatonin content in male rats is correlated with level of motor or running activity. The circadian rhythms in the two functions have been shown by Ralph and co-workers[834,835] to be phase-locked or synchronized, in continuous darkness

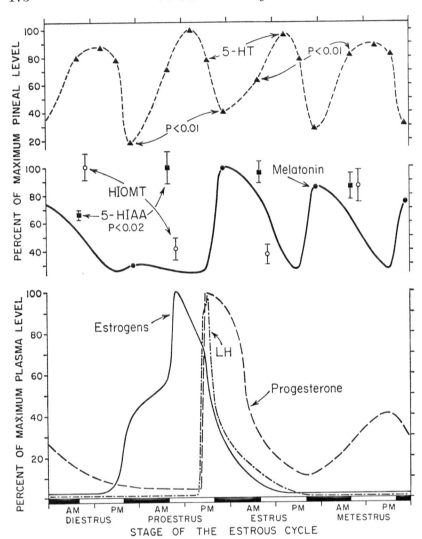

Figure 41. Suggested temporal phase relations of pineal contents of 5-hydroxytryptamine (▲, 5-HT), melatonin (●), 5-hydroxyindole-3-acetic acid (■, 5-HIAA) and hydroxyindole-*O*-methyltransferase (o), and of plasma estrogens, progesterone and luteinizing hormone (LH) during the estrous cycle of female rats. (Data for pineal contents from references 782,784 and 1084; data on plasma hormone levels adapted from references 508, 989, and 1043.)

(DD) and as well as in normal day-night light (LD) cycles. The highest nocturnal pineal melatonin content in female rats was found by Quay following vaginal proestrus (Fig. 41),[784] the time of greatest motor activity during the estrous cycle. (3) Ovariectomy of the infant (twenty-eight-day old) rat leads to significantly increased pineal HIOMT activity by twenty-five days later. When combined with injections of estradiol (50 μg) one and three days before autopsy, no increase in pineal HIOMT occurs.[17] Estradiol (10 μg) depresses pineal HIOMT activity in the mature female also.[1084] Although pineal melatonin content on a circadian basis is phase-locked to locomotor activity, in relation to the estrous cycle it is apparently negatively affected by plasma estrogen (Fig. 41). These estrous cycle plots of pineal indoleamines and HIOMT must be considered preliminary since relatively few points in time have been monitored. It is still apparent, however, that during the transition from diestrus to proestrus, significant differences or changes occur in pineal 5-HT and 5-HIAA as well as in HIOMT and melatonin.

Weiss and Crayton[1043] in studies on hormonal regulation of pineal adenyl cyclase have shown that physiological ovarian secretion of estradiol can influence the NE-mediated stimulation of pineal adenyl cyclase. Ovariectomy increases and estradiol decreases the stimulatory effect of NE on pineal adenyl cyclase. The action of estrogens does not appear to work via changes in gonadotropins since hypophysectomy fails to antagonize the stimulatory effect of ovariectomy, and also fails to modify the inhibitory effects of treatment with estradiol. NE was found by Weiss and Crayton to activate the pineal adenyl cyclase of rats in all stages of the estrous cycle except proestrus, when estrogen levels are highest (Fig. 41). Chronically administered progesterone has no effect on pineal adenyl cyclase activity.[1043] But an alteration of pineal HIOMT has been claimed to occur during the first part of pseudopregnancy.[1022] Testosterone administration to either male or female rats fails to alter pineal adenyl cyclase activity.

There is no evidence for any endocrine gland having a specific trophic effect on the pineal gland's indoleamine metabolism or synthesis of melatonin. In adult males hypophysectomy was found to have no effect on pineal content of HIOMT, although weights of whole body, reproductive accessory organs and pineal gland decreased.[994]

Dietary and Pharmacological Effects

Effects of dietary changes and of treatments with drugs on pineal levels of 5-HT, rhythmicity and metabolism have been investigated primarily with the aim of revealing mechanisms and controlling factors in the normal daily patterns of change. Other potential purposes include evaluation of possible pineal side-effects of aminergic and psychoactive drugs, and pineal changes that might accompany certain disease states or metabolic disorders. These concerns unfortunately have yet gained little attention.

Of dietary constituents, tryptophan is most important for studies on pineal indoleamines. It is at the same time the first amino acid shown to be indispensible nutritionally, and the first found to be toxic when fed in excess. Dietary levels of 2 percent or more cause adverse effects in rats. The concentration of 5-HT in pineal, brain and many other tissues is increased by a high tryptophan content in the food and is decreased by a high content of phenylalanine.[368,783] The pineal gland is notable for the magnitude of its increase in 5-HT when the dietary tryptophan content is high. In comparison with the hypothalamus, for example, the percent increase in pineal 5-HT is twice as great (Fig. 42). The depression of 5-HT content by phenylalanine is similar in magnitude in the two tissues.[783] A daily rhythm in plasma tryptophan occurs in man[1088] and laboratory mammals[915] and depends on the food intake.[272] Although the pineal's 5-HT content can be increased by acute as well as chronic tryptophan loading, the increment or percent change differs according to time of the day or night.[925,929,1101] Suppression of the circadian rhythm in pineal 5-HT results. The same is true when 5-HTP is injected. Pineal 5-HT content is increased, but the increment is greater at night than during the day.[739,925] The injection of 5-HT itself does not lead to any change in pineal 5-HT content in the normal animal,[782,785] but does increase

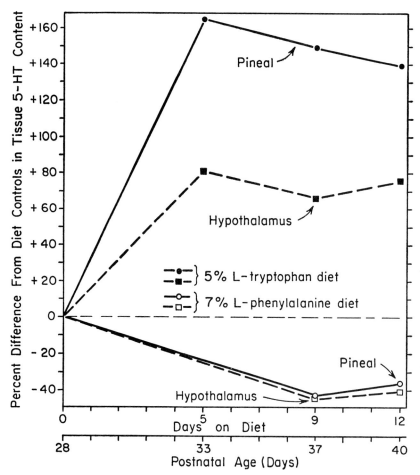

Figure 42. Comparisons of changes in pineal and hypothalamic 5-HT produced by excess dietary levels of tryptophan and phenylalanine. Animals were killed at the same time during the midafternoon of the daily photoperiod (data of Quay[783]).

it in animals that have been superior cervical ganglionectomized.[739]

Rats given 2.5 percent NaCl have been reported to have a lower pineal content of 5-HT (59 ± 9 ng/pineal) than controls (76 ± 5) killed at the same time.[96] A difference in the opposite direction was reported in the whole brain 5-HT contents of the same animals. The complex effects of different patterns and levels of feeding on brain synthesis and turnover of 5-HT[744] render difficult the interpretation of chronic and extreme nutritional experiments with brain and pineal indoleamines.

Drugs affecting particular enzymes in monoamine synthesis and metabolism have been the agents most frequently used in manipulations of pineal chemistry. Most of these are inhibitors and the enzymatic specificity of most is either imperfectly known or depends upon dosage to a significant degree. Inhibition of pineal tryptophan hydroxylase has been accomplished with α-propyl-dopacetamide (H22/54)[258] and more commonly with p-chlorophenylalanine.[120,435,915] A marked decrease in parenchymal 5-HT and slight if any decrease, at least at first, in pineal nerve ending 5-HT occurs. Mescaline has been found to stimulate pineal synthesis of 5-HT in organ cultures, apparently through stimulation of tryptophan-5-hydroxylase.[896] Inhibitors of the decarboxylation of 5-HTP, similarly to what is observed with the inhibitors of tryptophan hydroxylase, generally lead to decrease and loss of parenchymal 5-HT and slight or slow effects on nerve 5-HT.[258,423]

Injections of monoamine oxidase inhibitors have had much more diverse effects, although superficial perusal of the research reports may suggest consistency in results. A potent and relatively long-lasting but imperfectly specific[747] inhibitor, β-phenylisopropylhydrazine (Catron) was studied first and was found to block the nocturnal fall in pineal 5-HT but was variable in its effectiveness in increasing daytime 5-HT, probably due to differences in dosages nad postinjection times.[794,823,925,929] Fluorescence microscopy after nialamide showed increased NE in pineal nerves but no change in the parenchyma.[258,709] The combination of 5-HT administration with nialamide led to further increase in pineal nerve fluorescence, which was now indicative of an increased content of 5-HT.[709] The MAO inhibitor clorgyline discriminates between enzymes in the rat pineal. Type A, in pineal nerves and active on 5-HT, is very sensitive to the drug. Type B, comprising 85 percent of the pineal MAO and inactive on 5-HT, is relatively insensitive to clorgyline.[332] Harmine, long known as an inhibitor of MAO, has been found to stimulate pineal N-acetyltransferase activity *in vitro* and cause increased production of melatonin.[504]

Drugs inhibiting steps in the synthesis or breakdown of pineal catecholamines sometimes have little of any effect on the organ's indoleamines, and sometimes have profound effects. Pyrogallol, an inhibitor of catechol-O-methyltransferase is an example of the former[258] and α-methyl-*p*-tyrosine (α-MPT) is an example of the latter. α-MPT inhibits tyrosine hydroxylase, the rate-limiting step in the biosynthesis of NE. It also causes an increase in pineal 5-HT content.[1101]

Inhibitors of nucleic acid and protein synthesis have been employed most effectively in studies of stimulatory and biosynthetic control mechanisms in pineal glands in organ culture. Actinomycin D partially inhibits the daytime rise in pineal 5-HT *in vivo*[929] and cycloheximide prevents the synthesis *in vitro* of 5-HT, 5-HIAA and melatonin from labeled tryptophan.[53]

Another major assemblage of drugs that affect pineal indoleamines contains agents that counteract or block adrenergic neurons or their receptors. In addition to drugs that, (1) specifically inhibit the function of adrenergic nerves (antiadrenergic, *sensu strictu*) we will include here((2) those that block adrenergic receptors, (3) those that deplete monoamines from their adrenergic and related storage sites, and (4) those that destroy sympathetic nerve terminals. Guanethidine and bretylium are drugs that depress postganglionic adrenergic nerves and that have been used for this purpose in studies on the control of pineal indoleamines. Neither affects pineal 5-HT's nighttime or daytime levels during a normal photoperiod (LD) cycle, but bretylium blocks the elevation of pineal 5-HTP decarboxylase that occurs with continuous light.[925,928] Comparisons of the effects on the pineal by α- and β-adrenergic blocking drugs, especially *in vitro*, support the concept that the pineal receptor for NE is of the β rather than of the α type.[940,1040,1091] *Beta* blocking agents prevent NE-induced enhancement of pineal adenyl cyclase activity and block the stimulation by NE of the conversion of tryptophan to melatonin. Depleters of monoamine stores differ in their relative effects and specificity. Reserpine causes a loss of NE and 5-HT from pineal nerve endings and abolishes the circadian rhythm in parenchymal 5-HT content; the daily peak is lowered and the trough is raised. [112,709,925] Oxypertine at optimal and lower doses produces a differential depletion of NE and dopamine in rat brain with slight if any effect on 5-HT. Electron microscopy of treated rat brains and pineal glands suggests that the same result occurs in the two organs. [66] Slight to great reductions in pineal nerve monoamines have been produced also with α-methyl-m-tyrosine (α-MMT) and m-tyrosine. [709] The sympatholytic drug 6-hydroxydopamine (6-OHDA) has been used to destroy pineal sympathetic nerve fibers, but the probable effects on pineal indoleamine metabolism have not yet been explored. [250]

Other drugs that have been tested for possible effects on pineal indoleamines are psychopharmacologic agents of diverse kinds and relations. Desmethylimipramine, an antidepressant, depletes 5-HT from pineal nerves and should be a good agent for the testing of the interaction of NE and 5-HT in the nerve ending-pinealocyte control mechanisms. [435] However, in other studies, concerning widespread effects through the body, it causes a supersensitization of peripheral receptor sites for epinephrine and NE and may have an anticholinergic action as well. [436] Known anticholinergic drugs affect pineal indoleamine metabolism, but it is not known whether their actions are indirect by way of effects in the central nervous system or in the periphery. N-Methyl-3-piperidyl benzilate, the anticholinergic drug studied most extensively for its pineal effects, disrupts the pineal's circadian rhythms, including that in 5-HT content and alters pineal HIOMT activity. [618] Atropine methyl bromide inhibits the rise in pineal HIOMT in continuous darkness. But when accompanied by oxotremorine oxalate, a cholinomimetic, the higher levels of HIOMT in DD are restored. In normal LD conditions, oxotremorine causes a higher pineal HIOMT activity than that obtained after atropine. The results led Wartman and co-workers to conclude that cholinergic mechanisms are involved in the effect of darkness on pineal HIOMT.[1029]

The possible effect of morphine on pineal indole metabolism has been studied *in vitro*. This was prompted by the early finding that development of tolerance and physical dependence to morphine in the rat is associated with a concomitant acceleration of brain synthesis of 5-HT. However, rat pineal glands in culture, either with or without NE, failed to show modifications in synthesis of 5-HT, melatonin or protein in the presence of morphine.[895]

EFFECTS OF 5-METHOXYINDOLES

5-Methoxyindoles are currently the recipients of the most attention among pineal indoleamines and their derivatives as possible hormones. Excluded from consideration here are compounds which are transient metabolic intermediates (5-HTP, *N*-acetylserotonin, and (?) 5-hydroxytryptophol), biologically inactive products (5-HIAA and 5-MIAA), uncertain products (*beta*-carbolines), and 5-HT, whose plasma levels are the result of synthesis and release primarily from the intestinal mucosa. Most investigations on possible hormonal activities of pineal indole derivatives have concentrated on melatonin. 5-Methoxytryptophol merits consideration also, but has received relatively little attention. 5-Methoxytryptamine remains problematical as a normal pineal product in mammals. There is better evidence for it in birds. Thus, except where noted otherwise, the following review is mostly about the fates and actions of melatonin in the mammalian body.

Tissue Uptake, Turnover and Excretion

Radioactive melatonin injected into the tail veins of adult rats appears within one minute in all examined tissues. Its rapid and significant occurrence in the brain by this time indicates that there is little hindrance to its crossing the blood-brain barrier. One minute after intravenous administration chemically unmodified melatonin accounts for 70–80 percent of the labeled compounds present in diverse tissues, with the exception of liver and plasma. After thirty minutes, unmodified melatonin accounts for 35–50 percent of the total radioactivity in most tissues. About two thirds of the radioactivity found at this time in adrenal gland and brain is melatonin, whereas only 10–20 percent of that in liver and plasma is unmodified melatonin.[515] Study of the disappearance of radioactive melatonin from similarly (iv) injected mice shows at least two phases in the disappearance curve for whole body melatonin. The rapid decrease within the first ten minutes approximates a half-life of two minutes. After forty minutes the rate of melatonin's disappearance corresponds to a half-life of about thirty-five minutes. This suggests that a portion of the administered melatonin is protected from destruction, perhaps through either or both binding and solubility in lipid depots.[515] Further studies on the fate of administered radioactive melatonin using sucrose density gradients for the separation of subcellular fractions have shown 90–95 percent of the radioactivity in the rat ovary and adrenal gland after one hour is in the supernatant fraction, 2–3 percent in the mitochondrial fraction, and little or none was found in the other particulate material (excluding the pellet).[1082]

The relative uptake of administered melatonin by the ovaries and other organs has been used as evidence supporting a hormonal action of melatonin on the ovary. This is based on the fact that in the few cases in which tissue uptake of physiologic doses of hormones has been investigated, the known target organs appear to have a preferential uptake. Examples are uterine and vaginal uptake and retention of estradiol,[437] and cardiac, splenic and uterine concentration of catecholamines.[1051] It is of course not essential that an organ selectively concentrate a hormone in order for it to be acted on by it. Table LII summarizes the results from a survey of organ uptake of melatonin. It is interesting that pineal gland and the iris-choroid structures of the eye had outstanding uptakes as well as did ovary and several endocrine glands. Pineal uptake of melatonin was studied also *in*

TABLE LII

Organ distribution of H^3-melatonin one hour after intravenous administration of 750 or 100 μc (200 μc/μmole) to cats. Data of Wurtman et al.[1082]

Organ or Tissue	Mean μg/100g
Pineal Gland	25.9
Iris-choroid	6.25
Ovary	5.63
Pituitary Gland	2.92
Sympathetic Chain	2.59
Peripheral Nerve	2.23
Testes	1.88
Thyroid Gland	1.75
Adrenal Gland	1.52
Kidney	1.31
Uterus	1.25
Liver	1.08
Pancreas	0.90
Salivary Glands	0.75
Spleen	0.74
Plasma	*0.61*
Heart	0.56
Skin	0.51
Brain	0.48
Diaphragm	0.27
Adipose tissue	0.24

vitro with fresh bovine pineal slices in Krebs-Ringer bicarbonate buffer at 37°C with 0.5 μg ^{3}H-melatonin. After one hour a 1.5–4 fold concentration of melatonin was found in the pineal slices as compared with the medium. Subcellular fractionation studies showed 97.4 percent of the radioactivity in the supernatant fraction and almost all of the radioactive material present was unchanged melatonin.[1082]

Anton-Tay and Wurtman[33] have studied the uptake of ^{3}H-melatonin by brain regions from both intraventricular and intravenous injections. While appreciable uptake is shown by diverse regions following either route of administration, a greater concentration or uptake characterized the hypothalamus in these studies.

Light and drugs have been shown to affect the concentration of administered melatonin by specific tissues. Continuous light for five weeks caused a significant decrease in ovarian melatonin concentration in rats but did not affect cardiac levels.[1082] Pineal levels were lower also but the low counts of radioactivity did not allow meaningful statistical evaluation.

Rats treated chronically with phenobarbital had lower levels of melatonin uptake in the brain, and those given chlorpromazine had higher than normal brain uptake.[1072] These drug effects are likely to be due to changes in the liver's rate of metabolism of the administered melatonin. All of the phenothiazines which have been tested (chlorpromazine, promethazine and promazine) elevate brain and blood levels of administered melatonin. Imipramine raised the brain level but did not affect that of blood, while desmethylimipramine and amphetamine failed to cause changes in melatonin uptake by either.[1074] Reserpine given thirty minutes before melatonin caused a significant fall in melatonin uptake by brain and heart but did not affect that by the ovaries. Although both 5-HT and 5-MT (Fig. 31) are structurally similar to melatonin, neither altered the accumulation of melatonin by tissues.[1072]

Melatonin is completely metabolized in the body. A hepatic microsomal enzyme that hydroxylates melatonin in position 6 is responsible for the major pathway. This is followed by conjugation with sulfate (70–80 percent) or glucuronic acid (5 percent) and excretion in the urine. Only traces (to 2 percent) of administered melatonin appear in the urine as 5-methoxyindole acetic acid (5-MIAA).[514,515,528,529]

These results from laboratory mice, rats and rabbits can be supplemented by findings from five schizophrenic and non-schizophrenic volunteer patients.[442] In man as in rats over 90 percent of the radioactivity resulting from administered [β-^{14}C] melatonin was recovered in the first twenty-four hour urine sample and the remaining 10 percent in the next twenty-four hour sample. Table LIII summarizes the partial identifications and measurements of the excreted metabolites of melatonin. It is to be hoped that with improved gas chromatographic and mass spectrometric methods now available, metabolites of endogenous melatonin will be studied.

Responses to Melatonin and Congenors

The relative potency of melatonin and related compounds has been studied in standard preparations involving contrac-

TABLE LIII

Urinary metabolites (percent) from melatonin administered to male human mental patients and laboratory rats.[442]

Subject	6-OH Melatonin	6-Sulfate	6-Glucuronide	Unidentified
Patients				
Schizophrenia A	1.5	59.4	24.4	14.6
B	1.6	61.3	27.2	8.8
C	1.2	65.0	24.6	8.9
Huntington's chorea	2.3	79.0	13.0	0.9
Unspecified brain damage	3.8	65.0	24.2	3.7
Rats	6.8	60.0	29.5	3.7

tion by smooth muscle, antidiuretic activity, and other responses.[111,310,948] Melatonin has a slight oxytocic effect at high dosage, no effect on blood pressure and is a competitive inhibitor of some of the smooth muscle contractions elicited by 5-HT. The latter include responses of isolated rat duodenum,[965] rat uterus[386] and cat trachea.[830] The great potency of melatonin as a blancher of amphibian melanocytes depends on both the 5-methoxy and the N-acetyl groups. However, the N-acetyl group reduces melatonin's activity as compared with that of congenors tested on smooth muscle and blood pressure.[310]

Surprisingly limited use has been made of melatonin and related compounds in studies of molecular mechanisms and cellular responses *in vitro*. Some of the most interesting cellular materials and responses are from lower organisms and have been reviewed previously.[796] Among adult vertebrate cell systems, amphibian skin preparations have provided the most interesting results. Melatonin not only inhibits the frog skin's darkening response to MSH, but also inhibits the rise in c-AMP (Fig. 43).[1,851] Melatonin differs from NE in this system in that its effects can not be blocked by previous treatment with α-adrenergic blocking drugs. This has been taken to mean that melatonin probably interacts with receptors distinct from but related to adrenergic α-receptors. But the means by which these receptors suppress cellular accumulation of cyclic-AMP remains unknown.[851] The effects of melatonin *in vitro* have been studied also using the release of

Pineal Chemistry

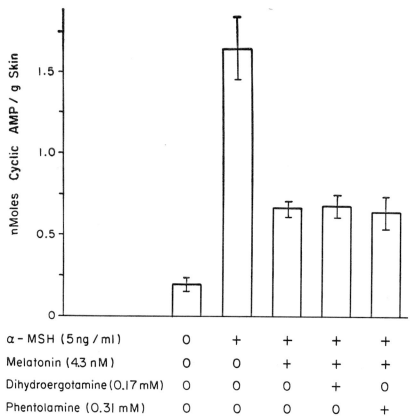

Figure 43. The lowering of cyclic-AMP in frog skin *in vitro* by melatonin. Melatonin counteracts the effect of α-MSH, and, unlike norepinephrine, is not blocked in the effect by the α-adrenergic blocking agents. (Adapted from Abe *et al.*[1])

glycerol by rat epididymal adipose tissue as the end point measurement.[1001] Melatonin in this system does not interfere with glycerol release when the latter is stimulated by α- or β-MSH but is inhibitory in the presence of ACTH. Both melatonin and 6-hydroxymelatonin cause an increase in glycerol and free fatty acid release in the presence of epinephrine but do not in its absence. Differences are detectable between the responses obtained with these compounds and with 5-HT, *N*-acetylserotonin and 5-MT, but the findings do not suggest that melatonin or its congenors have a role in the mediation of lipolysis in adipose tissue.

An overwhelming majority of the published investigations on the effects of melatonin and related compounds in mammals has depended upon administrations *in vivo*. While interesting and probably physiologically significant results have been obtained, these are sometimes obscured by contradictory findings, technical problems and alternative possible interpretations. Some sources of these problems may include: (1) Variations in purity or potency of the melatonin samples used for injection.[974] (2) Inadequate control injected animals.[240] (3) Potentiation of a melatonin effect may be necessary in the form of an appropriate conditioning length of photoperiod or of administration at a particular time of the daily physiological cycle,[277] or in terms of necessary tissue levels of other hormones (as noted in the previous paragraph). (4) The effect may be transitory and not coincide in time with the arbitrary moment selected by the investigator for its measurement. (5) The effect may be indirect, by way of the nervous system or other systems whose mediation of a melatonin effect may be suppressed by incidental ambient environmental conditions or physiological states. (6) The effect may not be specific to melatonin but occur following administration of other agents, such as sympathomimetics. This becomes a concern especially when the minimum effective dose, or other tested dose, is high. The relevance of the last four of these considerations will become apparent in the following paragraphs. It can be noted at the outset that various parenteral routes of administration of melatonin and related compounds have been employed successfully, from the early use by Wurtman and coworkers of subcutaneous and intraperitoneal injections[1071,1076] to the chronic subcutaneous implantations of melatonin in beeswax by Rust and Meyer.[874]

Presumptive target organs responding *in vivo* to melatonin can be arranged schematically to illustrate some of the possible hypothetical routes by which melatonin could conceivably have its demonstrated effects (Fig. 44). Although many reports assume or imply only direct effects (1 → 8 on right side of Fig. 44) for administered melatonin, indirect nervous system and humoral routes (left side of Fig. 44) are gradually receiving more attention.

Target Organs

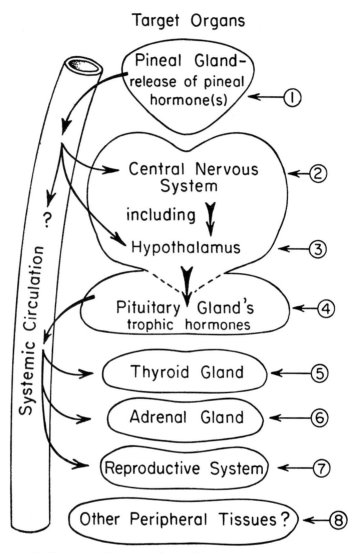

Figure 44. Heuristic diagram of possible routes of mediation (left side) of the effects of parenterally administered melatonin. Primary sites of direct or indirect effects form a hierarchy and are numbered (1–8) in the order of their discussion in the text.

One of the neglected pathways by which melatonin may possibly have its effects is via the pineal gland itself. It has been suggested that as an alternative hypothesis to pineal methoxyindoles being themselves hormones, these pineal products could possibly function as chemical messengers within pineal tissue,[791,803] perhaps influencing the release into the bloodstream of one or more pineal compounds of truly or exclusively hormonal nature. Since *in vivo* tests of melatonin's effects have seldom if ever included pinealectomized control subjects, and are infrequently supported by similar effects *in vitro*, this theoretical possibility remains worthy of consideration. Mammalian pineal glands *in vivo* as well as *in vitro* have an exceptional capacity for concentrating melatonin (Table LII). Three changes have been reported in the pineal glands of rats following administration of melatonin: (1) Under continuous light (LL) but not under normal day-night conditions (LD), a daily dose of 150 μg reversed slightly the light-induced depletion of lipid from the pinealocytes.[233] (2) In normal day-night conditions (LD) melatonin (50 μg subcutaneously) suppressed the pineal's circadian rhythm in 5-HT if administered at the eighth hour of the daily light period but not if injected six hours later.[277] (3) Melatonin (10^{-3} and 10^{-5} M) *in vitro* increased uptake by bovine pineal slices of ^{125}I-thyroxine. 5-HT, TSH, and aldosterone had no effect on pineal uptake and NE at concentrations of 10^{-5} and 10^{-6} M decreased pineal uptake.[144] These last two sets of experiments with melatonin support the notion that one site of melatonin's physiological action is within the pineal organ. It remains to be determined whether melatonin modifies pineal synthesis or release of presumptive protein or polypeptide hormones.

Melatonin and related compounds can cause various changes in the central nervous system and in behavior. Some of these can be characterized, at least superficially, as induction of sleep. Responses of this nature were obtained with hypothalamic implants of 15–30 μg melatonin in cats[597] and with intraperitoneal injection of melatonin, tryptophol, 5-hydroxytryptophol and 5-methoxytryptophol in mice.[80,262] Results of the same general sort have been claimed by Anton-Tay *et al.*[30] following administration of various doses of melatonin to human subjects. Normal subjects showed increases in EEG alpha activity, sleep, imagery and feelings of well-being and elation. Epileptic patients had "a decrease in paroxistic elements" and two parkinsonians receiving 1.2 g orally for four weeks had "a striking improvement" in their symptoms. This last finding in parkinsonian patients is obscure in terms of its possible mechanism, but it is perhaps paralleled by the blocking action of melatonin on the adventitious body movements induced in mice by L-DOPA.[177]

Experimental administrations of melatonin and congenors either systemically or as implants in hypothalamus or lower brainstem have provided evidence for the hypothesis that the antihypophyseal and antigonadal actions of some of these compounds are mediated by way of these lower brain centers. Especially noteworthy are the brain implantation studies of Fraschini and co-workers[291,294,295,667] and the subcutaneous implantations of melatonin in weasels by Rust and Meyer.[874] Several neurochemical changes have been reported in rats and rabbits that had received intraperitoneal injections of melatonin. Hypothalamic and cerebral γ-amino-butyric acid (GABA) increased; midbrain 5-HT increased as cerebro-cortical 5-HT decreased; and brain pyridoxal kinase activity increased.[29,31] These changes all occurred within an hour or two and disappeared by several hours later. Melatonin and to a lesser extent 5-methoxytryptophol reversed the depressing effect of pinealectomy on the thiamine diphosphate-phosphohydrolase activity of the rat hypothalamic supraoptic and paraventricular neurosecretory nuclei, according to recent experiments of deVries.[215,216] Other investigations in the same laboratory have shown that the level of this enzyme activity in these nuclei is directly proportional to the level of circulating pituitary gonadotropins. Therefore, on this system, melatonin's effect is similar to that seen following increases in circulating gonadotropin.[951,952] A suggested and tentative pattern of routes and mechanisms by which secreted or administered pineal 5-methoxyindoles may cause this and related hypothalamic effects is diagrammed in Figure 45.

Complex, and often subtle, behavioral changes have been reported as results of injections of melatonin. These include: (1) improvement of learning ability in experimental phenyl-

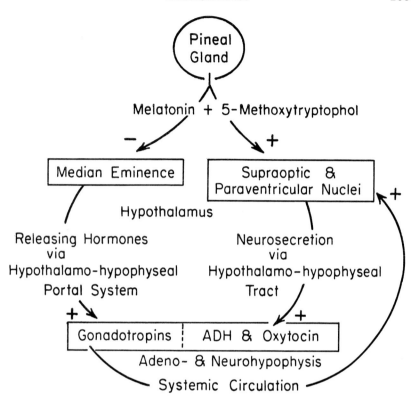

Figure 45. Suggested routes and mechanisms of the effect of pineal 5-methoxyindoles on the hypothalamus.

ketonuric mice;[1066] (2) decreased wheel-running activity by food-deprived rats;[1062] (3) rate changes in operant behavior of pigeons;[891] and (4) stabilization and synchronization of 24-hour rhythms in food and fluid intake and urine volume of thymectomized rats.[363]

Effects of melatonin on the pituitary and its dependent endocrine glands can be reviewed in the logical order shown in Figure 44. Analyses of pituitary glands after treatment with melatonin have suggested no effect on secretion of ACTH,[452] usually an antagonistic effect on gonadotropin secretion,[8,295,667,969] a decrease in MSH content[476] and an increase in 5-HT content of the pars intermedia.[746] Other findings by Kastin *et al.* are consistent with their idea that the lowered pituitary MSH found after darkness[477] may be mediated by melatonin. Pineal output of melatonin increases and pituitary content of MSH decreases during darkness.[477] Removal of the pineal gland leads to elevation of pituitary MSH.[474] Questions remain concerning the specificity of action and possible interactions of monoamines in the mediation of these pituitary effects of melatonin and related compounds.

Injection of rodents with melatonin usually leads to signs of thyroid inhibition, but opinions vary as to whether this is a direct effect or whether it is mediated through higher centers.[89,196,208-210,410,656,678,717,842,910-912] An inhibitory action of melatonin on the adrenal gland has been claimed by several groups of workers, and where adrenal subdivisions are specified, the cortex is the part concerned.[196,319,342,911,1000] Although melatonin has been reported to reverse the adrenal enlargement following unilateral adrenalectomy this action in female mice was shared by 5-HT, N-acetylserotonin, 5-hydroxytryptophol, 5-methoxytryptophol and 5-HIAA.[1000] Melatonin added (5 μg/ml) to incubations of adrenal tissue has been found to not affect 3-β-ol-dehydrogenase activity but it reduced the production of $\triangle^4$-3-ketonic corticosteriods from endogenous precursors and the response of the cortex to ACTH. From these results Giordano and coworkers[319] concluded that melatonin acts directly on the adrenal cortex and inhibits the enzyme activity that catalyzes the conversion of cholesterol to pregnenolone. Again the question remains concerning the specificity of the response and the dose/response relationship.

The reproductive organs comprise the most frequently studied presumptive targets of melatonin and other constituents of pineal extracts. Antigonadal effects of melatonin injections were first demonstrated and studied in an extensive manner by Wurtman and co-workers.[1071 1076] Although a number of laboratories have confirmed and added to these results,[8,158,193,242,290,404,487,488,629,661,874,911,935,1002,1077] others have had difficulty in obtaining gonadal effects with melatonin.[209,233,461,527,933] While technical factors, such as potency of preparation[974] or dose level,[869] or potentiating circumstances of photic environment or day[1003] or time of day,[277] may possibly be responsible for the variation, evidence is incomplete and mostly circumstantial. Some of the reproductive effects of melatonin are shared by 5-methoxytryptophol,[172,390,613] as well as some of its precursors (5-HTP, 5-HT) which cannot be considered to be hormones.[209,1002,1003] A comprehensive study has yet to be made on the relations of molecular structure among monoamines and indoles to their gonadal activity. Furthermore, antigonadotropic activity also resides in non-melatonin fractions of bovine and human pineal extracts. The active material is in the molecular range of small polypeptides.[102,231,601,966] For other points of view and information on other aspects of melatonin's reproductive effects the reader is referred to recent reviews dealing with the physiological relations of the pineal to the reproductive system.[292,666,801,840,1080]

A few other systems have been studied in mammals following administration of melatonin. Although subcutaneous injections of melatonin to rats failed to modify milk ejection,[646] chronic implantations of melatonin in the rabbit median eminence lowered milk yield.[894] However, this effect was relatively non-specific since it was shared by 5-HT, dopamine and NE. The best evidence indicates that mammalian melanocytes both *in vivo* and *in vitro* are refractory to melatonin,[167,411,493,606,837,845,921] unlike the melanin-bearing cells of many fishes and amphibians. Melatonin and pinealectomy can, however, affect hair growth and pigmentation in some lower mammals.[410,874] But these effects are probably by way of the hypothalamo-hypophyseal endocrine system. Melatonin has no effect on the growth of tumors in rats,[420] although at various times enhanced tumor growth has been claimed following pinealectomy.[191,192,674]

EFFECTS OF BETA-CARBOLINES

The natural occurrence and production of β-carbolines in pineal tissue is still uncertain. Nevertheless, the psychopharmacologic potency of many of these compounds provokes

TABLE LIV

Concentrations (M) required for 50 percent inhibition of bovine liver monoamine oxidase *in vitro* by some beta-carbolines and iproniazid. Compounds I through III are suspected to occur in pineal tissue; their structures are shown in Figure 32 (p. 153).

Compounds	Tyramine[610]	Substrate Tryptamine[396]
I 6-hydroxytetrahydroharman	7.5×10^{-3}	
II 6-Methoxytetrahydroharman	5.0×10^{-5}	6.3×10^{-3}
III 6-Methoxyharmalan	4.5×10^{-7}	
IV 6-Methoxytetrahydro-β-carboline		1.3×10^{-3}
Iproniazid	4.75×10^{-10}	2.5×10^{-5}

a disproportionate interest in them, their possible mammalian biosynthesis and diverse effects. The specific β-carbolines suspected to occur in the pineal gland are shown in Figure 32. They are competitive inhibitors of monoamine oxidase (Table LIV). Their structural relatives can inhibit cholinesterases[312] and the uptake of NE by slices of cerebral cortex.[875] 6-Methoxytetrahydro-β-carboline can elevate brain levels of 5-HT,[614] and this is apparently not due to inhibition of monoamine oxidase nor through a direct action on the brain.[401] There is, however, an increase in the bound fraction of brain 5-HT.[400] 6-Methoxytetrahydroharman causes behavioral disturbances in rats at doses as low as 0.008 mM/kg.[612] The toxic syndrome elicited by various β-carbolines in laboratory animals has been known for many years and is characterized by excitation, tremors and convulsions.[302]

CONCLUSIONS

1. Indoleamines and their derivatives are the pineal compounds that have received the most interest and investigation in recent years.

2. Among these compounds, melatonin and related 5-methoxy derivatives of 5-HT have been intensively studied as possible pineal hormones with effects on brain, pituitary gland and dependent peripheral endocrine and reproductive organs. Many investigators are coming to believe that at least some of these effects are secondary to a primary effect of melatonin on the central nervous system, perhaps especially

in the hypothalamus. The possibility remains, however, that melatonin and the related pineal indoleamines have humoral functions within the pineal gland itself.

3. Supporting a truly hormonal status for melatonin are the findings that: (a) in mammals the final enzymatic pathway for the synthesis of melatonin is localized to the pineal gland; (b) melatonin is found in the blood of normal animals but not those that have been pinealectomized; (c) melatonin is rapidly taken up from the bloodstream by various tissues leading to tissue concentrations greater than that of plasma in ovary and endocrine organs by one hour after intravenous injection; (d) its turnover is otherwise rapid and the resulting hepatic metabolites (6-hydroxymelatonin and conjugates) are biologically inactive; (e) responses primarily of an inhibitory nature are elicited in some of the endocrine glands and parts of the reproductive system. Effects on the central nervous system and behavior are still of uncertain chemical specificity. Although some of the reported effects of melatonin are opposite to those of pinealectomy, demonstration of melatonin's efficacy in attempted replacement therapy following pinealectomy is incomplete.

4. Pineal indoleamines and many of the pineal activities related to their biosynthesis and metabolism have a circadian rhythmicity with remarkable amplitude and precision of timing related to the daily times of environmental onset of light and darkness. This rhythmicity depends upon, and is under the control of, the sympathetic innervation of the pineal gland. But before this innervation reaches the pinealocytes during postnatal development an independent circadian rhythm in pineal 5-HT is demonstrable. Norepinephrine's actions on pinealocyte metabolism in culture confirm the essential role of this neurotransmitter and the sympathetic innervation of the adult organ.

5. In adults, but apparently not in infants, the lateral eyes are required for the responses of the pineal's indoleamine rhythms to changes in environmental illumination. Photic information affecting pineal indoleamine rhythms is transmitted from lateral eyes to brain by the inferior accessory optic

tract, and passes from brain to pineal gland via the superior cervical sympathetic ganglia.

6. Dietary contents of tryptophan and phenylalanine can raise and lower respectively the pineal content of 5-HT. Acute pharmacological loading with either tryptophan or 5-HTP raises pineal 5-HT content and suppresses the circadian rhythm in this constituent. The rhythm in 5-HT is not affected by hypophysectomy, thyroidectomy and adrenalectomy. Although no endocrine gland has any specific trophic action on the pineal gland and its indoleamines, physiological secretion of estradiol decreases and ovariectomy increases the stimulatory effect of NE on pineal adenyl cyclase. Adenyl cyclase in turn has an important metabolic role in the circadian rhythms of particular pineal enzymes involved in the synthesis of the precursors of melatonin.

Chapter Eight

CATECHOLAMINES

PINEAL CATECHOLAMINES AND
THEIR METABOLIC RELATIONS

MAMMALIAN PINEAL GLANDS contain at least three cate-- cholamines, DOPA (= 3,4-dihydroxyphenylalanine), dopamine (DA) and norepinephrine (NE) (Table LV). Their precursors, phenylalanine and tyrosine, and also octopamine have been identified and measured in pineal tissue (Tables XXXV and LV). Norepinephrine, as the neurotransmitter at peripheral and pineal sympathetic nerve endings, is generally held to be the physiologically active and significant member of this series, with the others important as precursors and sometimes active as sympathomimetics.[46,1015,1016] However, recent knowledge about the individualistic central distribution and functional relations of dopamine, and new findings concerning octopamine in sympathetic nerves suggest that these compounds may be transmitters also, or co-transmitters.[648,650] Experiments testing the significance of NE in the regulation of pineal metabolism have demonstrated a pre-eminent role for this neurotransmitter in the daily rhythmic and other changes. This is especially clear in the case of pineal indoleamine metabolism, as discussed in the previous chapter. Possible regulatory contributions by dopamine and octopamine in pineal tissue remain to be explored. The relatively very high concentrations of dopamine (Table LV) encourage such an investigation.

All of the enzymatic steps for the synthesis of norepinephrine from phenylalanine or tyrosine occur in pineal tissue (Fig. 46). Recent experiments show that the

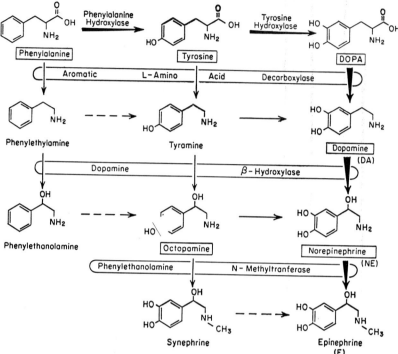

Figure 46. Biosynthetic pathways of catecholamines in the mammalian body. Heavy arrows show the primary paths; slender arrows show two of the demonstrated secondary paths; and dashed-line arrows indicate *in vitro* or theoretically possible routes. Compounds whose names appear in boxes have been identified and measured in pineal tissue (see Tables XXXV and LV). With the exception of phenylethanolamine-N-methyltransferase, the enzymes named here have all been demonstrated in mammalian pineal glands.

TABLE LV

Pineal content of catecholamines (μg/g tissue) in rat and man.

Species	Compound				References
	DOPA	Dopamine	Octopamine	Norepinephrine	
Man	0.04	0.50	—	0.10	878,880.
Rat	—	34.3 ± 10.9	0.6*	2.8–10.6	650,731,738,1073.

* = per pineal gland

rat pineal gland contains a phenylalanine hydroxylating system and that the tyrosine present in the tissue is not due to blood-borne transport of tyrosine from the liver to the pineal gland.[61] It is thought, however, that the pineal system for hydroxylating phenylalanine may involve tryptophan hydroxylase and may not be identical to that found in the brainstem.[61] In addition, tyrosine hydroxylase is found in large amounts in pineal tissue.[604] It has a marked substrate specificity and is generally thought to be the usual rate-limiting step in the biosynthesis of NE. The synthesis of NE in the pineal gland from phenylalanine or tyrosine takes place within the sympathetic nerve endings. Although it was once thought that tyrosine hydroxylase occurs in a particulate fraction, recent studies show it to be mainly in the soluble fraction[535] and to be not usually membrane bound.[671]

The decarboxylation of DOPA to form dopamine, the next step in the biosynthesis of NE, occurs also in the cytoplasm of sympathetic nerve endings. The responsible enzyme, aromatic L-amino acid decarboxylase, is thought by some to have a relatively broad specificity for L-amino acids.[574] It is present in high concentration in pineal tissue[924] and is increased following the denervation of the gland.[738,928] Pyridoxal phosphate is a cofactor for this enzyme; it is tightly bound to the apoenzyme as a Schiff's base.

The β-hydroxylation of dopamine to form NE occurs through the agency of another enzyme having a relatively broad substrate specificity. Dopamine β-hydroxylase acts on those compounds having a benzene ring with a side chain of two or three carbon atoms terminating in an amino group. It is associated with the chromaffin granules in the adrenal medulla[1008] and with the analogous catecholamine-containing granules or vesicles in sympathetic nerve endings.[534] It is in part bound to the granule membrane and occurs in part in the soluble contents of the granule. It requires ascorbic acid for activity and *in vitro* requires in addition other cofactors, including fumarate or acetate, catalase and ATP. Since it is a copper-containing enzyme, there are available various pharmacologic inhibitors, most of which contain thiol groups and act by binding enzyme Cu++. Disulfiram (tetraethylthiuram) is one such that is potent both *in vivo* and *in vitro*.[329,670] There are present in most tissues endogenous inhibitors of dopamine-β-hydroxylase. These also act by complexing with the Cu++ of the enzyme.

Insofar as known, in no species does the pineal gland have the capacity to N-methylate NE to form epinephrine. The required enzyme, phenylethanolamine-N-methyltransferase, is highly localized in the adrenal medulla, with small amounts occurring in brain and heart.[45]

Biosynthesis *in situ* is not the only way by which NE in sympathetic nerve endings is acquired by pineal and other sympathetically innervated organs. Uptake and binding of NE from the extracellular fluid and the circulation is a functionally important mechanism. Several kinds of studies have shown the pineal gland's sympathetic nerve endings to have selective uptake of NE. Wolfe *et al.*[1057,1058] demonstrated that tritiated NE is taken up from the circulation by the rat pineal gland and is selectively concentrated in the nerve endings in the vicinity of the granulated (dense core) vesicles. Unfixed pineal glands from such studies showed that the ^{3}H-NE was within the *microsomal fraction*, when homogenates in isotonic sucrose were subjected to ultracentrifugation over a continuous density gradient.[750] This fraction or zone was considered by the investigators to be similar to that which contains the granulated (dense core) vesicles in other organs.[1080] Isolated pineal glands from cats have been shown by Dengler and coworkers to be able to take up labeled DL-NE to a concentration of about 25x that in the medium.[207] A lower concentration ratio (4x) was found for pineal glands from calves. Uptake of NE was inhibited by reserpine and ouabain, and required an active carrier mechanism. About 30 percent of the total isotope taken up by calf pineal slices was unchanged NE, and the remainder was in the form of acidic products of oxidative deamination by monoamine oxidase (Fig. 47). In general, when isotopically labeled NE is injected into an experimental animal, it persists in sympathetically

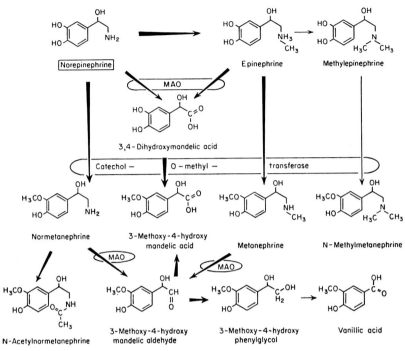

Figure 47. Primary pathways of metabolism of norepinephrine and epinephrine in the mammalian body. Norepinephrine and the enzymes most concerned in its metabolism, monoamine oxidase (MAO) and catechol-O-methyltransferase, are found in pineal tissue.

innervated tissues for many hours, in fact, for long after its physiological actions have ended.[1051] This implies that uptake and binding of NE by nerve endings is a significant means for short term inactivation of the free transmitter.

The fates of pineal NE (Fig. 47) are more complex than its biosynthesis, although but two enzymes, monoamine oxidase (MAO) and catechol-O-methyltransferase (COMT) are the important enzymatic participants in its metabolism. The turnover of NE in the nerve endings is rapid but not homogeneous; small amounts are released spontaneously[385] and larger amounts are released upon stimulation of the nerve. The released *free* NE has four possible fates (Fig. 48). Although some of it interacts with receptor sites in vascular

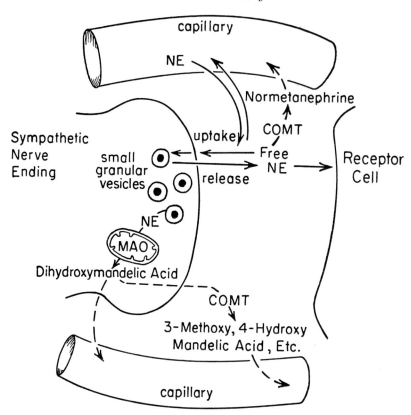

Figure 48. Fates of norepinephrine (NE) in, and released from, sympathetic nerve endings, such as those found in the pineal gland. COMT = catechol-*O*-methyltransferase, MAO = monoamine oxidase.

smooth muscle or pinealocytes, most of it is taken up again by the sympathetic nerve ending and stored in the dense core vesicles. Alternatively some passes into capillaries as *free* NE and some is rendered physiologically inert as normetanephrine by COMT before passing into the bloodstream. Besides the fates occurring after release, much of the NE within the nerve ending is destined to be destroyed before release. In this instance the monamine oxidase within the nerve terminals converts it to physiologically inactive metabolites.[513] Denervation of the rat pineal gland by superior cervical ganglionectomy leads to a reduction or loss of this MAO activity within the terminals.[930] As noted earlier, a

TABLE LVI

Mean uptake of ^{3}H-norepinephrine by organ and brain slices *in vitro* from cynomolgus monkeys (*Macaca irus*), expressed as tissue: medium ratios after twenty minute incubations with 0.2 nmoles (4.2 c/mmole) ^{3}H-NE in 2 ml Krebs-Henseleit bicarbonate buffer saturated with 95% O_2, 5% CO_2.[311]

Organ or Brain Region	Mean ± Standard Error
Pineal	13.16 ± 1.16
Posterior Pituitary	1.27
Anterior Pituitary	1.20
Brain Regions	
Putamen	8.58 ± 0.66
Head of Caudate Nucleus	7.46 ± 0.33
Amygdaloid Nucleus	6.00
Hypothalamus	
Mammillary Body	3.30 ± 0.94
Supraoptic Nucleus	3.17 ± 0.50
Paraventricular Area	2.31 ± 0.37
Medial Geniculate Body	2.75 ± 0.77
Ala Cinerea	2.40 ± 0.48
Septal Nuclei	2.30 ± 0.96
Insular Cerebral Cortex	2.16
Other regions	0.67 to 1.96

specific form of MAO, enzyme A, is found in the sympathetic nerves, including those of man, and a different form of MAO, enzyme B, is found in the pinealocytes.[333]

Pineal tissue has a remarkable capacity for uptake and concentration of various amines, either from the surrounding medium *in vitro* or from the normal circulation *in vivo*. Gfeller *et al.*[311] showed that in comparison with thirty-nine brain regions and anterior and posterior parts of the pituitary gland, slices of the monkey (*Macaca irus*) pineal gland have nearly twice as great a concentrating ability for ^{3}H-NE during a twenty-minute incubation (Table LVI). Uptake of epinephrine from the blood *in vivo* has been demonstrated by Steinman *et al.*,[939] who administered ^{3}H-epinephrine to adult male rats under ether anesthesia (Tables LVII and LVIII). The tissue concentrations of ^{3}H-epinephrine and its metabolites were determined after perfusion of the intracranial vessels with isotonic saline solution. At either ten or sixty minutes after intravenous injection the ratio of pineal:brain concentration of ^{3}H-epinephrine was 150:1; after intraventricular (lateral cerebral) administration it was 2:1. These and the differences

TABLE LVII

Mean organ uptake of ^{3}H-epinephrine at ten minutes after intravenous injection of 2.10 μg (116 μc) to male rats anesthetized with ether.[939]

Organ	ng ^{3}H-E/g tissue*
Pineal	37 5
Pituitary	3.18
Brain Regions	
Hypothalamus	0.306
Mes- + Diencephalon	0.212
Pons + Medulla	0.214
Cerebral Cortex	0.163

* N = 3.

TABLE LVIII

Percentages of ^{3}H-epinephrine and its metabolites occurring in rat pineal, pituitary and whole brain one hour after intravenous (IV) (2.10 μg, 116 μc) or intraventricular (IC) (44 ng, 2.13 μc) administration of ^{3}H-epinephrine to male rats under ether anesthesia.[939]

Labeled Compound	Pineal		Pituitary		Brain	
	IV	IC	IV	IC	IV	IC
Epinephrine	82.1	45.3	44.5	32.4	25.7	41.6
Metanephrine	1.24	12.1	17.2	10.6	22.4	5.4
3-Methoxy, 4-Hydroxy Mandelic Acid	0.73	6.25	12.4	9.8	25.6	3.8
3,4-Dihydroxy- Mandelic Acid + Dihydroxyphenylglycol	0.08	2.46	0.12	12.6	0.04	2.6
Conjugated Metabolites	2.46	19.8	6.30	26.7	9.3	43.8
Total Activity (dpm × 10^{-5}/g tissue/min.)	55.0	5.82	2.81	1.23	1.13	3.26

shown in Table LVII can be attributed in part to the effect of the blood brain barrier for epinephrine[1032] and the relative lack of such a barrier in pineal and pituitary glands. Nevertheless, the marked uptake by pineal as well as certain other organs and brain regions suggests that epinephrine released from the adrenal medulla under stress may be taken up by, and have significant effects in, these structures. It is therefore of interest to examine the metabolites of epinephrine found after uptake. A comparison of these is summarized in Table LVII, again taken from the data of Steinman and co-workers.[939] The pineal gland is notable on the basis of two differences vis-a-vis pituitary gland and brain—retention of a greater portion of the epinephrine in a chemically unmodified form, and a relatively small content of 3-methoxy derivatives. This raises questions, still unanswered, about the turnover kinetics of epinephrine in pineal tissue and the availability of a compartment that is relatively protected from the activity of catechol-*O*-methyltransferase.

LOCALIZATIONS

Catecholamines have been localized microscopically within particular pineal structures by means of three techniques, fluorescence histochemistry, radioautography and electron microscopy. Subcellular fractionation techniques are available also for localization of these compounds within pineal cells and organelles, but they have been relatively little used since the amount of tissue required is greater, at least by standard methods.

The fluorescence histochemical method of Falck and Hillarp[256] for catecholamines and tryptamines has been utilized most effectively in revealing the pineal localizations of these compounds. The details and chemical specificity of the method have been presented and evaluated elsewhere.[176,249,257,365,443] By this method, primary catecholamines in a protein matrix or layer are rapidly and quantitatively condensed with formaldehyde in a Pictet-Spengler reaction to form 1,2,3,4-tetrahydroisoquinoline. This in turn is rapidly dehydrogenated by formaldehyde to its corresponding 3,4-dehydroisoquinoline, which has a greenish fluorescence. Tryptamines, such as 5-HT and 5-MT, and their precursor 5-HTP, are similarly converted by formaldehyde to yellow fluorescent 3,4-dehydro-β-carbolines. In one of a number of recent modifications of the general method, selective demonstration of NE has been proposed on the basis of cleavage by periodic acid of the -C-C- bond at the 3,4-position of the tetrahydroisoquinoline derivative of NE only, and not of DOPA, dopamine or epinephrine. The formation of these tetrahydro compounds or intermediates of the various fluorescent amine products can be controlled as a reverisible process by borohydride reduction.[175,176,668] This enables not only specific cleavages at this step, but also the distinguishing of specific fluorescence from so-called non-specific fluorescence or autofluorescent sources within tissue slices.

Owman and his colleagues at Lund have made the most extensive fluorescence histochemical studies of pineal catecholamines and tryptamines in mammals.[112,113,707,710] Other investigators using the same method have added observations concerning developmental changes, species differences and the effects of drugs.[86,422,586,588,984] It is difficult to decide upon the significance of the very great species differences observed in the amounts and localizations of catecholamines and tryptamines within the mammalian pineal gland. Factors such as the unspecified time of day or season, the method of handling and killing, and technical differences in the preparation and reaction of the tissue can all be involved. It must be appreciated also that when the fluorescence emission is intense, a spectrally green fluorescence of a concentrated site of catecholamine may appear yellow to the unaided sensory system of the investigator. Thus microspectrofluorometry is a necessary adjunct to the chemical interpretation of results from the method with pineal tissue.

For the purposes of the present discussion, the most important findings concerning pineal catecholamines revealed by fluorescence histochemistry are the restricted localization of catecholamines to the pineal nerve fibers and endings, and their displacement or commingling at these sites with 5-HT.[707-709] These observations form part of the basis for the mechanism postulated here of the adult rat pineal's twenty-four hour rhythms in catechol- and indoleamines. The sympathetic nerve fibers and endings within the rat pineal gland lose their fluorescence following either bilateral cervical sympathectomy[707] or chemical sympathectomy with 6-hydroxydopamine.[250]

Electron microscopic radioautography has shown that rat pineal uptake *in vivo* of tritiated NE occurs only in non-myelinated nerve axons and endings which contain granular vesicles.[139,963,1057,1058] Reserpine administration leads to the loss of the labeled material at these sites. The same sites are equally capable of taking up and storing labeled amine after injection of ³H-5-HTP.[67,963] Two hours after iv injection of ³H-5-HTP, 43 percent of the silver grains, accrued from the radioactivity in the tissue slices, lie over nerve endings. Over the pinealocytes, comprising a much greater volume of the tissue, a proportionally smaller number (53%) of silver grains are found. Moreover, the perivascular and extracellular spaces, which comprise in the rat pineal a larger percentage in volume than the nerve endings, have only about 4 percent of the silver grains.[67]

Axons and nerve endings within mammalian pineals are shown by electron microscopy to contain vesicles, or a so-called plurivesicular component.[211] Numerous reports have been made on these and other vesicular structures in adrenergic and other kinds of nerve endings and presynaptic formations in various parts of the nervous system. At the present time this bewildering array of ultrastructural vesicles appears to be divisible into three general types.[121] Within all three types of vesicles, some have a dense, granular or electron-dense core, and some do not. (1) Synaptic vesicles, *sensu strictu*, are those vesicles 300–600 Å in diameter and which constitute 90–95 percent of all vesicular structures seen in central and peripheral nerve terminals, including those of the mammalian pineal gland. Those synaptic vesicles that have a dense or granular core are believed to be the ones involved in the binding and storage of monoamines such as NE and 5-HT, while the agranular or core-less synaptic vesicles are, by exclusion, believed to be associated with all transmitters other than monoamines. (2) A vesicle of about twice (= 1000 Å) the diameter of the usual synaptic vesicle is also associated with nerve terminals storing monoamines, including those in the pineal gland.[123] However, it is found as well in various neurons of uncertain transmitter type, in some ganglia, brain regions and in the adrenal medulla. (3) The third kind of vesicle, and the second one of the larger size (800–1200 Å), provisionally includes such probably diverse structures as the large granular vesicles of pinealocytes,[730] neurosecretory granules of the hypothalamo-hypophyseal system and chromaffin granules. The granular material within vesicles of this kind has some of the staining reactions seen in the synaptic apparatus of neurons, suggesting for this and other reasons that the granularity or electron opacity of the core results from a major portion of the content being proteinaceous. Electron microscopy of pineal complexes from lower vertebrates through mammals suggests the presence of a consistent pattern of vesicle types and localizations.[171,695] Small and large granular vesicles which experimentally demonstrate content or uptake of monoamines are found in the nerve endings and axons. Larger granular vesicles (vesicle type 3) which demonstrate no clear evidence of monoamine content[737] are found in the pinealocytes. This last type of granular vesicle will be considered again in relation to pineal proteins.

Extensive correlative ultrastructural, biochemical, cytochemical and pharmacological studies, especially by Pellegrino de Iraldi and her co-workers in Argentina, have shown that the small granular vesicles of the rat pineal's nerve endings and fibers constitute the storage sites of catechol- and indoleamines within the neuronal compartment. These studies have led to the definition of two subcompartments within the small granular vesicles, the *central core* and between it and the surrounding membrane a *matrix*, having different staining properties (Fig. 56, Table LIX).[736,737] Experiments have demonstrated that both catechol- and indoleamines are localized in the central core. However, the possibility is not excluded that 5-HT and NE have different biochemical storage sites within the core at the molecular level. Drugs that have different degrees of chemical selectivity in their action of depleting, releasing or displacing NE, 5-HT and selected monoamines in adrenergic nerve endings have the effects to be expected on the small granular vesicles within the pineal nerve endings (Table LX). Pyrogallol, an inhibitor of COMT, does not modify the granulated vesicles nor does it protect them from the action of reserpine, whereas administration of the MAO-inhibitor iproniazid prior to reserpine does protect the pineal's small granular vesicles from degranulation.[731] Either single or chronic injections of

TABLE LIX

Relative staining intensity of core and matrix of rat pineal adrenergic nerve vesicles by different fixation-staining procedures for electron microscopy (adapted primarily from Pellegrino de Iraldi and Suburo[735,736]). OsO4 = osmium tetroxide alone; GA + OsO4 = glutaraldehyde followed by OsO4; WT = Wood's technique[1063] for catechol- and indoleamines; ZIO = Champy-Maillet mixtures having an appropriate content of zinc iodide; + + + = most intensely stained or electron dense; O − + = minimally stained or electron translucent.

	OsO$_4$	GA + OsO$_4$	WT	ZIO
Core	+ + +	+ + +	+ +	+
Matrix	O–+	O–+	O–+	+ +·+

TABLE LX

Effects of amine depleting, releasing and displacing drugs on number, size and/or staining intensity of presumptive amine storage sites in small granular vesicles of rat pineal adrenergic nerve endings. $\doteq$ = no distinct change; ($\downarrow$) = slight reduction; $\downarrow$ = marked or great reduction; $\downarrow_o$ = reduction to near absence.

Drug Biochemical Effect	Staining Technique* and Vesicle Site					
	OsO$_4$ Core	GA + OsO$_4$ Core	WT Core	ZIO Core	Matrix	References
Reserpine 5-HT, NE & DA $\downarrow$	$\downarrow$	$\downarrow$	$\downarrow$	$\downarrow$	$\downarrow$	222,223,370,435, 731–733.
p-Chlorophenylalanine 5-HT $\downarrow$ (NE & DA $\doteq$)	$\doteq$	$\downarrow$	$\downarrow$	$\downarrow$	($\downarrow$)	120,222,734,735, 745,902.
Oxypertine NE $\downarrow$; 5–HT$\doteq$ or ($\downarrow$)	$\downarrow$			$\downarrow$		66,222,370,735, 736.
Tyramine 1 NE pool $\downarrow$ & 5-HT($\downarrow$)?						735,736.
Acute	$\doteq$		($\downarrow$)	$\downarrow$	($\downarrow$) or $\doteq$	
Chronic	$\downarrow$		$\downarrow$	$\downarrow_o$	$\downarrow_o$	

* See Table LIX for abbreviation key of staining techniques.

iproniazid increase the proportions of vesicles that are granulated and the average sizes of both vesicles and granules. Angiotensin is also reported to cause an increase in the pineal's granular vesicles in the nerve endings.[716] The effects of other drugs on the vesicles have been reported, but where interpretation is possible they belong to the categories already mentioned.[125-127,222,360,370,846,902] Exposure of rats for two or four days to −6° to −8°C led to an increase in the zinc iodide-osmium (ZIO) reacting material in the pineal synaptic vesicles.[525] Unfortunately, the results from practically all of the experiments modifying the granular synaptic vesicles are unaccompanied by information on the ambient photic or photoperiod conditions and timing. Therefore, the findings offer little opportunity to interpret the biochemical (NE or 5-HT) or circadian phase (night or day) of the reported responses.

PHYSIOLOGICAL AND PHARMACOLOGICAL CHANGES

Circadian Rhythms and Effects of Light and Darkness

Since circadian rhythms in adult rat pineal 5-HT and HIOMT depend upon an intact sympathetic innervation, it was reasoned that there might be a related daily change in the NE content of the gland. Wurtman and Axelrod[1073] found this to be so (Fig. 49). Although the amplitude of the rhythm is not great, available data points are particularly interesting, suggesting that pineal NE content falls during the daily light phase (day) and rises during the dark phase (night). Unfortunately relatively less experimental work has been done on this pineal rhythm as compared with that for 5-HT. However, Moore and coworkers[652,1083] have shown that blinding (bilateral enucleation), bilateral section of the inferior accessory optic tract (Fig. 39), or unilateral enucleation and ipsilateral section of the tract lead to loss of the adult rat pineal's rhythm in NE. The resulting pineal content of NE remains at a level intermediate to the normal daily maximum and minimum. Superior cervical ganglionectomy leads to nearly complete disappearance of pineal NE in the rat,[738] thus preventing the possibility of studying the influence of the postganglionic sympathetic fibers on the rhythm in NE. Decentralization, cutting the connections between the spinal cord and the upper part of the sympathetic trunk, however, leads to a reduction of about 50 percent. Although it remains to be determined whether the latter operation modifies the rhythm in pineal NE, on the basis of the results from sectioning the inferior accessory optic tract one would expect it also to abolish the rhythm. The presumption is that the neural and sympathetic connections with the central nervous system are necessary

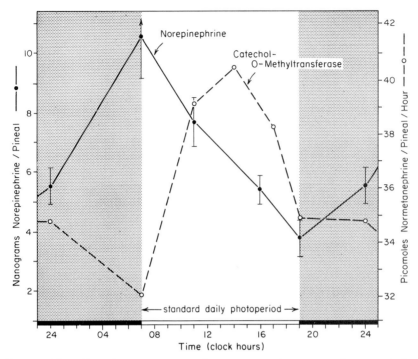

Figure 49. Pineal contents of norepinephrine and catechol-O-methyltransferase in adult rats according to timing in relation to a standard daily period of light. (Adapted from Wurtman and Axelrod[1073] and Bäckström and Wetterberg.[60])

for the transmittal to the adult pineal of both photic information and information from a master *oscillator* (clock) system in the brain.

The circadian rhythm in pineal content of NE could be mediated within the pineal organ by one or more of several mechanisms: changes in rates of synthesis, release, metabolism, uptake and binding. The possibility of increased pineal synthesis of NE at night is supported by the finding of increased pineal tyrosine hydroxylase activity at that time.[604] Since the rate of NE synthesis *in vivo* is generally thought to be controlled by this enzyme,[559] increased tissue content or activity of tyrosine hydroxylase could represent a basis for increased NE synthesis.[51] Investigations on possible twenty-four hour changes in pineal decarboxylation of DOPA or β-hydroxylation of dopamine have not been reported. Similarly there is no direct evidence for twenty-four hour changes in pineal release, uptake and binding of NE. However, there is some evidence that enzymic machinery for pineal metabolism of NE follows a twenty-four hour rhythmicity. Although *in vitro* studies have failed to demonstrate any such rhythmicity in pineal MAO,[925] Bäckström and Wetterberg[60] have shown pineal catechol-*O*-methyltransferase (COMT) activity to rise during the day and to be at a low level through the night (Fig. 49). They observed also that in continuous light, pineal COMT activity remained at the high level seen near midday in animals subjected to daily light (day) and dark (night) (LD) phases. There was, therefore, no evidence of a twenty-four hour rhythm in the pineal enzyme when the animals were in continuous light. It remains to be demonstrated whether the daytime fall in pineal NE requires COMT. In another organ, the uterus, the rise and fall of catecholamine content during the estrous cycle cannot be explained on the basis of changes in uterine COMT, although rat uterine COMT activity is greatest during estrus and is increased by administration of estrogen.[318]

A preliminary and probably incomplete explanation of the mechanism of the pineal's twenty-four hour rhythm in NE can be proposed at this time. This explanation represents a refinement and extension of an earlier and similar proposal by Wurtman and co-workers.[1083] It is based primarily upon two phenomena, the dependence of the rate of synthesis of NE in sympathetically innervated organs upon the rate at which nerve impulses reach the sympathetic endings,[649] and the triggering actions of daily onset of light and darkness on compartmental shifts in pineal biogenic amines. During the night, when the rat is behaviorally most active, sympathetic activity might be expected to be greatest, leading to increased synthesis and storage of NE in the pineal's sympathetic nerve endings. At the onset of light there is physiological as well as biochemical evidence of release of NE within the pineal. A pronounced and sudden pineal vasoconstriction occurs at this time.[818,819] Subsequently during the day, 5-HT accumulates within the pineal sympathetic nerve terminals, presumably occupying sites that might have held NE. With the onset of darkness this stored 5-HT is released from the endings and enhanced availability of binding sites for NE occurs. Since tyrosine hydroxylase is inhibited by catecholamines such as NE and dopamine,[992] the postulated increased availability of binding sites at nightfall may minimize the levels of free catecholamines within the nerve terminals and thereby reduce endogenous inhibition of tyrosine hydroxylase and NE synthesis within the pineal nerve endings. A summarizing diagram of this mechanism is presented in Figure 50. Interrelations of the adult pineal's twenty-four hour rhythm in NE with indoleamines and other related metabolites were summarized in Figure 36 (p. 158).

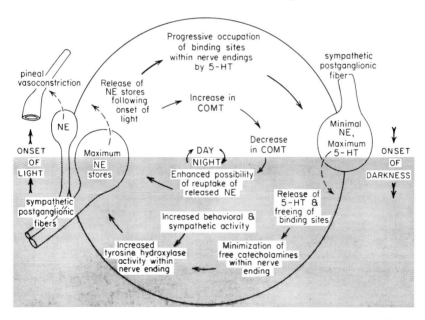

Figure 50. Postulated mechanism of the adult rat pineal gland's 24-hour clock, which depends on both sympathetic innervation and daily phases of light and darkness. COMT = catechol-*O*-methyltransferase, 5-HT = 5-hydroxytryptamine, NE = norepinephrine.

Developmental Changes

Catecholamines and cellular mechanisms for their syn-thesis, storage and uptake appear early in the developing rat pineal gland. In animals two hours old, catecholamine-containing nerves are detectable by fluorescence histochemis-try in the pineal capsule, particularly at the apex and dorsum of the gland below the vena cerebri magna. By twenty-four hours after birth a few adrenergic bundles have penetrated the pineal and by a day later adrenergic terminals containing catecholamines occur around blood vessels and among pinealocytes in some regions.[585,586] Adult density of adrener-gic nerves occurs within the pineal between two and three weeks after birth.[581]

The developmental course of the granular synaptic vesicles within the pineal nerves follows a pattern consistent with that described for the nerves and nerve endings. Small num-bers of small granular vesicles (500 Å) are seen by a few hours after birth. They increase greatly in number during the first two weeks postnatally, while the number of large (1000 Å) granular vesicles, although first appearing a little earlier, remain in the range observed in the adult from the day of birth. With the increase in numbers of small granular vesicles there is also an increase in the proportion of small granular vesicles to agranular vesicles, from which type they appear to develop (Fig. 51). Some of the large granular vesicles found within the pineal nerve terminals seem to develop through a similar process. But most of them, according to Machado,[581] originate through pinching off from sacs and tubules of smooth endoplasmic reticulum which had accumulated granular material (Fig. 51). However, Pellegrino de Iraldi and DeRobertis[732] have suggested that these vesicles form by the dilatation and pinching off of the ends of neurotubules. It appears, however, that at least part of the large granular vesicles and much of the material of the small granular vesicles (granules + ? membranes) are formed locally in the peripheral axons and nerve terminals. By eight to ten days after birth the pineal catecholamine-containing innerva-tion is functional and is able to convey photic information

SMOOTH ENDOPLASMIC RETICULUM

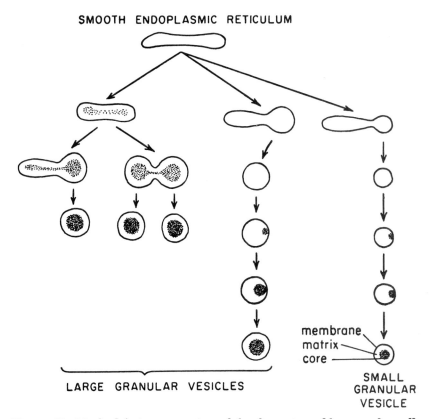

LARGE GRANULAR VESICLES

SMALL
GRANULAR
VESICLE

Figure 51. Machado's interpretation of the formation of large and small granular vesicles in pineal adrenergic nerve fibers and endings. (Modified from Machado.[581])

to the gland.[581,654] The twenty-four hour rhythm in NE content appears distinctly by ten days of age.[654]

Biochemically detectable amounts of dopamine and NE appear in rat pineal glands a little more slowly than the cellular structures for their storage. This is likely to be due at least partly to the lesser sensitivity of the biochemical measurements. Hyyppä[422] found that pineal dopamine was not measurable before ten days after birth, at which time the amount per gland was 4 ng. At thirty days it was 10 ng and at sixty days 12 ng. Considering the remarkable dopamine concentrations attained by adult rat pineals (Table LV), this rate of

TABLE LXI

Developmental changes in pineal norepinephrine content (ng/pineal) in rats kept either in constant lighting conditions from birth (six to fourteen day old groups) or in such conditions for seven days prior to autopsy. DD = constant darkness; LL = constant light; P = probability values for LL versus DD comparisons based on a two-tailed t test.*

Postnatal Age (Days)	Mean Norepinephrine Content/Pineal		P
	LL	DD	
6	6.1 ± 0.2	· 5.9 ± 0.7	> 0.05
10	1.9 ± 0.9	4.5 ± 0.3	< 0.01
14	1.3 ± 0.1	4.3 ± 0.1	< 0.001
85	2.2 ± 0.2	13.4 ± 0.3	< 0.001

* Data of Moore and Smith.[654]

developmental increase seems slow. Rat pineal NE content was found by Moore and Smith[654] to be not measurable at one day after birth, but was so at six days, when it was 6.1 ± 0.2 ng/pineal in animals raised in constant light and 5.9 ± 0.7 ng/pineal in animals in constant darkness. Measurements at later stages showed first a decline and then a rise in pineal NE under conditions of constant light or darkness (Table LXI). It will be interesting to determine if the developmental pattern of pineal catecholamine increase is modulated by the interactions of indoleamines and catecholamines at the binding sites within the pineal nerve fibers.

Pharmacological Effects

It has been demonstrated in various ways, discussed in this and the preceding chapter, that displacement of NE by 5-HT at binding sites within pineal nerve terminals occurs as a normal and circadian process. The converse is also demonstrably true. A selective increase of pineal NE occurs as a consequence of pineal nerve ending depletion of 5-HT with either *p*-chlorophenylalanine or desmethylimipramine.[435] This pineal increase in NE was not affected by decentralization of both superior cervical ganglia, and did not occur in other sympathetically innervated organs. The release of NE from other sympathetically innervated organs by 5-HT has been observed, however.[273] The pineal increase in NE con-

TABLE LXII

Effects of administration of a monoamine oxidase inhibitor (Nialamide, 500 mg/kg, ip) and L-DOPA (100 mg/kg, sc) on pineal catecholamine contents (mean ± standard error, μg/g tissue), of normal (NL), bilaterally superior cervical decentralized (DC) and bilaterally superior cervical ganglionectomized (SG) adult rats.*

Animal Group	Dopamine		Norepinephrine	
	Not Injected	DOPA + Nialamide	Not Injected	DOPA + Nialamide
NL	34.4 ± 10.9	183.7 ± 23.1	13.96 ± 1.96	23.16 ± 3.22
DC	36.2 ± 12.8	122.0 ± 45.7	7.63 ± 1.05	7.13 ± 0.69
SG	33.6 ± 7.4	72.3 ± 22.8	1.12 ± 0.31	1.25 ± 0.35

* From Zieher and Pellegrino de Iraldi.[1097]

tent following depletion of 5-HT probably results from an enhancement of NE synthesis triggered by disappearance of 5-HT from the small granular vesicles, as discussed previously as an important event associated with the daily onset of darkness (Fig. 50). The interactions of monoamines at the binding sites within pineal nerve terminals probably can account for many of the pharmacological results reported for modification of pineal catecholamine as well as indoleamine contents. As shown by Zieher and Pellegrino de Iraldi[1097] the increases in pineal contents of dopamine and NE by L-DOPA and a monoamine oxidase inhibitor depend to different degrees on the integrity of the sympathetic innervation from the superior cervical ganglia and the connections between the central nervous system and the anterior part of the sympathetic chains (Table LXII). The dopamine pool in contrast with that containing NE appears to be relatively much less affected in its pharmacological responses following modification of the sympathetic innervation.

Among the more interesting and incompletely explored pharmacological manipulations of the pineal gland and its catecholamines is that employing nerve growth factor and its antiserum. Administration of the nerve growth factor antiserum to rats *in utero* reduces by 90 percent adult pineal uptake *in vivo* of tritiated NE.[892] No effects on the pineal gland have been reported following early experimental administration of nerve growth factor. However, the descrip-

tion of a forgotten human case of nearly a century ago suggests
that such effects may occur. In 1878 Cunningham reported
a human case of hypertrophy of the sympathetic nervous system accompanied by a pineal gland of twice normal size and
tumors of the submaxillary and parotid glands.[187] The salivary
glands are now known to be a good source of the nerve growth
factor. Along with its known trophic effect on the sympathetic
nervous system[555] can it possibly similarly affect the pineal
gland?

The effects of NE and other catecholamines on other chemical constituents of pineal tissue are considered under the
chapters covering the affected compounds.

CONCLUSIONS

1. Mammalian pineal glands have measurable quantities
of DOPA, dopamine (DA), octopamine, and norepinephrine
(NE). Also present are the amino acid precursors,
phenylalanine and tyrosine, and the enzymes for synthesis
of NE and its precursors from either phenylalanine or tyrosine.

2. Although pineal tissue does not contain any unique
catecholamine or unusual enzyme active on these compounds,
its contents of NE and especially of DA are relatively great,
and characteristics of its turnover and control of NE are distinctive.

3. Fluorescence histochemistry, radioautography and
electron microscopy of pharmacologically modified pineal
glands concur in the localization and uptake of NE and probably its precursors in the sympathetic fibers and terminals
and their small (500 Å) granular vesicles.

4. The pineal is apparently unsurpassed in its ability to
take up and concentrate from either the blood *in vivo* or a
culture medium *in vitro*, NE and epinephrine and probably
other related amines. In comparison with pituitary gland and
brain, pineal uptake and concentration of epinephrine is distinctive in that a greater proportion is chemically unmodified
and relatively little is 3-methoxylated.

5. Circadian rhythms occur in rat pineal NE, tyrosine hy-

droxylase and catechol-*O*-methyltransferase. A daily rise in pineal NE content occurs through the night and a progressive fall occurs through the time of light. This rhythm is detectable by ten days after birth and depends on the presence of the lateral eyes, the inferior accessory optic tract and the pineal's sympathetic innervation.

6. The circadian rhythm in pineal NE can be explained primarily on the basis of: (a) the dependence of the rate of synthesis of NE on the rate of arrival of nerve impulses in the sympathetic axon and terminal, and (b) the triggering actions of daily onset of light and darkness on compartmental shifts of NE and 5-HT in the small granular vesicles of the sympathetic endings.

7. The ontogeny of the catecholamine-containing nerve fibers and their granular synaptic vesicles occurs earlier and more rapidly than the developmental increase in pineal content of DA and NE.

8. Many of the pharmacological changes that can be made in pineal content of NE can be interpreted as results of mutual interactions and displacements at binding sites within the pineal's adrenergic nerve terminals and their small granular synaptic vesicles. Modifications of pineal DA content in such experiments, however, depend less than those of pineal NE content on the integrity of the sympathetic innervation. Not only is the functional significance of the pineal's large DA concentration not clear, but a major fraction of pineal DA may occur in an extraneuronal compartment.

9. Pineal NE as the neurotransmitter of its sympathetic innervation has a crucial role in the mediation of pineal biochemical circadian rhythms in adult mammals. Fragmentary evidence suggests as well a possibly more general trophic influence on the pineal of either or both its sympathetic innervation and the nerve growth factor contributing to the control of the development of the sympathetic system.

Chapter Nine

NUCLEOTIDES AND NUCLEIC ACIDS

NUCLEIC ACIDS HOLD great interest as genetic materials. But in pineal tissue only relatively elementary and quantitative information is available concerning these compounds. This information nevertheless can serve as a guide in the detection and evaluation of changes in cellular biosynthetic activity and in numbers and concentrations of cells.

Partial hydrolysis of nucleic acid yields nucleosides and nucleotides. Nucleotides and their derivatives participate in many of the most important metabolic events within pineal cells. In some of these metabolic transformations they have critical roles in the mediation of the effects of neurotransmitter and probably other humoral compounds, and probably in the control of levels of activity along particular pathways.

NUCLEOTIDES AND DERIVATIVES

Adenosine

Nucleotides are phosphoric esters of nucleosides. The latter are compounds in which ribose or deoxribose is conjugated to a purine or pyrimidine base. An example nucleoside of interest in pineal research is adenosine, in which adenine is linked to ribose (Fig. 52). Rats injected with adenosine show vasodilation within the pineal gland.[771,772] This is a general phenomenon. Adenosine, adenosine monophosphate (AMP), adenosine diphosphate (ADP) and adenosine triphosphate (ATP) are potent vasodilators in most of the body's vascular beds.[350] Other nucleotides and nucleotide derivatives are inactive. The hypothesis that these active and widespread compounds participate in local tissue regulation

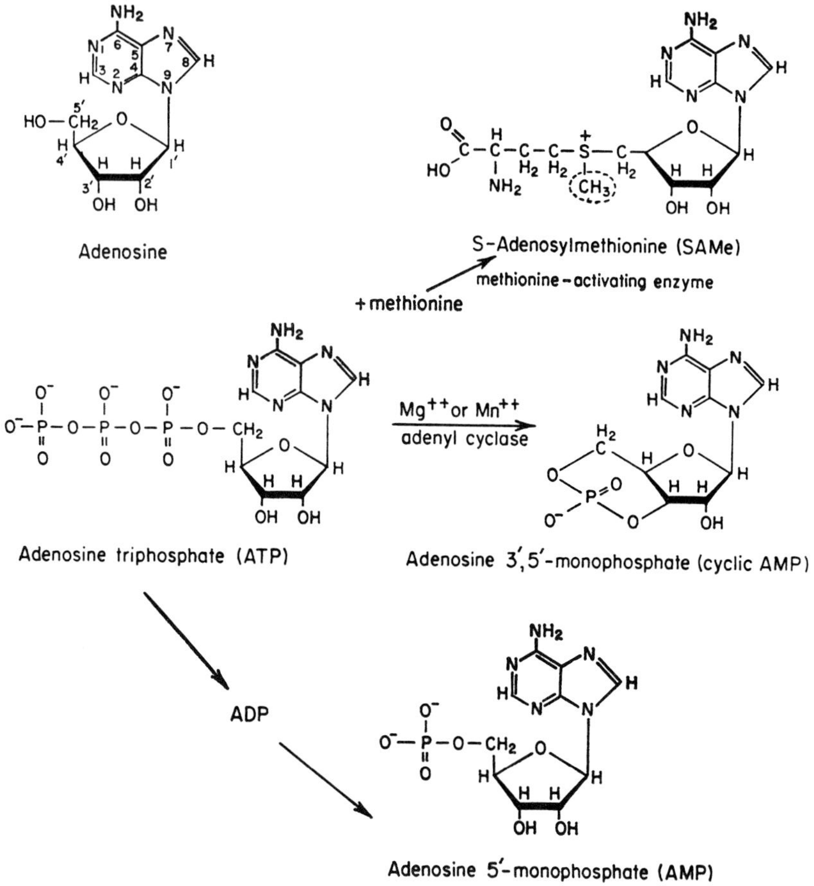

Figure 52. Structures and relations of pineal adenine nucleotides and derivatives.

of blood flow is difficult to support in most tissues studied thus far. On the other hand, experimental studies appear to firmly link adenosine to regulation of coronary circulation, during alterations in both blood flow and metabolism.[350] Equivalent studies and even measurement of tissue concentrations of adenosine are not yet available for the pineal gland.

Adenosine Triphosphate (ATP)

Adenosine triphosphate (ATP) is a high energy phosphate compound (Fig. 52) in which free energy available from cellular oxidative reactions is captured for later use. The energy contained in ATP is then available for a multitude of endergonic processes within the body.

Adult rat pineal ATP has been measured by Quay using the luminescence produced in the presence of firefly lantern extract.[781] The pineal tissue concentrations obtained (mean = 1.39 $\mu\mu$moles/g) were slightly greater than those reported in rat brain and peripheral nerve, but markedly lower than those reported in rat liver and skeletal muscle. Twenty-two weeks of continuous white light failed to modify pineal ATP content in adult male rats.[781] Future studies on pineal ATP and other nucleotides will have the advantage of improved methods and model investigations on brain ATP where restriction of oxygen supply can lead very rapidly to breakdown of energy rich tissue phosphates.[455]

Pineal hydrolysis of ATP and a variety of other nucleotides has been studied with cytochemical methods. The localizations observed of adenosine triphosphatase (ATPase) and other phosphatases are important indicators of the places within the pineal cells and tissues where major energy transformations and utilizations may be taking place. Stefănescu-Gavăt has reported intense ATPase activities (pH 9.4 and 7.2) within bovine pineals, in the cytoplasm and nucleus of pinealocytes, and in neuroglial and endothelial cells.[938] In the pineal gland of the squirrel monkey (*Saimiri sciureus*) on the other hand, Manocha reported mild to moderate ATPase activity in pinealocytes and moderately strong activity in pineal neurons.[593] Human pineal glands obtained at autopsies of twenty-one to eighty-two year old individuals three to eight hours postmortem showed marked ATPase activity primarily in the walls of pineal blood vessels.[92] These observations by Bayerová and Bayer are supported by the results of Torack and Barrnett studying the fine localization of nucleoside phosphatase activity in pineal gland and brain of rats.[978,979] Although a wide variety of nucleoside phosphate esters, including ATP, were used as substrates, at least by the light microscope the enzyme localizations were similar. In the pineal gland, the capillary endothelial cells contained numerous foci of enzyme activity within pinocytic vesicles.

Activity was also found at the interface between pinealocytes and what were tentatively identified as neuroglia. This enzymic localization was similar to that observed at the surface between Sertoli cells and developing spermatozoa in rat testis. The possibility was hence suggested that these pineal glial cells may possess a *nurse* or nutritive function in relation to the pinealocytes. Although this is the only enzymatic evidence that has appeared concerning such an intercellular relationship within pineal tissue, cytological and cytochemical studies have sometimes given the impression of a pattern of pairing between *light cells* and *dark cells* or *type I* and *type II cells*.[778,786] In these cases the dark or *type II cells* are respectively more heavily stained and more reactive to the acid hematein technique for phospholipids, and the light or *type I cells* are respectively more lightly stained by histological methods and have a greater number of lipid droplets and less acid hematein reaction in the surrounding cytoplasmic matrix. The dark or *type II cells* are more glioid in general structure than the light or *type I* pinealocytes.

Adenosine 3',5'-monophosphate (c-AMP)

Cyclic-AMP was discovered by Sutherland and Rall as the intracellular mediator of the hepatic glycogenolytic effect of epinephrine and glucagon.[949] Diverse and numerous recent investigations show that neural transmission and operation of many parts of the endocrine system share a common mechanism of biochemical mediation at the cellular level. Cyclic-AMP is an important component in this mechanism. Other components are calcium ions, intracellular microtubules, microfilaments, secretory vesicles and protein kinases.[836] It has been proposed that all of the wide variety of effects elicited by c-AMP are mediated through regulation of the activity of protein kinases. It now appears likely that most if not all effects of c-AMP are brought about through the phosphorylation of key cellular proteins by ATP catalyzed by c-AMP-dependent protein kinase. Very little is known, however, about the substrate (receptor) proteins in these reactions.[338]

Ebadi and co-workers have measured c-AMP in pineal and other tissues from rats.[225,227] In comparison with brain regions and pituitary gland the pineal had the greatest concentration of c-AMP (58 $\mu\mu$moles/mg protein).[228] A five-fold daily rhythm was found also in pineal c-AMP in adult male rats conditioned to a standardized daily photoperiod twelve hours in length (LD 12:12). Ten hours after onset of light pineal c-AMP concentration was 185 ± 24 and ten hours after the onset of darkness it was 32 ± 4 $\mu\mu$moles/mg protein. In blinded animals pineal c-AMP content was the same at the two times of the day and resembled that obtained in normal animals ten hours after the start of darkness.[225a,226]

Fontana and Lovenberg have found and partially characterized a cyclic-AMP-dependent protein kinase in bovine pineal tissue.[282] The pineal enzyme showed properties very similar to those of c-AMP-dependent protein kinases obtained from other tissues. However, the pineal enzyme appeared to prefer as substrates proteins with a high arginine content. The enzyme system was shown to consist of two proteins, a kinase and c-AMP-binding protein. The kinase is active primarily in the phosphorylation of histones and was suggested to function in the control of the twenty-four hour rhythms of the enzyme activities in the biosynthetic pathway leading to melatonin. Cyclic-AMP stimulation of the protein kinase appeared to work by means of the ability of the cyclic nucleotide to dissociate the c-AMP-dependent protein kinase into a form independent of the cyclic nucleotide and a protein that can bind cyclic nucleotide. Partial reversibility was found in this dissociation, since following removal of c-AMP from the binding proteins, reassociation can occur between the binding protein and the protein kinase that is free of cyclic-AMP. The cyclic nucleotide-binding protein inhibits the activity of the protein kinase that is free of the cyclic nucleotide and this inhibition can be relieved by the addition of c-AMP.

In the chapter on pineal indoleamines the stimulatory effects of c-AMP on the biosynthesis of melatonin were noted and diagrammed (Fig. 36). In this work a derivative of cyclic-

AMP, $N^6,O^{2'}$-dibutyryl cyclic-AMP, was used instead of c-AMP itself due to its greater potency, ease of penetration, and lesser susceptibility to degradation by cyclic nucleotide phosphodiesterase. The mechanism of action of dibutyryl cyclic-AMP is still not entirely clear.[495] At least in some cellular systems the effects of the two cyclic nucelotides are distinctly different.[934] Furthermore, Klein and Berg have shown the dibutyryl cyclic-AMP inhibits cyclic nucleotide phosphodiesterase in cultures not only of pineal but of other tissue as well.[495] Nevertheless, the use of dibutyryl cyclic-AMP by Shein and Wurtman, Klein and Weller, and Berg *et al.* has been instructive concerning the probable mediation of the stimulatory effects of NE on melatonin biosynthesis via c-AMP or a related pineal constituent.[105,106,495,503,897,898] Dibutyryl cyclic-AMP also causes a rise in pineal incorporation of ^{32}P into phospholipids *in vitro* and it is suggested that endogenous c-AMP mediates the similar response observed in the presence of NE.[107] Investigators planning studies with dibutyryl cyclic-AMP should note that it will decompose to the N^6-monobutyryl derivative, c-AMP and butyrate in several buffers or during storage in solution. Decomposition is most rapid in Krebs-Ringer bicarbonate buffer.[953]

Pineal synthesis of c-AMP from ATP depends upon the activity of the enzyme adenyl cyclase (Fig. 52). Experimental evidence has been obtained supporting belief that changed pineal c-AMP levels brought about by neurotransmitters and hormones are the result of changes in the activity of pineal adenyl cyclase. Enzyme activity *in vitro* is increased three to six-fold by the addition of L-NE and is also enhanced by L-epinephrine and L-isoproterenol. But it is not affected by D-NE, DL-dehydroxymandelic acid, DL-normetanephrine, dopamine, tyramine, D-amphetamine or L-phenylephrine. 5-HT and histamine, which have been shown to increase formation of c-AMP in other tissues, do not do so in pineal tissue. 5-HT (at 10^{-3} M), however, can inhibit the stimulation of pineal adenyl cyclase by L-NE (at 10^{-4} M).[940,1038,1040] This may be another component of the interaction or antagonism of NE and 5-HT within the pineal gland which is responsible for the biochemical 24-hour rhythmicity (Fig. 36). Polypeptide hormones such as glucagon, ACTH and LH, which enhance content of c-AMP in liver, adrenal cortex and corpus luteum respectively, fail to affect pineal adenyl cyclase. Drugs such as guanethidine, cocaine and desmethylimipramine, which modify sympathetic responses through actions at adrenergic terminals, also fail to change pineal adenyl cyclase activity. But the *beta* adrenergic blocking drugs, propranolol and dichloroisoproterenol, antagonize the NE-induced stimulation of pineal adenyl cyclase. The *alpha* blockers, phenoxybenzamine and phentolamine are much less effective. Therefore, pharmacologically rat pineal adenyl cyclase behaves in its responses like a postjunctional *beta* adrenergic receptor.[1040] Denervation of the rat pineal gland by superior cervical ganglionectomy does not reduce pineal adenyl cyclase significantly, but it does increase its sensitivity to the stimulatory effects of L-NE.[1039] Pineal adenyl cyclase's response to L-NE is also rendered more sensitive by exposure of the animal to continuous light for nine days.[1038]

A hormonally based sexual difference in stimulation of rat pineal adenyl cyclase by L-NE has been demonstrated by Weiss and Crayton.[1042-1044] NE was found to stimulate pineal adenyl cyclase of males to a greater extent than that of females, and in females it stimulated it during all stages of the estrous cycle except proestrus, the stage at which estrogen levels are greatest (Fig. 41). Gonadectomy in males had no effect on pineal adenyl cyclase activity but in females it increased slightly the stimulatory effect of L-NE. Neither testosterone nor progesterone administration affected pineal adenyl cyclase activity, but administration of estradiol for two days to ovariectomized rats inhibited the activation of pineal adenyl cyclase by either L-NE or sodium fluoride. No inhibition occurred when estradiol was injected one hour before sacrifice or when it was added *in vitro*. Since hypophysectomy failed to alter the effects either of ovariectomy or of administration of estradiol, the action of estrogens on the pineal adenyl cyclase system were not brought about through release of pituitary gonadotropins. Instead, these and findings discussed in Chapter Seven are consistent with the hypothesis that interactions between estrogens and biogenic amines in the regulation of pineal adenyl cyclase activity and synthesis of melatonin contribute to the timed proestrous pulse of LH release during the estrous cycle. Thus through the course of the estrous cycle a hormonal cycle involving the pineal gland and its adenyl cyclase activity can be suggested: pituitary → ovary → pineal → (hypothalamus) → pituitary   (see Fig. 41).

S-Adenosylmethionine (SAMe)

S-Adenosylmethionine is the methyl donor in many transmethylation reactions in mammalian tissues. Within the pineal gland it is the methyl donor for the methylation of various biogenic amines through the action of specific methyltransferases. It undoubtedly performs a similar function in the methylation of other kinds of substrates, such as RNA, DNA and others, by other and still unstudied methyltransferases in pineal tissue. SAMe is formed from methionine and ATP in the presence of a methionine-activating enzyme (Fig. 52), which is widely distributed in tissues. Although this enzyme has apparently not yet been measured in the pineal gland, the levels of its product, SAMe, have been measured in pineal tissue. This has been done by Baldessarini and Kopin using isotope dilution of SAMe-methyl-^{14}C by unlabeled tissue SAMe and estimation of the specific activity of the diluted SAMe-methyl-^{14}C by the enzymatic formation of melatonin-methoxy-^{14}C-acetyl-^{3}H from the methyl donor and N-acetylserotonin-acetyl-[3]H.[76,77] Highest levels of SAMe were found in adrenal (48.0 ± 10.0, pineal gland (38.4 ± 2.7) and liver (28.8 ± 1.5 μg/g tissue) among the organs and brain regions analyzed. Brain (10–12 μg/g) and serum (0.47 ± 0.02 μg/g) levels were much lower. S-Adenosylhomocysteine, which can be formed either from homocysteine or by the loss of the active methyl group from SAMe (Fig. 26), inhibits the methylation of biogenic amines.[199] Its levels in pineal tissue have not been measured.

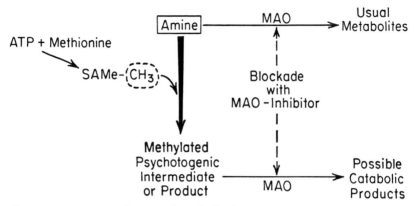

Figure 53. Suggested means by which abnormal levels of psychotogenic methylated amines might be produced through loading with methionine and blockade of monoamine oxidase (MAO) (modified from Baldessarini[75]).

Factors that modify tissue levels of SAMe have been studied in rat liver and brain but not in the pineal gland. Methionine loading increases SAMe and tends to protect tissues from depletion of SAMe such as can occur after inhibition of monoamine oxidase. Baldessarini has provided results that are consistent with the proposal that inhibition of MAO coupled with methionine loading favors transmethylation.[75] Enhanced methylation of biogenic amines with blockade of routes dependent on MAO may lead to abnormal levels of psychotogenic intermediates or products, such as are believed by some investigators to be responsible for some of the effects seen in schizophrenia (Fig. 53). The extent to which pineal synthesis of 5-methoxytryptamine or β-carboline derivatives can be increased by this means remains to be determined.

Conditions that lower rat tissue contents of SAMe include normal maturation and administration of methyl acceptors, MAO inhibitors, chlorpromazine, and imipramine. Pyrogallol, tropolone and purpurogallin lower tissue SAMe and are methyl acceptors. The known inhibitory action of pyrogallol and tropolone on methyl transferases may occur partly through the lowering of levels of SAMe. The effect of chlorpromazine on tissue content of SAMe may be by way of decreased utilization of ATP and decreased formation of SAMe from ATP.

The effect of imipramine on neural tissue content of SAMe may be produced through the decreased uptake of amines and their therefore greater exposure to methyltransferases than to intracellular oxidases, thus increasing the utilization of SAMe.[75]

NUCLEIC ACIDS

Nucleic acids are composed of pentose sugars joined with phosphate and with purine or pyrimidine bases. Within cells they are associated with basic proteins to form nucleoproteins. Pineal nucleic acids are currently known only in terms of localizations and quantitative changes shown by the two major categories, deoxyribonucleic acid (DNA) and ribonucleic acid (RNA). As in other kinds of mammalian cells, DNA in pineal cells is at least mostly nuclear and chromosomal, therein forming essential genetic material. Also as in other kinds of cells, pineal RNA is both nuclear and cytoplasmic and has important roles in intracellular transmission of chemical information and regulation of protein synthesis. Certainly one of the most interesting and important chapters in pineal chemistry to be written by future investigators is that dealing with kinds, activities and functions of RNA.

Cytochemistry

Cytochemical studies on pineal nucleic acids have for many years employed more or less specific staining coupled with hydrolysis and with digestion by deoxyribonuclease and ribonuclease in order to improve the chemical specificity. Examination of pineal tissue sections so prepared for study by light microscopy has usually revealed appreciable RNA in the cytoplasm and in some of the nucleoli of the pinealocytes. Wislocki and Dempsey showed that basophilia of both of these parts of macaque (*Macaca mulatta*, one to three years old) pineals was absent if the tissue sections had been treated previously with ribonuclease.[1053] Similar studies were made subsequently on pineal glands from men[91,376] and from domestic mammals,[376,622] and on those from rats that had been submitted to surgical or other treatments. Thus cytoplasmic basophilia of pinealocytes was decreased in rats kept in continuous light for eight weeks, as compared with those in continuous darkness,[867] and was increased after either bilateral adrenal enucleation[470] or splenctomy.[983] However, in all of these studies only visual comparisons were made in the evaluation of cytoplasmic basophilia and RNA content. The significance of work of this kind would be increased greatly through the use of microscopic spectrophotometry for the measurements, such as has been employed by Nováková *et al.* in their studies on the nucleic acid content of developing pineal glands.[691]

Electron microscopy of mammalian pineal tissue has provided evidence of RNA through the relative distributions and density of ribosomes within both pinealocytes and astrocyte-like neuroglia. In cat pinealocytes most of the ribosomes are scattered throughout the cytoplasm either singly or in small groups. While in the pineal astrocytes of the same species, more of the ribosomes are associated with rough endoplasmic reticulum. Ribosomes are seen also in the glial cell processes.[1026] Some evidence of probable changes in RNA contents of rat pinealocytes has been proposed and can be gleaned from electron micrographs of pineal glands from animals that have been given drugs[143] or that have been castrated or hypophysectomized.[165,886] A particularly marked increase in numbers of ribosomes within pinealocytes has been claimed following castration.[165]

Electron microscopy of the pinealocyte-like principal tumor cells of an ectopic pinealoma from a seven year old girl, also showed ribosomes, some free and some on the granular endoplasmic reticula.[644]

Developmental Changes

In a study on the uptake and incorporation of ^{14}C-uridine into RNA of rat brain regions, MacKinnon and Simpson observed in "neonates" (one to five days postnatal age) that the pineal gland was among those brain regions and associated structures having the greatest activity.[590] Nováková and co-workers using quantitative cytophotometry estimated relative contents of DNA and RNA in pineal tissue sections from male rats from one to 365 days of age. The pinealocyte DNA content remained constant through the first year of life and was consistent with the maintenance of the diploid number of chromosomes through this period. Pinealocyte content of RNA on the other hand showed variations at particular ages. From one to fifteen days a decline in RNA content occurred, followed by a rise which reached a maximum around the fortieth day. The RNA content appeared to remain high from the time of weaning through the period of adolescence or early maturation (up to the sixtieth day). Thereafter it gradually decreased.[691]

Circadian Rhythms and Effects of Light and Darkness

A circadian rhythm in rat pineal content of RNA has been found by three groups of investigators. The highest levels occur during the day and the lowest are at night, except in the first study, in which animals were injected either with an anticholinergic drug or the saline solution vehicle alone.[618] It is probable that the rhythm was distorted by the handling and the injections. The most extensive data on pineal RNA contents in undisturbed rats has been provided by Nir and co-workers.[685] Consistent with the very low level of mitotic activity in the adult pineal gland,[825,826] no significant diurnal changes were found in pineal DNA in either males or females. But a distinct circadian or 24-hour rhythm was shown by pineal RNA content (Fig. 54). This was much more distinct in males than in females, probably because of the increased variation due to hormonal influences in the latter. The phasic relationships of the RNA rhythm in most respects fit well with what would be expected metabolically from related pineal biochemical and cytological rhythms. The rises and peaks in nuclear and nucleolar sizes as well as RNA content precede those in protein content (Fig. 54). In relation to the timing of the peak in RNA, that of nucleolar size seems a little tardy. There is no explanation for this. On the other hand, the early daily rise in RNA corresponds well with the time of daily increase in pineal 5-HT, and the peak in protein

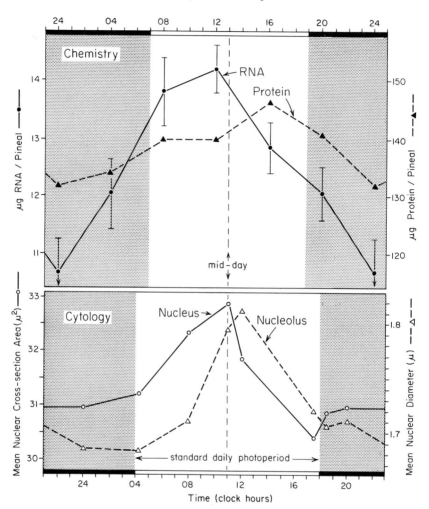

Figure 54. Circadian rhythms of pineal RNA, protein, and pinealocyte nuclear and nucleolar sizes in adult male rats. (RNA and protein plots from data of Nir *et al.*[685]; nuclear and nucleolar plots taken from data of Quay and Renzoni[826] for medullary pinealocytes.)

content (and presumably synthesis) follows closely on the heels of both stimulated uptake of amino acids by NE (Fig. 36) and the peak in RNA content. Since the daily rise in pineal RNA content seems to start well before the onset of light (Fig. 54), one might wonder whether this indicates a biochemical release or stimulation of RNA synthesis during

TABLE LXIII

Pinealocyte RNA content* in ninety day old male rats killed either during the solar day (11:00) or during the solar night (23:00), following continuous light (LL) or continuous darkness (DD) from birth or exposure to a normal day-night lighting (LD) regime.†

Time	LD	Group LL	DD
11:00	‡ 106.9 ± 4.5	139.9 ± 3.9	98.0 ± 17.7
23:00	96.7 ± 4.2	119.2 ± 4.7	91.6 ± 15.4

* Arbitrary cytophotometry units.
† From Nováková *et al.*[692]
‡ Mean ± standard deviation (N = 15 pinealocytes from each of 4 animals/sample; 4 × 15 = 60).

darkness, such as might conceivably be mediated through depletion of 5-HT or synthesis and release of melatonin within the pineal parenchyma. Available data, however, do not provide support for such a hypothesis at this time.

Exposure of weanling female rats to continuous light (LD 24:0) for ten days or longer was found by Nir *et al.* to cause a 20 percent reduction in the pineal RNA content.[683] Matched groups exposed to continuous darkness (LD 0:24) were not significantly different from controls exposed to a daily photoperiod twelve hours in length (LD 12:12). Neither continuous light nor continuous darkness affected pineal DNA content. Amount of DNA per gland increased at the same rate during development under the three lighting conditions from twenty-one to fifty-one days of age. Using rats of a different sex and strain and starting treatment from birth Nováková *et al.* obtained different results in pineal RNA following continuous light. Their study differed also in that RNA was determined cytophotometrically in individual pinealocytes rather than biochemically in pooled whole pineal glands. In this case, the rats living in continuous light (LD 24:0) for ninety days were reported to have higher RNA content during the solar day than during the solar night and the day values were also higher than those of the daylight period in control (LD 12:12) rats. The solar night RNA values in the continuously lighted group were also higher than those found at the corresponding time in the controls (Table LXIII). When rats that had been raised in continuous darkness were exposed to daylight for

TABLE LXIV

Effect of a single subcutaneous injection of 10 μg 17β-estradiol on pineal RNA, DNA and protein of thirty-one day old female rats.*

Chemical Constituent	† Hours post Injection		
Injection Group	15	18	24
DNA			
Estradiol	‡ 6.7 ± 0.5	7.7 ± 0.5	6.2 ± 0.2
		P<0.02	
Control	6.4 ± 0.3	6.6 ± 0.3	6.4 ± 0.2
RNA			
Estradiol	8.3 ± 0.4	9.4 ± 0.3	8.6 ± 0.3
		P < 0.05	
Control	7.9 ± 0.2	8.3 ± 0.3	8.4 ± 0.3
Protein			
Estradiol	91.5 ± 3.4	97.1 ± 3.6	103.0 ± 2.2
			P < 0.05
Control	96.5 ± 1.3	94.6 ± 3.5	94.6 ± 2.2

* From Nir *et al.*[688]
† All animals killed between 09:00 and 11:00 (daily photoperiod = 07:00—19:00)
‡ All values are mean μg/pineal ± standard error of the mean (N = 15–20/group)

ten to sixty minutes pinealocyte RNA content was little changed. Only when they had experienced one day of normal (LD) lighting did their pinealocyte RNA contents attain the levels seen in control (LD) animals. Thus light in this situation activates increase in pinealocyte RNA. The relationship is therefore similar to that observed between light and retinal ganglion cells.[692]

Hormonal Effects

Nir and coworkers have provided data that suggests that a single injection of 10 μg estradiol can increase briefly pineal DNA, RNA and protein in twenty-one or thirty-one day old female rats (Table LXIV).[688] No change occurred in pineal nucleic acids or protein of twenty-one day old females that had received seven daily injections of 5 μg estradiol. The effects of the single injection are easier to understand in the case of pineal RNA and protein content than for DNA. An increase in DNA content would not be expected to be so short-lived and would be expected to lead to, or be reflected in, an increase in cell number. In earlier work, Quay and Levine were unable to influence either pineal mitotic activity or pineal volume with injections of 17β-estradiol in immature rats.[825] If estradiol affects pineal nucleic acids and protein metabolism at physiological levels, changes in the pineal features should be observable during the estrous cycle. Nir and coworkers have presented data of this sort. Pineal DNA, as to be expected, was constant through the four stages of the cycle, but both RNA and protein contents seemed to have peaks at diestrus. However, statistical significance could not be established due to high variance. Earlier work of Nir *et al.*[685] might also in a preliminary way be used to suggest that estrogens or related hormonal influences may decrease pineal RNA and protein contents. This is based on the fact that they found significantly lower pineal RNA and protein contents, but similar DNA contents, in females as compared with males. Furthermore, the circadian rhythms in pineal RNA and protein were of lower amplitude in females and the variation within samples was evidently greater. An inhibitory action of estradiol on pineal RNA and protein synthesis would be consistent with estradiol's inhibition of the activation of pineal adenyl cyclase by NE, discussed above in the section on cyclic-AMP. As in the studies on the pineal adenyl cyclase system, *in vitro* rather than *in vivo* experiments are apt to be more informative concerning hormonal effects on pineal RNA and protein synthesis. Experiments *in vivo* are not only beset with the vagaries of indirect paths of hormonal action but also, in the case of the pineal gland, with the problems of controlling the release of, and activations by, the endogenous amines of the gland.

CONCLUSIONS

1. Adenosine, and possibly as well, related nucleotides, may contribute to the control of the pineal gland's vascular flow, as in certain other parts of the body.

2. Pineal hydrolysis of ATP through cytochemical methods has been demonstrated within diverse cells and at various locations by different investigators. But strongest pineal ATPase activities in man and other species are recorded from capillary endothelia. Mild to moderate ATPase activity is

often reported in pinealocytes or at the interface between these *light cells* and presumptive neuroglia or *dark cells,* which may, therefore, have a nutritive function.

3. Pineal concentrations of c-AMP are greater than those of brain regions and pituitary gland, and follow a light-dependent circadian rhythm with a peak value near the end of the daily period of light more than five times that of the night-time nadir.

4. *In vitro* studies with the c-AMP analogue, dibutyryl cyclic-AMP, indicate that c-AMP has a major role within the pineal gland in mediating the effects of NE and other humoral agents on the pineal's synthetic activities. An important part of this regulatory metabolic system is a c-AMP-dependent kinase, which in pineal tissue has both similarities and differences in comparison with like enzymes in other tissues.

5. Pineal synthesis of c-AMP from ATP depends upon adenyl cyclase, which in the pineal gland is stimulated by either L-norepinephrine (NE) or L-epinephrine. The fact that this effect is inhibited by 5-HT adds support to the concept that interactions or antagonisms of NE and 5-HT are responsible for the generation of the pineal biochemical 24-hour rhythms.

6. Estradiol inhibits the activation of pineal adenyl cyclase by NE. This and other findings are consistent with the hypothesis that interactions between estrogens and biogenic amines within pineal tissue are important in the regulation of pineal adenyl cyclase activity and the metabolic sequelae stimulated by c-AMP.

7. The pineal gland is among the organs having the highest concentrations of S-adenosylmethionine (SAMe), the natural methyl donor in many or most transmethylation reactions. It is likely that the control of some of these reactions within the pineal gland *in vivo* is significantly influenced by the regulation of the contents of SAMe and related compounds. But this remains to be fully investigated, although it is relevant to experimental evaluation of possible biochemical origins of some kinds of mental disease.

8. Rat pinealocyte and whole pineal DNA contents remain

stable through the first year of postnatal life, but RNA contents have significant changes correlated with age as well as light-dependent circadian, and possibly estrous, cyclic changes. The morning rise in pineal RNA content is associated with increases in mean pinealocyte nuclear and nucleolar sizes and precedes the circadian crest in protein content. The probable contributions of pineal biogenic amine interactions and hormonal effects to regulation of pineal rhythms in RNA and protein synthesis are still poorly understood.

Chapter Ten

PROTEINS—OUTLINE OF ENZYMES

ENZYMES FOUND IN pineal tissue are of great interest for the understanding of pineal synthetic activities and the associated metabolic control mechanisms. Scattered reports on pineal enzymes have never been brought together and reviewed except to a very limited extent or with the exception of mostly histochemical results.[41,344]

Enzyme activities of mammalian pineal tissue are outlined here according to the nomenclature of the Commission on Enzymes of the International Union of Biochemistry,[278] and in the case of "new" enzymes according to the working rules devised by the Commission.[85] The systematic name of each enzyme follows the numerical designation. In parentheses are the trivial names, followed by any other synonyms used in pineal references. The aims of this review are to provide a concise survey of the major features in pineal enzymology, and to enable easy reference to fragmentary and often redundant literature on the subject.

1. OXIDOREDUCTASES
1.1 Acting on the CH-OH group of donors
1.1.1 With NAD or NADP as acceptor

1.1.1.1 *Alcohol:NAD oxidoreductase* (Alcohol dehydrogenase).

A measurable level of activity could not be demonstrated in lamb pineals.[968]

1.1.1.27 *L-Lactate:NAD oxidoreductase* (Lactate dehydrogenase).

Strong LDH activity has been shown generally throughout rat and monkey pineal tissue,[79,595] and moderate activity in a human pinealoma.[479] In the rat maximal pineal activity occurs at proestrus and the minimum at late diestrus.[266]

1.1.1.30 *D-3-Hydroxybutyrate:NAD oxidoreductase* (3-Hydroxybutyrate dehydrogenase)

In rat pineals continuous light diminishes and continuous darkness augments this enzyme activity.[131] Moderate activity has been observed in a human pinealoma.[479]

1.1.1.37 *L-Malate:NAD oxidoreductase* (Malate dehydrogenase)

Weak activity has been observed cytochemically in adult rat pineals *de vivo* and moderate activity in infant pineals *in vitro*.[79,634] In the latter instance activity was shown in the cytoplasm of pinealocytes and was increased, especially around the nucleus, following treatment with thyroxine. Moderate activity has been found in human pinealoma.[479]

1.1.1.41 *L-Isocitrate:NAD oxidoreductase-decarboxylating* (Isocitrate dehydrogenase)

Very strong activity in the cytoplasm of infant rat pinealocytes has been shown cytochemically *in vitro*, especially after treatment with thyroxine.[634]

Moderate activity has been found in human pinealoma.[479]

1.1.1.49 *D-Glucose-6-phosphate:NADP oxidoreductase* (Glucose-6-phosphate dehydrogenase)

Moderate to intense activity has been observed cytochemically in adult rat pineals, but investigators differ on whether pineal activity is similar to or greater than that in neighboring or related structures, such as the habenular nuclei, ependyma and various circumventricular organs.[2,79] A moderate reduction in pineal activity occurs in fetal guinea pigs as they develop toward the adult condition.[1012] Moderate activity has been seen in a human pinealoma.[479]

1.1.2 With a cytochrome as acceptor

1.1.2.1 *L-Glycerol-3-phosphate:cytochrome* c *oxidoreductase* (Glycerolphosphate dehydrogenase)

Ungulate pinealocytes cytochemically show strong activity, which is greater than that of other diencephalic structures.[40]

In rat pineal glands continuous light decreases, and continuous darkness increases the activity.[131] Strong activity has been found in human pinealoma.[479]

1.2 Acting on the aldehyde- or keto-group of donors

1.2.1.16 *Succinate-semialdehyde:NAD(P) oxidoreductase* (Succinate semialdehyde dehydrogenase)

In human brains obtained six to twenty-four hours post-mortem moderate activity (102 mmoles/kg/hour) was measured in the pineal gland; pineal activity was greater than that of diverse areas of white matter, and was less than that of diverse areas of gray matter, including hypothalamus (225 mmoles/kg/hour). This suggests that the γ-aminobutyrate pathway is less prominent in pineal tissue than in these latter brain regions.[640]

1.3 Acting on the CH-CH group of donors

1.3.99.1 *Succinate:(acceptor) oxidoreductase* (Succinate dehydrogenase, SDH).

Cytochemical appraisals of pineal SDH activity vary widely in their descriptions of levels observed, from weak to strong.[40,79,131,133,541,904,1012] These discrepancies can not be accounted for on the basis of different species of mammals used, rather they can probably be attributed to conditions of incubation and to the physiological status of the animal at the time of death. A lack of significant differences between species, or between animals of different adaptations has been observed.[774] Quantitative studies with minced rat pineals and 2,3,5-triphenyl-2H-tetrazolium as the acceptor have shown (a)Al^{+++} and Ca^{++} promote and Cu^{++}, malonate, iodine and hydroquinone inhibit activity; (b) activity more than doubles in both sexes during the first six weeks postnatally, followed in about a year by a gradual decrease; (c) pineal activity equals 50 percent of that of liver, 75 percent of choroid plexus of ventricle IV, 90 percent of cerebral cortex (area 18), and 160 percent of hypophyseal posterior lobe.[773] Significant changes in rat pineal SDH follow modification of the sympathetic system by pharmacological means: (a) injection of norepinephrine (NE) increases the activity measured one to eight hours later; (b) dibenamine alone may depress activity after eighteen to nineteen hours, but when it is followed by NE, or 5-HT or any one of several sympathomimetic amines it potentiates increased activity; (c) the monamine oxidase inhibitor, Marsilid, alone can increase activity after eighteen to twenty hours, but when it is followed by NE or DOPA it potentiates decrease in pineal SDH.[773] Although no significant changes were produced *in vivo* by modifications in thyroid, adrenal cortical and gonadal endocrines,[773] it has been claimed recently that there is variation correlated with the estrous cycle. Thus maximal activity was found during late estrus and minimal activity during metestrus; intermediate levels characterized diestrus and proestrus.[266] A cir-

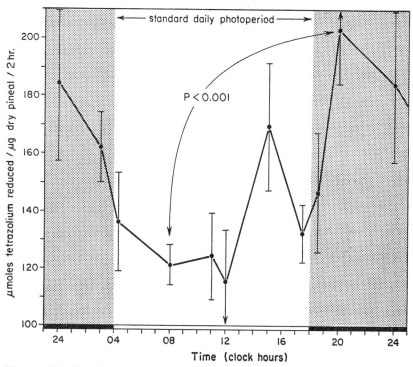

Figure 55. Circadian rhythm in pineal succinic dehydrogenase activity. Each point represents the mean (± standard error) of eight to ten separately incubated adult Long-Evans ♀ rat pineal glands taken September 23 to October 6. (Method of Quay.[773])

cadian rhythm occurs in rat pineal SDH activity, with a basal (minimum) level during the hours of light followed by a rapid increase near the daily start of darkness (Fig. 55).[820] Continuous light depresses the activity,[131,781] and continuous darkness has been reported to increase it.[131] The depression by continuous light can be blocked by blinding, and a partial block occurs after bilateral cutting of the nervi conarii (Table LXV).[781] The incompleteness of the latter blockade is probably due to either or both possible partial regeneration of the sectioned sympathetic fibers, or survival of vascular or minor sympathetic fibers supplying the organ. Strong enzyme activity has been reported in a human pinealoma.[479]

1.4 Acting on the CH-NH$_2$ group of donors

1.4.1.2 *L-Glutamate: NAD oxidoreductase-deaminating* (Glutamate dehydrogenase)

Little if any enzyme activity was found cytochemically in lamb and rat pineal glands.[781,968] In both young and old individuals of the latter species, neither continuous light (LL) nor continuous darkness (DD) had any effect on apparent activity.[781] However, moderate activity was found in a human pinealoma.[489]

1.4.3.4. *Monoamine: oxygen oxidoreductase-deaminating* (Monoamine oxidase, MAO).

Different levels of activity have been obtained cytochemically and biochemically depending on the species, substrate, incubation conditions, and perhaps other factors.[40,314,388,595,702,905,917] The magnitude of species differences is well illustrated by the studies of Håkanson and Owman (Table LXVI).[357] As noted earlier, comparably great species differences occur in pineal contents of the substrate monoamines. But correlations between relative MAO activity and monoamine stores are not evident.[357] As noted earlier, two monoamine oxidases have been found in pineal tissue, including that of man,[333] one in sympathetic nerve fibers (Type A) and another in pineal-specific tissue—presumably associated with the pinealocytes (Type B). Type A acts on tyramine and 5-HT, is readily inhibited by clorgyline (0.1 μM),

TABLE LXV

Effect of continuous light (LL) on rat pineal succinic dehydrogenase activity and effects of bilateral section of the optic nerves or of the nervi conarii 1–2 mm from the pineal gland.*

Experiment		Lighting		
Surgery	N	LL+	LD (control)+	P
1				
Optic nerves cut	8–10	177 ± 13	190 ± 6	n.s.
Not operated	10–12	145 ± 5	200 ± 9	<0.001
2				
Nervi conarii cut	11	124 ± 4	159 ± 8	<0.01
Sham-operated	10–12	109 ± 7	163 ± 6	<0.001

* From Quay.[781]
† Animals were killed alternately during mid-morning.
Values are mean ± standard error, μmoles tetrazolium reduced/μg pineal dry weight/two hours.

TABLE LXVI

Species comparisons of pineal monoamine oxidase activity according to two techniques.*

Species	MAO Activities		
	Biochemical† Mean ± Se	(N)	Cytochemical‡ Visual Estimate
Cow	2070 ± 390	(7)	+ + + +
Rat (intact)	1300 ± 220	(11)	+ + + +
Rat (sympathectomized)	1020 ± 70	(5)	+ + + +
Rabbit (intact)	1100 ± 170	(14)	+ + + +
Rabbit (sympathectomized)	420 ± 90	(5)	+ +
Man	1120 ± 150	(6)	+ +
Cat (intact)	80 ± 10	(9)	+
Cat (sympathectomized)	40 ± 10	(6)	0 → (+)

* From Håkanson and Owman.[357]
† With 5-HT as substrate and incubation at 37° 1 hr in 0.1 M pH 6.8 phosphate buffer; results expressed as CPM of 5-HIAA (1μg 5-HIAA = 20,000 CPM).
‡ With tryptamine as substrate, tetrazolium salt as the reduction indicator (electron acceptor?), and incubation at 37° in 0.1 M pH 7.6 phosphate buffer; results expressed as nil—0, very low—(+), low— + , moderate— + + , high— + + +, and very high — + + + +.

is easily inactivated by trypsin and is relatively heat-stable; about 15% of pineal MAO is of this type and is barely detectable after bilateral superior cervical ganglionectomy.[332,356,357,930] Type B acts on tyramine with a higher apparent K_m (Table LXVII), does not act on 5-HT, is less readily inhibited by clorgyline (0.1mM), is not readily inac-

TABLE LXVII

Michaelis constants for monoamine oxidase(s) of rat superior cervical ganglion and pineal gland.*

| | Apparent K_m for: | | |
| | Tyramine (mM) | | 5-Hydroxytryptamine (mM) |
Tissue	Enzyme A	Enzyme B	Enzyme A
Ganglion	0.10	0.87†	0.43
Pineal Gland		0.76	0.58
		0.43‡	

* From Yang *et al.*[1096]
† Determined in the presence of 0.1 mM clorgyline.
‡ Crude mitochondrial fraction was frozen and thawed thrice and then dialysed against 67 mM, pH 7.2 phosphate buffer.

tivated by trypsin and is heat-labile.[1096] Low MAO activity found by Mori *et al.* in three human pineal tumors might have been due to the single substrate tested, tryptamine.[658] However, by another and more sensitive technique employing radioactive tryptamine, Vogel *et al.* found in human brains pineal MAO activity comparable in level to that found in a number of gray regions, but distinctly less than that found in hypothalamus.[1010]

Rat pineal MAO activity attains adult levels by 10 days after birth following a postnatal rise of about 50 percent.[1102] Human pineal MAO activity has been studied in relation to age changes and pathology.[705,1075] Little if any change with age was found in group comparisons ranging in age from three to twelve years to fifty-five to seventy years (N = 25).[1075] Postmortem changes at room temperature in rabbit pineal MAO activity were found to be very slight at least for eight hours.[705]

At least with tryptamine as substrate rat pineal MAO activity is not affected significantly by either continuous light (LL) or continuous darkness (DD).[930] Increase in rat pineal MAO activity following injection of gonadotropin (HCG) has been claimed.[982]

1.6 Acting on NADH₂ or NADPH₂ as donor

1.6.99.1 *NADPH₂:(acceptor) oxidoreductase* (NADPH₂ diaphorase)

This enzyme, studied cytochemically in guinea pig pineals,

has the same general distribution in pinealocytes as the following enzyme, but a somewhat stronger reaction has been shown, and it extended outward within the smallest cytoplasmic extensions. The changes in level of activity with pregnancy and reproductive ablations, and the lack of significant changes with various hormonal treatments follows the same pattern as described for guinea pig NADH-diaphorase below.[1012]

1.6.99.3 *NADH$_2$ (acceptor) oxidoreductase* (Reduced NAD dehydrogenase, NADH-diaphorase, diaphorase).

Cytochemically this enzyme activity has been shown to be strong in the pinealocytes and weak in the glia of human pineal glands.[92] The enzyme has been demonstrated in guinea pig pinealocytes, which show lobular differences in apparent level of activity both in fetal and adult animals. Increase in activity in pineals of this species has been reported to occur in pregnant females during the second half of gestation; fetectomy did not affect the activity, but it reverted to "normal" levels by two days after parturition or oophorectomy or hysterectomy. No detectable histochemically shown changes in enzyme activity were found in pineals of normal guinea pigs following two weeks of any one of a number of hormonal treatments (chorionic gonadotropin, estradiol, progesterone, placental tissue or gonadectomy).[1012] In rat pineals this enzyme is lowered by continuous light (LL) and raised by continuous darkness (DD).[131]

1.9 Acting on haem groups of donors

1.9.3.1 *Cytochrome* c: *oxidoreductase* (Cytochrome oxioxidase).

Cytochemically this enzyme in rat pineals has been reported to be decreased by continuous light (LL) and increased by continuous darkness (DD).[131]

1.14 Other enzymes using O$_2$ as oxidant

1.14.3.1 *L-Phenylalanine, dihydrobiopterin:oxygen oxidoreductase 4-hydroxylating* (Phenylalanine 4-hydroxylase)

Bagchi and Zarycki[61] have presented evidence for the presence of a phenylalanine hydroxylating system in the rat pineal gland leading to the formation of tyrosine. The presence of tyrosine in pineal tissue, therefore, is not necessarily due to the hemal transport of tyrosine from the liver, where phenylalanine 4-hydroxylase activity is well known. *In vivo* administration of *p*-chlorophenylalanine incompletely blocked the liver enzyme, but strongly blocked the pineal tyrosine-forming system. The pineal hydroxylating system may at least largely involve tryptophan hydroxylase and may be different from that found in brain.[61]

1.14.3.a *L-Tyrosine, tetrahydropteridine: oxygen oxidoreductase 3-hydroxylating* (Tyrosine 3-hydroxylase).

This enzyme is usually considered to be the rate-limiting one for the synthesis of norepinephrine in various tissues.[559] In kitten pineal glands this enzyme activity follows a nearly linear 3-fold increase postnatally from day two to fifty.[603] It is present in relatively large concentration in adult pineal glands, and follows a circadian rhythm with the peak activity at nighttime and the trough during the daylight hours.[604] In human postmortem samples tyrosine hydroxylase activity has been compared in brain regions and pineal glands. Wide individual variation occurred, but pineal activity was intermediate in relation to that of putamen, globus pallidus and head of candate nucleus on the maximal extreme and frontal cortex, thalamus and hypothalamus on the minimal extreme. The concentration in human pineals (N = 2) was about half that in rat pineals (N = 5).[1010]

1.14.3.b *L-Tryptophan, tetrahydropteridine: oxygen oxidoreductase 5-hydroxylating* (Tryptophan 5-hydroxylase).

This enzyme is generally considered to be the rate-limiting one in the biosynthesis of 5-hydroxytryptamine (5-HT) (Fig. 31).[354, 572, 943] It has been found in rat, beef and human pineal glands, and has been claimed to be in higher concentrations in pineal gland than in any other tissue.[100, 572] As a very labile enzyme, it poses difficulties for isolation and study. The pineal enzyme is also responsible in this tissue for hydroxylat-

TABLE LXVIII
Tryptophan- and phenylalanine-hydroxylating activities compared between beef pineal glands and rat brainstem.*

Enzyme source Selective omissions	Tryptophan hydroxylated‡	Phenylalanine hydroxylated‡
Beef pineal: Complete system†	3.8	3.0
—Fe^{++}|	2.4	2.9
—$DMPH_4$	0.17	< 0.01
—O_2	0.25	0.15
Rat brainstem: Complete system†	1.18	< 0.01
—Fe^{++}	1.17	< 0.01
—$DMPH_4$	0.07	< 0.01
—O_2	0.01	< 0.01

* From Jequier et al.[438]
† = 0.2–0.4 ml partially purified enzyme, 0.25 M Tris-acetate buffer (pH 7.5), 1mM $DMPH_4$ (= 2-amino-4-hydroxy-6, 7-dimethyl-5,6,7,8 tetrahydropteridine), and 0.1 mM ferrous ammonium sulfate in a total volume of 0.3–0.5 ml.
‡ mμmoles substrate hydroxylated/mg protein.

ing phenylalanine, whereas brain tryptophan hydroxylase has no detectable activity toward phenylalanine (Table LXVIII).[100,438] The pineal enzyme requires a reduced pteridine and oxygen and is inhibited by p-chlorophenylalanine (pCPA).[572] Further studies with this inhibitor have provided additional evidence for the pineal and brain enzymes being different. Although it depletes pineal 5-HT, pCPA does not inactivate pineal tryptophan hydroxylase. But it lowers the affinity of the enzyme for the substrate, presumably by competitive inhibition. Under normal conditions, the pineal of pCPA-treated rats cannot synthesize 5-HT because the Km of pineal tryptophan hydroxylase in pCPA-treated rats is much higher than the concentration of L-tryptophan. Loading the animal with L-tryptophan overcomes the inhibition by pCPA.[200] Diverse catechol compounds, including norepinephrine (NE) [76% inhibition at $10^{-4}M$], inhibit the tryptophan hydroxylases from beef pineal and rat brainstem, presumably due to their chelating ability toward iron.[438] However, studies with rat pineal organ cultures have indicated that dibutyryl adenosine 3′,5′ monophosphate and NE accelerate synthesis of 5-HT through an action at the hydroxylation of tryptophan. In this situation, the stimulatory action of NE is mediated by cyclic-AMP.[898]

TABLE LXIX

Comparisons of hydroxyindole-O-methyltransferase activities in retinas and pineal glands of diverse vertebrate animals.*

Species	Tissue	
	Pineal Gland†	Retina†
Fish:		
Salmo gairdneri (trout)	1,492.→2,249.	172.
Hesperoleucus symmetricus (roach)	484.→1,920.	—
Amphibians:		
Rana pipiens (frog)	58.6‡	111.4
Bufo marinus (toad)	63.6‡	55.3
Necturus maculosus (mud puppy)	4.6‡	31.8
Reptiles:		
Pseudemys scripta (turtle)	432.	29.0
Cnemidophorus lemniscatus (lizard)	6,651.	5.4
Iguana iguana (lizard)	1,237.	6.3
Natrix vallida (snake)	2,903.	0.0
Birds:		
Gallus (leghorn chickens)	914.	20.3
Zenaidura macroura (mourning dove)	5,721.	13.3
Junco oreganus (Oregon junco)	15,669.	0.0
Zonotrichia atricapilla (golden-crowned sparrow)	8,830.	0.9
Melospiza melodia (song sparrow)	9,642.	0.3

* Data from Quay[788] and Hafeez and Quay.[353]

† Results are mean mμmoles melatonin formed/g/hr with N-acetylserotonin as substrate, ^{14}C-methyl-S-adenosylmethionine as methyl donor and with phosphate buffer at pH 7.9.

‡ Pineal region of brain incubated (eg. pineal + adjacent brain tissue).

2. TRANSFERASES

2.1 Transferring one-carbon groups

2.1.1.4   *S-Adenosylmethionine: N-acetylserotonin-O-methyl-transferase* (Acetylserotonin methyltransferase, ASMT, Hydroxyindole-O-methyltransferase, HIOMT).

A pineal enzyme O-methylating N-acetylserotonin to form melatonin was first discovered, purified and studied by Axelrod and Weissbach.[56, 57] This type of enzyme activity has been found in the pineal glands of all examined vertebrates from fish to amphibians, reptiles, birds and mammals (Table LXIX).[52,74,353,790] In the course of evolution pineal HIOMT activity appears to have increased and similar enzymatic activity of other organs, and especially brain and retina has decreased (Table LXIX).[790] However, in at least one mammalian species, the rat, significant HIOMT activity has been

TABLE LXX

Differentiating properties of hydroxyindole-O-methyltransferase (HIOMT) activity in three tissues of rats.*

Property	Pineal	Retina	Harderian Gland
Optimum pH	7.5–8.4	7.5–8.4	7.3–7.9
Effect of freezing & storage @ 20°C	65% reduction (5 days)	65% reduction (5 days)	stable (2 mos.)
Effect of divalent cations†	none	none	stimulation
K_m for S-adenosylmethionine	0.9×10^{-5}M	1.0×10^{-5}M	0.3×10^{-3}M
K_m for N-acetylserotonin	0.4×10^{-5}M	0.9×10^{-5}M	1.2×10^{-3}M
Relative O-methylation of substrates:			
N-acetylserotonin (set at 100)	100	100	100
5-hydroxytryptophal	14	15	11
5-HT	14	13	16
5-HIAA	11	14	17
% Inhibition by compounds at 10^{-4}M:			
Melatonin	2%	3%	0
N-3,4-dichlorobenzoyl-5-bromotryptamine	57%	54%	21%
N-benzoyl-5-bromotryptamine	62%	57%	19%

* From Cardinali and Wurtman.[149]

† As demonstrated by opposing effects of EDTA $(10^{-3}$M) and Mg^{++} $(10^{-3}$M).

found in retina and Harderian gland as well as in the pineal.[147, 149, 672a, 1009] There are differences in the properties or behaviors of the enzyme activities from the three tissues (Table LXX). It is clear that the pineal and retinal enzymes are either identical or very similar, and differ markedly from the Harderian gland enzyme. Species differences in the properties of HIOMT are widespread. These range from the pronounced differences between birds and mammals (Table LXXI) to differences in substrate specificity seen within each of these groups (Tables LXXII-LXXIV). Postmortem decline of pineal HIOMT activity at room temperature is slow; in whole rats percent changes observed are: 3 min (zero time) -0, 1 hr-5 percent, 3 hrs. -35 percent, 6 hrs -40 percent and 12 hrs -57 percent.[827] Studies on physiological controls and effects on pineal HIOMT activity in any species should be preceded by investigation of possible species peculiarities in the enzyme's properties.[815, 828]

Bovine pineal gland HIOMT has been isolated in pure form and studied in detail by Axelrod and Weissbach[57], Jackson and Lovenberg[433] and by Karahasanoğlu and Özand.[468]

TABLE LXXI

Differentiating properties of pineal hydroxyindole-O-methyltransferase
from cows and Japanese quail
(*Coturnix coturnix japonica*).[*]

Property	Cow	Quail
Electrophoretic mobility[†]	slower	faster
Heat stability (51°C, 3 min)	65% reduction	98% reduction
K_m (with 2.5×10^{-9}M SAMe, & varying concentrations of N-Acetylserotonin)	$51.0 \pm 5.8\ \mu$M	$4.8 \pm 0.65\ \mu$M
Substrate specificity:[‡]		
N-Acetylserotonin	1.42	1.63
5-Hydroxytryptamine	0.07	1.75
Bufotenine	0.05	0.51
5-hydroxytryptophol	0.25	2.38
6-hydroxy-N-acetyltryptamine	0.007	0.24
4-hydroxy-N-acetyltryptamine	0.007	0.30

[*] Data of Axelrod and Lauber,[49] and Axelrod and Vesell.[55]
[†] On starch block, in 0.05M pH 8.6 sodium barbital buffer at 4°C.
[‡] Results expressed as mμmoles product formed/mg pineal tissue, from incubations in pH 7.9 phosphate buffer, 1 mμmole ^{14}C-SAMe and 0.1 μmole substrate.

The smallest unit molecular weight is about 21,800 or 39,000 depending on investigator, but higher molecular weight aggregates occur and differ in degree in their properties (Table LXXV). The separation by DEAE-Sephadex chromatography of two peaks of activity of the lowest molecular weight enzyme suggests that it exists also in at least two different charged molecular species. However, these proteins ("A and B") appear to be identical in all other examined physical and chemical properties.[433]

It has been suggested that the circadian changes sometimes observed in the pineal activity of the enzyme might be due to an association-dissociation phenomenon.[433] It is interesting that this rather sluggish enzyme represents a significant portion (4%) of the soluble proteins in the pineal gland. Rather marked changes in rate of protein synthesis or degradation would have to occur if circadian changes in pineal HIOMT activity are to be explained by changes in amount of enzyme present. Other aspects of circadian changes and physiological controls in pineal HIOMT activity are discussed in the chapter on indoleamines.

TABLE LXXII

O-and N-methyltransferase activities of avian pineal glands*

Species	Enzyme: HIOMT Substrate: N-Acetylserotonin	5-HT	HNMT Histamine	PNMT Normetanephrine	COMT NE
Japanese quail	1.53	1.42	1.04	1.01	0.12
Turkey	2.30	0.46	0.18	0.06	0.03
Duck (Kahki-Campbell)	4.21	0.33	0.29	0.06	0.25
Chicken (leghorn)	5.11	1.20	0.68	0.12	0.17
Pigeon	0.73	0.02	0.22	0.05	0.04

* Data of Axelrod and Lauber[49]; results expressed as mμmole of ^{14}C-methylated product/mg pineal tissue from incubations as described in footnote to Table LXXI; HIOMT = hydroxyindole-O-methyltransferase, HNMT = histamine methyltransferase, PNMT = phenylethanolamine-N-methyltransferase, and COMT = catechol-O-methyltransferase.

TABLE LXXIII

Comparison of different mammalian species in the relative activity of their
pineal hydroxyindole-O-methyltransferase with N-acetylserotonin as substrate.°

Species	N	Mean ± Se
Monkey (*Macaca mulatta*)	3	42,524. ± 8,481.
Sheep (*Ovis aries*):		
castrate males	6	36,473. ± 12,003.
intact females	30	23,579. ± 1,351.
Beef (*Bos taurus*)	4	20,602. ± 2,012.
Raccoon (*Procyon lotor*)	3	13,518. ± 3,851.
Rat (*Rattus norvegicus*)	13	4,139. ± 334.
Cat (*Felis catus*)	2	871. ± 29.

° Data of Quay and Smart[827]; results expressed as net CPM of ^{14}C-melatonin
formed/mg tissue/hour in incubations similar to those described in footnote to
Table LXXI.

Tryptic digests of bovine HIOMT have yielded about 30 peptides. Three or four contain tryptophan. The amino acid composition of bovine pineal HIOMT is shown in Table LXXVI. An unusually great leucine content (52/336 residues) and the large amount of this enzyme protein in pineal tissues should facilitate study of its biosynthesis and molecular control mechanisms.[433] Substrate binding and comparative structure-activity relationships of inhibitors have been investigated by Ho and coworkers.[392-399] They have designated the structure shown in Figure 56 as that of the ideal inhibitor or pineal HIOMT and they have as well studied its metabolism and identified its products.[392]

In rats, pineal HIOMT activity is the last one to appear during development of enzymes in the pathway from tryptophan to melatonin. Activity was barely detectable at 6 days after birth and was only 10 percent of adult levels by twelve days. Adult activity levels were attained by thirty-four days.[1102] In human pineals HIOMT activity has been studied in relation to age and pathology.[705,1075] Great individual variability was observed and only slight if any decrease with age was found in sample groups from three to twelve to fifty-five to seventy years in age. The enzyme activity is maintained during viral neoplastic transformation of hamster pineal cells *in vitro*[1049] and can serve as a marker for pinealoma metastases in man.[168,1085]

TABLE LXXIV

Substrate specificity of pineal hydroxyindole-O-methyltransferase from different mammalian species.*

Substrate	Beef (Bos taurus)	Sheep (Ovis aries) ♂	Sheep (Ovis aries) ♀	Raccoon (Procyon lotor)	Rat (Rattus norvegicus)	Cat (Felis catus)	Monkey (Macaca mulatta)
N-Acetylserotonin	100.0	100.0	100.0	100.0	100.0	100.0	100.0
N-Acetyl-6-methoxyserotonin	64.5	101.1	83.9	101.7	64.3	110.7	17.8
5-Hydroxytryptophol	9.5	8.7	6.4	6.6	0.5	0	2.2
5-Hydroxyindole	8.7	3.1	4.3	15.7	1.4	0	1.0
5-Hydroxy-6-methoxytryptamine	4.5	5.6	—	14.1	0	0	0
6-Hydroxytetrahydroharman	2.6	2.9	1.3	0	0	0	0
Bufotenine	0.7	0	—	2.7	0	0	0
5-Hydroxytryptamine	0.4	1.4	—	0.8	0	0	0

* Data of Quay and Smart[837]; incubation conditions were similar to those described in footnote to Table LXXI; activities expressed as percent of that observed with N-acetylserotonin as substrate; see Table LXXIII for relative absolute values with N-acetylserotonin as substrate.

TABLE LXXV

Kinetic characteristics of different polymers of purified
bovine pineal hydroxyindole-*O*-methyltransferase.[*]

Molecular Weight	K_m for N-acetylserotonin $(\times 10^6 M)$	K_m for SAMe[†] $(\times 10^7 M)$	% Inhibition by S-adenosyl-homocysteine	Substrate activation (V_2/V_1)	OAA[‡] activation (V_2/V_1)
250,000	16.9	6.7	38	2.63	1.80
250,000–					
225,000	13.9	5.6	,48	3.22	2.45
197,500	13.9	5.0	46	3.40	3.27
180,000	7.3	4.6	77	4.40	3.33
150,000	9.7	3.6	81	4.65	2.72
125,300	9.5	1.6	83	3.00	2.34
100,000	7.4	1.5	80	2.36	2.55
83,000	5.9	2.3	78	1.87	2.20
65,700	6.8	2.8	58	1.56	2.25
48,200	11.1	5.0	63	1.41	2.25

[*] Data of Karahasanoğlu and Özand.[468]
[†] SAMe = S-adenosylmethionine.
[‡] OAA = *cis*-oxaloacetic acid-potassium *cis*-oxaloacetate buffer.

TABLE LXXVI

Amino acid composition of bovine pineal
hydroxyindole-*O*-methyltransferase.[*]

Amino acid	Estimated number of residues[†]
Lysine	10
Histidine	6
Arginine	26
Aspartic acid	26
Threonine	15
Serine	24
Glutamic acid	40
Proline	14
Glycine	35
Alanine	38
Half-cysteine	10
Valine	25
Methionine	4
Isoleucine	10
Leucine	52
Tyrosine	15
Phenylalanine	15
Tryptophan	3–4

[*] Data of Jackson and Lovenberg.[433]
[†] Determined using an enzyme molecular weight of 39,000.

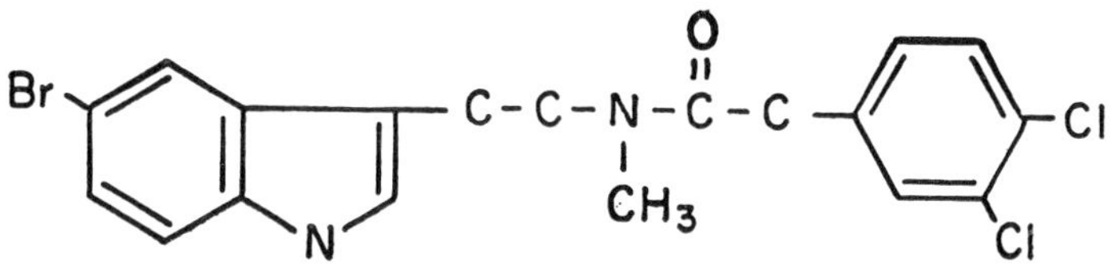

Figure 56. Structure of the ideal inhibitor of HIOMT (hydroxyindole-*O*-methyltransferase).[392]

X-rays as well as environmental light in the visible range are inhibitory for this enzyme *in vivo* in mammalian pineal glands.[83,241,243] In addition to the physiological control mechanisms discussed in the chapter on indoleamines, complex control mechanisms have been examined and reviewed by Heller.[378] In avian pineal glands besides the effects of light discussed earlier,[59,669,789,793,806] there are seasonal changes in HIOMT activity.[82]

2.1.1.6 *S-Adrenosylmethionine: catechol-O-methyltransferase* (Catechol methyltransferase, catechol-*O*-methyltransferase, COMT).

COMT activity has been found in various organs including pineal glands from birds (Table LXXII) and mammals and also in red blood cells.[47] Norepinephrine is the usual substrate, and it is transformed to normetanephrine. This enzyme's activity in monkey pineals (0.02 μ mole product/g/90 min) is very much less than that found in either the neuro- or adenohypophysis of the same species (1.46 and 3.20 μmole product/g/hr respectively.[50] In human tissue samples pineal COMT activity is of the same order of magnitude as that of various brain regions, but it is approximately a half of that observed in rat brain.[1010] The circadian rhythm in rat pineal COMT (Fig. 49) and its correlates and controls were discussed in the chapter on catecholamines.

2.1.1.8 *S-Adenosylmethionine: histamine-N-methyltransferase* (Histamine-*N*-methyltransferase, HNMT, imidazole-*N*-methyltransferase).

HNMT has been detected and measured in avian (Table LXXII), monkey and human pineal glands but could not be detected in rat pineal glands taken at three times over a 24-

hour period.[50,60,1075] It is found in human erythrocytes also, but not in those of rats.[47] It seems possible that species differences in pineal HNMT may be related in part to the presence of mast cells in avian, monkey and human pineal glands and their absence in those of rats. Monkey pineal activity is comparable to that of adenohypophysis and is about one fourth to one third that of neurohypophysis.[50] Human pineal samples from three to twelve to fifty-five to seventy years in age show little if any significant change in HNMT activity with age.[1075]

2.1.1.a *S-Adenosylmethionine: phenylethanolamine-N-methyltransferase*   (Phenylethanolamine-N-methyltransferase, PNMT).

PNMT activity is highly localized in mammals to the adrenal medulla where it is responsible for the conversion of norepinephrine to epinephrine.[45] It has been detected, nevertheless, in avian pineal glands (Table LXXII) and might possibly occur in the pineals of some other submammalian vertebrates on the basis of the wider tissue occurrence in these of epinephrine content and its possible local biosynthesis.

2.1.1.b *S-Adenosylmethionine: H_2O-methyltransferase* (Methanol-forming enzyme).

This enzyme was first noted in mammalian pituitary glands[48] but has since been found in erythrocytes and apparently in mammalian pineal gland and various other tissues.[47,60,159] A low enzyme activity found in rat pineal glands was quantitatively about the same at three times of the day.[60] It is reported lacking in human pinealomas and has been suggested along with hydroxyindole-O-methyltransferase as a useful indicator in the differential identification of pituitary and pineal tumor metastases.[927] A physiological significance for this enzyme remains to be demonstrated.

2.3 Acyltransferases

2.3.1.5 *Acetyl-CoA: arylamine-N-acetyltransferase* (Serotonin-N-acetyltransferase).

This enzyme is present in many organs, including the pineal gland, but its properties are primarily known from the liver enzyme.[1031] The pineal enzyme is of especial interest due to its essential, and perhaps rate-limiting, status for the synthesis of melatonin. It catalyzes the formation of the precursor of melatonin, *N*-acetylserotonin from 5-hydroxytryptamine. The characteristics, cyclic changes, and controls of this pineal enzyme activity have been discussed in the chapter on indoleamines. It is detectable in rat pineal glands as early as four days before birth and attains adult levels by the end of the third week after birth. At this time nocturnal values are more than 30 times greater than daytime values.[245,494] Since no such circadian rhythm in this enzyme activity is found in other tissues, questions arise as to whether the pineal enzyme has different properties, or whether the rhythm in the pineal enzyme can be explained solely on the basis of a pineal specific control mechanism, or a combination of these. In any case, this pineal enzymatic system offers one of the best models for diverse kinds of studies on the molecular basis of neuronal control mechanisms and the synthesis of enzyme molecules.[198]

2.3.1.6 *Acetyl-CoA: choline-O-acetyltransferase* (Choline acetyltransferase, choline acetylase, ChAc).

This enzyme is responsible for the synthesis of the transmitter acetylcholine, and is therefore important in evaluations of the origin(s) and control of low levels of acetylcholine found in pineal glands of some species. However, through the body the enzyme occurs not only in some neurons, but also in red blood cells and some tissues that are without neural elements. Low levels of this enzyme activity have been measured in rat, bovine, monkey and human pineal samples.[254,531,591,855] In the rat's superior cervical ganglia, cutting of the spinal nerve connections ("decentralization") leads to great reduction in ChAc activity. But in rat pineal glands neither superior cervical ganglionectomy nor decentralization cause significant changes (Table LXXVII). These results have been interpreted as indicating an only minimal parasympathetic innervation for the rat pineal gland and that practically all of the pineal ChAc may reside in tissues and cells other than neurons or their fibers.[855] However, nerve fibers with acetylcholine esterase activity have been demonstrated cytochemically in

TABLE LXXVII

Choline acetyltransferase (ChAc), acetylcholine esterase (AChE) and cholinesterase (ChE) activities of superior cervical ganglia and pineal glands in normal and operated rats.[*]

Tissue Operation[†]	ChAc Mean ± Se	% difference	AChE Mean ± Se	% difference	ChE Mean ± Se	% difference
Ganglia						
Controls	159.0 ± 33.7		10.76 ± 1.40		2.29 ± 0.11	
Decentralized	4.5 ± 4.2	−97% §	5.10 ± 0.96	−53% §	1.33 ± 0.32	−42% §
Pineal Glands						
Controls	1.4 ± 0.4		0.18 ± 0.04		0.09 ± 0.01	
Ganglionectomied	1.3 ± 0.5	n.s. ¶	0.10 ± 0.02	−44% §	0.06 ± 0.01	−33% ‖
Decentralized	1.4 ± 0.3	n.s.	0.19 ± 0.04	n.s.	0.08 ± 0.01	n.s.

[*] Results from Rodriguez de Lores Arnaiz and Pellegrino de Iraldi[855], expressed as μmole (AChE & ChE) or nmole (ChAc) of product formed/mg tissue protein/hr at 37°C.
[†] Decentralized = afferent fibers to the superior cervical ganglia cut; ganglionectomied = bilateral removal of the superior cervical ganglia; both operations performed seven days prior to sacrifice.
§ P < 0.001
‖ P < 0.01
¶ n.s. = difference not statistically significant.

pineal glands of rats and other species (see enzyme 3.1.1.7).

2.3.1.? (Thiolesterase or acyltransferase)

An enzyme which attacks thiolacetic acid has been demonstrated to be highly active in hamster pinealocytes, by means of electron microscope cytochemistry. Structural localization of the product of enzyme activity was "on membranes of mitochondria of pinealocytes and axons and on lysosome-like dense bodies in pinealocytes".[741]

2.4 Glycosyltransferases

2.4.1.1 *α -1,4-Glucan: orthophosphate glucosyltransferase* (α-Glucan phosphorylase, glycogen phosphorylase, phosphorylase a).

A moderate to strong histochemical reaction denoting this enzyme activity was found by Shimizu and Okada[906] in one day old rat pineal glands. The enzyme activity was diminished in older glands to an apparent absence in those from adults. In subsequent studies on the specificity of the method used, that of Takeuchi and Kuriaki, it has been found capable of demonstrating amylo-1,4-1,6-transglyco-sylase (a β-glucosidase, E.C. 3.2.1.21) as well as phosphorylase.[244,957] Adult pineal phosphorylase content should be reexamined with biochemical methods.

2.6 Transferring nitrogenous groups

2.6.1.1 *L-Aspartate: 2-oxoglutarate aminotransferase* (Aspartate aminotransferase, glutamic-oxaloacetic trans-aminase).

This enzyme has been found in lamb pineal glands at about the same concentration as in epithalamus and cerebral cortex.[967,968] Porcine pineal glands have been shown to have a high content of this transaminase, and a content considerably greater than that of the following transaminase(E.C. 2.6.1.2).[450]

2.6.1.2 *L-Alanine: 2-oxoglutarate aminotransferase* (Alanine aminotransferase, glutamic-pyruvic trans-aminase).

Lamb pineal glands have about the same concentration of this enzyme as cerebral cortex and epithalamus, and in all three the concentration or level of activity is about half that shown for the previous enzyme (E.C. 2.6.1.1).[967,968] A lower content has been reported also in porcine pineals, brains and pituitary glands.[450]

2.6.1.5 *L-Tyrosine: 2-oxoglutarate aminotransferase* (Tyrosine aminotransferase).

The transamination of tyrosine assumes importance from the possible participation of this reaction in the regulation of biosynthesis of catecholamines. This might occur by modification of tissue levels of tyrosine available for hydroxylation. This enzyme has been found in much higher concentration in sheep pineal glands than in diverse brain regions, of which only selected high, intermediate and low examples are noted in Table LXXVIII.[1030]

2.1.1.19 *4-Aminobutyrate: 2-oxoglutarate aminotransferase* (Aminobutyrate aminotransferase, γ-aminobutyrate-α-oxyglutarate transaminase, GABA-T).

This enzyme activity as studied in human pineal glands and brain regions contrasts markedly with the previous one in distribution of relative activities (Table LXXIX). The low pineal activity is consistent with a low pineal representation by the γ-aminobutyrate pathway and a low content of γ-aminobutyric acid (GABA).

2.7 Transferring phosphorus-containing groups

TABLE LXXVIII

Levels of tyrosine aminotransferase found in sheep pineal glands and brain regions.[*]

Source	μmoles product/g tissue/hr Mean $\pm$ Se[†]
Pineal gland	12.54 ± 1.35
Brain regions:	
Caudate nucleus	7.33 ± 0.12
Superior colliculus	7.06 ± 0.38
Thalamus	6.65 ± 0.33
Cerebral cortex	5.93 ± 0.26
Hypothalamus	5.43 ± 0.49
Medulla oblongata	2.81 ± 0.14

[*] Data from Webb and Gibb.[1030]
[†] N = 5–6 per source.

TABLE LXXIX

Levels of aminobutyrate aminotransferase found in
human pineal glands and brain regions.[*]

Source	μmoles produce/hr/:	
	g tissue[†]	g protein[†]
Pineal gland	33.8	646.
Brain regions:		
Corpus callosum	36.7	435.
Cerebral cortex	123.4–164.4[‡]	1686.–2063.[‡]
Hypothalamus	165.5	2282.
Central thalamus	175.9	1924.
Caudate nucleus	204.0	2227.

[*] Data from Sheridan *et al.*[900]
[†] Means from 5–6 subjects.
[‡] Range in means from different cortical regions.

2.7.1.a *Cyclic-AMP: protein phosphotransferase* (Cyclic
AMP-dependent protein kinase).

This enzyme consists of a regulatory protein (cyclic-AMP
binding) and a catalytic protein (protein kinase) that
phosphorylates histones when activated by c-AMP. The
pineal gland is a rich source of this enzyme system. Pineal
homogenates from rats and beef contain per mg protein
several times greater kinase activity than has been reported
for brain tissue.[282] It may function in the control of the circadian enzymatic changes in the pineal's melatonin biosynthetic
pathway, as discussed in the chapter on indoleamines.[283]

2.7.3.2 *ATP: creatine phosphotransferase* (Creatine kinase, creatine phosphokinase).

This enzyme activity has been found at moderate to high
levels in lamb pineal glands, but still at levels considerably
lower than those of cerebral cortex.[967,968]

3. HYDROLASES

3.1 Acting on ester bonds

3.1.1.3 Glycerol ester hydrolase (Lipase).

This enzyme hydrolyzes esters of glycerol or other alcohols
and long chain fatty acids. Pineal tissue contains lipolytic
protein[871] and lipase activity which has usually been studied
by means of histochemical procedures. A moderate to high
pineal lipase activity has been observed with Gomori Tween

methods.[131,133,753] The artificial (Tween) substrates are commercial detergents which consist of water soluble esters of long-chain fatty acids with polyglycols or polymannitols. True lipases have been found to hydrolyse esters of unsaturated fatty acids of this series, whereas other esterases in addition to true lipase hydrolyse the saturated members.[330] The method is currently not held in favor, due to the often patchy results, imperfect specificity and questionable relevance to actions on natural substrates.[724] Nevertheless, physiological changes in the pineal activity observed by means of this method are still noteworthy for reexamination if for no other reason. Continuous light and a salt-free diet have each been reported to lead to decreased rat pineal lipase activity, and continuous darkness and adrenalectony have each been reported to increase it.[131,599]

3.1.1.7 *Acetylcholine acetyl-hydrolase* (Acetylcholinesterase, AChE).

AChE has been taken as evidence of the cholinergic function of a neuron. In autonomic ganglia the action potential entering along preganglionic fibers is thought to release acetylcholine (ACh) from the synaptic vesicles in the terminations of the preganglionic fibers. This transmitter (ACh) then passes the synaptic cleft and combines with receptors on the postganglionic cell membrane, resulting in the propagation of an action potential along the postganglionic fiber. The polarized state of the postsynaptic membrane is restored by the rapid destruction of ACh by AChE. The presence of AChE in both pre- and postganglionic fibers of the parasympathetic system and in the preganglionic fibers of the sympathetic system is generally recognized. The variably and sometimes entirely cholinergic nature of some postganglionic fibers of the sympathetic system is less well appreciated. Occurrence of AChE in sympathetic postganglionic nerve fibers within the pineal glands of various mammals has been demonstrated by both histochemical and biochemical methods,[251,252,594,984] although early histochemical studies failed to find this enzyme in rat, rabbit, and ungulate pineals.[37,40,308] Removal of the superior cervical ganglia of the rat leads to loss or reduction of pineal AChE activity both histochemically and biochemically (Table LXXVII).[583,855] Chemical "sympathectomy" with 6-hydroxydopamine also destroys the AChE-containing fibers of the rat pineal gland.[250] In the pineal gland of the squirrel monkey (*Saimiri sciureus*) AChE activity has been reported to occur not only in the nerve fibers but also at mild to moderate levels of activity in neuron perikarya (peripheral postganglionic cell bodies?), pinealocytes, blood vessels and sinusoids.[594] Where tissue comparisons have been made, pineal AChE activity is less than that of brain regions.[967,968] No reports have been found concerning the possible occurrence of AChE in human pineal glands.

3.1.1.8. *Acylcholine acyl-hydrolase* (Cholinesterase, non-specific cholinesterase, butyryl cholinesterase, pseudocholinesterase, BuChE, ChE).

This enzyme has a wider tissue distribution than the preceding one and has been localized histochemically in neuroglia, capillary walls, some smooth muscle fibers and some other tissues as well as in the perikarya of some neurons, but here in low concentration.[6] The enzyme has been detected in bovine, rat and monkey pineal glands.[252,531,594,855] Rat pinealocytes have been reported to show histochemically a strong ChE activity after birth which disappears within two weeks.[583] In adult rats histochemically detectable ChE activity has been claimed to not occur in capillary walls and to occur only in nerve trunks lying outside of the organ.[252,444] However, biochemical incubations suggest that a low level of ChE activity remains in adult rat pineal glands and is partly dependent on the innervation from the superior cervical sympathetic ganglia (Table LXXVII).

3.1.1.a (Non-specific esterases).

This is an artificial category for a variety of histochemically demonstrable esterase activities having considerable overlap in substrate specificities and responses to inhibitors. Most of these have been studied primarily through their actions on naphtholic and indoxylic esters. They are usually found in either or both microsomal and lysosomal fractions depending on organ of origin.[142] Thiolacetic acid (CH_3COSH), another substrate used for this group, can be acted upon by cholinisterase as well as aliesterase (E.C. 3.1.1.1?) and possibly other types of esterases.[142] Table LXXX provides a summary of the diverse reactions reported in pineal glands, according to species and substrate.

TABLE LXXX

Summary of "non-specific esterase" activities reported in mammalian pineal glands.

Species Substrate(s)	Observations	References
Man		
Naphthol AS acetate	Chiefly in perivascular region and to slight extent in pinealocytes; not inhibited by E 600.*	92
Squirrel monkey		
α-Naphthyl acetate & Naphthol AS-LC acetate	Mild to moderate reaction in pinealocytes; moderately strong reaction in pineal neurons.	594
Rat		
β-Naphthol acetate	Moderate reaction in pineal.	541,1012
α-Naphthyl acetate and Naphthol AS acetate	Sharply localized reaction in caps on lipid droplets; present by 1 week after birth.	753
Naphthol acetate	Slight increase in pineal reaction following continuous light.	131
Thiolacetic acid	Moderate to strong reaction in pinealocytes and "interstitial" cells; eserine and E 600* inhibited the diffuse cytoplasm reaction in these but not the granular localized reaction; absent in pineal nerve fibers and endings.	37

* E 600 = diethyl-*p*-nitrophenyl phosphate.

3.1.1.b (Acetylsalicyclic acid esterase, "aspirin" esterase)
Thiéblot and coworkers have reported in pineal tissue enzyme activity of this nature at about the same level as in nervous tissue.[968]

3.1.3.1 *Orthophosphoric monoester phosphohydrolase*
(Alkaline phosphatase, alkaline phosphomonoesterase).
Alkaline phosphatase is one of the histochemically most frequently studied types of pineal enzyme activity. By light microscopy and newer methods pineal alkaline phosphatase in man and other mammals usually appears to be localized exclusively within and adjacent to the capillary

walls.[40,42,92,541,622,883,1012] But by electron microscopy intense activity was found within fibrocytes as well as endothelial cells in adult rat pineal glands; the pinealocytes were negative.[37] Human pineal glands of various ages were found by Machado and Machado to be completely negative for alkaline phosphatase activity, in contrast to the intensely positive and adjacent subcommissural organ.[584] In human pinealoma, however, strong alkaline phosphatase activity occurs.[479] Also, in the developing rat pineal gland Gardner noted the appearance of alkaline phosphatase reactive bipolar spongioblasts in 15-day-old embryos.[305] Wislocki and Leduc reported strong alkaline phosphatase activity within pinealocytes as well as blood vessels of young (1–3 years) monkey (*Macaca mulatta*) pineal glands.[1054] Different pineal localizations obtained in different species and by different investigators may possibly be due in part to different substrates used and to other technical differences. A comprehensive and detailed study of pineal phosphomonoesterases in at least one species is needed. It is now agreed that alkaline phosphatases from several different human tissues are distinctive in electrophoretic and enzymatic properties. Furthermore, there is no doubt that several different substrate-specific alkaline phosphatases exist.[725]

Physiological changes in rat pineal alkaline phosphatase include decrease and increase following respectively continuous light and continuous darkness;[131] and rise and fall during the estrous cycle. Maximal pineal activity was reported for early estrus and minimal activity for late estrus.[266]

3.1.3.2 *Orthophosphoric monoester phosphohydrolase* (Acid phosphatase, acid phosphomonoesterase).

Acid phosphatase activity is concentrated in the lysosomal fraction prepared from various mammalian organs. However, the lysosomal association is not absolute.[942] Cytoplasmic pleomorphic dense bodies in rat pinealocytes have a positive reaction for acid phosphase activity with β-glycerophosphate as substrate and have been identified as lysosomes. Their frequency of occurrence is greater in pineals of old animals (25 months) than in those from young adults (9 months old).

Administrations of either reserpine or nialamide failed to affect the relative numbers of lysosomes seen in the pinealocytes.[123,124] In monkey pinealocytes lysosomes are often most prominent and pleomorphic in the cytoplasmic terminals in the vicinity of capillaries.[1026] In rat pineal glands acid phosphatase-containing lysosomes have been seen also in fibrocytes, pericytes and endothelial cells.[37] They are seen as well in pineal neuroglia, especially abundantly in the astrocytes of cat pineal glands.[1026]

The above localizations of acid phosphatase activity in pineal glands appear to be more consistent as well as more precise than those reported from many light microscopic histochemical studies.[541,593,938] Nevertheless, the latter include some that report acid phosphatase primarily in the peripheral cytoplasm of pinealocytes and particularly in cell processes bordering on capillaries and sometimes in adjacent stromal cells.[40,42,133,1012] Moderate acid phosphatase activity has been shown histochemically in human pinealomas.[479]

Physiological changes in rat pineal acid phosphatase activity have been reported in relation to effects of light and in correlations with stages of the estrous cycle. Continuous light leads to an increase in activity and continuous darkness leads to little if any change.[131] The change caused in pineal acid phosphatase by continuous light is opposite to that shown by a wide variety of oxidative enzymes as well as of alkaline phosphatase. It can be suggested that increased pineal acid phosphatase occurs during inactive phases of pinealocyte activity, when secretory materials are being degraded by lysosomal activity. The testing of this hypothesis, however, remains to be undertaken, although it has a precedent or model in the cyclic changes in hypophyseal chromaphil lysosomal activity. Acid phosphatase activity in female rat pineal glands has been reported as maximal during early estrus and minimal during late estrus and metestrus.[266] This might be consistent with the idea that pineal synthetic activity is minimal during the former stage and recommences during the latter ones. However, unlike the enzymatic relations following continuous light, during the estrous cycle enzymatic maxima and minima for succinic dehydrogenase, alkaline phosphatase and acid phosphatase approach being synchronous.[266]

3.1.3.5 *5'-Ribonucleotide phosphohydrolase* (5'-Nucleo-tidase).

The pineal level of this enzyme activity in lambs has been reported to be similar to that of cerebral cortex.[967,968] A strong cytochemical reaction has been shown in bovine pineal glia and pinealocytes. In the latter the reaction was present in cytoplasm and nucleoli but not in the nucleoplasm.[938]

3.1.3.9 *D-Glucose-6-phosphate phosphohydrolase* (Glu-cose-6-phosphatase).

The histochemical localization of this enzyme activity in beef pineal glands is apparently similarly to that of the preced-ing enzyme.[938]

3.1.4.c *Adenosine 3',5'-monophosphate adenosine 5'-phosphate phosphohydrolase* (Adenosine 3',5'-mono-phosphate phosphodiesterase, cyclic nucleotide phosphodiesterase, PDE).

Through this enzyme's activity cyclic 3',5'-AMP (c-AMP) is converted to 5'-AMP. This is the only physiological pathway known for the termination of the action of c-AMP.[157] A microas-say method and a comparison of tissue levels have been pro-vided by Weiss and coworkers.[1045] Rat pineal levels of this enzyme (1.0 ± 0.1 nmoles c-AMP hydrolized/mg tissue/min.) were found to be less than those of brain regions, spleen and kidney, and to be greater than those of liver, stomach, lung, heart and submandibular gland. Multiple nucleotide phosphodiesterases are present in rat pineal tissue and separate out in both membrane and supernatant fractions. In bovine pineal homogenates, however, most of the enzyme is in the soluble fraction (Table LXXXI).[1041] Rat pineal activity is within the lower end of the range of activities observed in different parts of the central nervous system (Table LXXXII). Two K_m values (enzymes) have been identified in 1-day-old rat pineals. In the newborn almost all of the enzyme has a high K_m, whereas in the sixty-day-old animal there is a 1:1 ratio between a high and a low K_m enzyme. Thus it is the low K_m enzyme that increases during pineal development.[1037]

TABLE LXXXI

Subcellular distribution of adenyl cyclase and 3',5'-cyclic nucleotide phosphodiesterase in bovine pineal homogenates.°

Fraction	Adenyl cyclase R.S.A.†	% of Total‡	Phosphodiesterase R.S.A.†	% of Total‡
Whole homogenate	1.0	100	1.0	100
900 g Supernatant	1.2	65	1.7	83
900 g Sediment ("nuclei")	0.6	25	0.6	19
17,000 g Supernatant	0.1	3	1.7	50
17,000 g Sediment ("mitochondria")	3.4	50	0.4	20
100,000 g Supernatant	—	0	1.6	45
1,000,000 g Sediment ("microsomes")	0.1	1	1.0	3

° From Weiss and Costa[1041]; homogenates in 0.32 M sucrose containing MgSO₄ (3×10^{-3}M).

† R.S.A. = relative specific activity, amount of cyclic 3',5'-AMP formed or destroyed per quantity of protein per unit time compared with that of whole homogenate; for adenyl cyclase, $1 = 1.2$ μμmole c-AMP formed/mg protein/min; for phosphodiesterase, $1 = 11$ mμmole c-AMP hydrolyzed/mg protein/min.

‡ = Percent of total activity in whole homogenates; total activity = total protein in each fraction × relative specific activity.

Pineal cyclic nucleotide phosphodiesterase can be inhibited *in vitro* by either theophylline (to -35%) or dibutyryl cyclic-AMP (to -49%).[495] The importance of this pineal enzyme in the mechanisms regulating biosynthesis of indoleamines has been diagrammed (Fig. 36, p. 158) and discussed in the chapter concerning these compounds (p. 159–161).

TABLE LXXXII

Relative contents of adenyl cyclase and 3',5'-cyclic nucleotide phosphodiesterase in rat pineal glands and central nervous system.°

Tissue	Adenyl cyclase	Phosphodiesterase
Parietal cerebral cortex	0.28 ± 0.06	49 ± 2
Corpora quadrigemina	0.26 ± 0.04	11 ± 1
Olfactory bulb	0.25 ± 0.01	19 ± 2
Thalamus	0.24 ± 0.06	24 ± 2
Pineal gland	0.21 ± 0.02	10 ± 2
Hippocampus	0.20 ± 0.02	48 ± 3
Cerebellum	0.20 ± 0.04	7 ± 1
Septum & fornix	0.16 ± 0.03	30 ± 3
Hypothalamus	0.15 ± 0.04	25 ± 1
Caudate nucleus	0.14 ± 0.03	32 ± 2
Medulla oblongata	0.13 ± 0.02	11 ± 1
Pons	0.10 ± 0.02	11 ± 1
Spinal cord	0.08 ± 0.01	8 ± 1

° From Weiss and Costa[1041]; results expressed as mean ± standard error of the mean, for mμmoles of cyclic 3',5'-AMP formed (adenyl cyclase) or destroyed (phosphodiesterase)/mg protein/min. (N = 5 and 6 respectively).

3.1.6.1 *Aryl-sulphate sulphohydrolase* (Arylsulphatase).

Variably weak to moderate enzyme activity has been reported in rat pinealocytes studied by light microscopic histochemistry. By electron microscopy most of the pinealocyte activity was localized to lysosomes, with some occurring as well in the outer portions of the Golgi apparatus and the cisternae of the agranular endoplasmic reticulum. Activity was lacking in the granular and agranular vesicles. Lysosomes of endothelial cells, pericytes and fibroblasts as well as those of pinealocytes and "interstitial" cells were similarly strongly reactive.[37] The apparent enzyme activity in cultured rat pineal glands is increased by cortisol (1 mg/ml medium) perhaps by means of an action on lysosomes.[634]

3.2 Acting on glycosyl compounds

3.2.1.1 *α-1,4-Glucan 4-glucanohydrolase* (α-Amylase).

An enzyme activity of this type has been reported by Thiéblot *et al.* to occur in lamb pineal glands at a greater level of activity than in epithalamic and cerebral cortical tissues.[967,968]

3.2.1.20 *α-D-Glucoside glucohydrolase* (α-Glucosidase, maltase).

Lamb pineal tissue has been reported ineffective in the hydrolysis of methyl-α-D-glucoside.[968]

3.2.1.26 *β-D-Fructofuranosidase fructohydrolase* (β-Fructofuranosidase, sucrase, invertase).

An attempt to demonstrate this activity in lamb pineal tissue was unsuccessful.[968]

3.2.1.31 *β-D-Glucuronide glucuronohydrolase* (β-Glucuronidase).

β-Glucuronidase is another enzyme often associated with lysosomes.[942] Physiologically it is often related to steroid metabolism, and is found to increase in stimulated reproductive organs and accessory structures.[724] The activity in lamb pineal glands has been reported as about twice that in epithalamus and cerebral cortex.[967,968] The rat pineal gland shows a strong and evenly distributed histochemical reaction for this enzyme.[1024] Cultured newborn rat pineals show no effect following the addition of testosterone.[634] Moderate β-glucuronidase activity has been observed in human pinealomas.[479]

3.4 Acting on peptide bonds (= peptide hydrolases)

3.4.1.1 *L-Leucyl-peptide hydrolase* (Leucine aminopeptidase).

Strong leucine aminopeptidase activity has been found in pineal glands of various species, including man,[40,92,451,681,982] but has been reported as lacking in human pinealomas.[479] The activity is found within the pinealocytes and has been suggested as indicating a proteinaceous nature for the pineal's secretion.[681] The high level of this enzyme activity shown by lamb pineal tissue was found to be many times greater than that in epithalamus and cerebral cortex.[967,968] Rat pineal leucine aminopeptidase studied histochemically has been claimed to be increased by chronic administration of gonadotropin (HCG).[982]

3.4.–.– (Benzoylarginine-ethyl-esterase).

Incubations of lamb pineal tissue for enzymatic activity with this designation have been reported to be negative under diverse experimental conditions.[968]

3.5 Acting on C-N bonds, other than peptide bonds.

3.5.1.2 *L-Glutamine amidohydrolase* (Glutaminase).

An unsuccessful attempt to demonstrate this enzyme in lamb pineal glands has been reported.[968]

3.6 Acting on acid anhydride bonds

3.6.1.3 *ATP phosphohydrolase* (ATPase).

An ATPase activity has been found at equivalent levels in lamb pineal and brain. Histochemically the strongest activity within mammalian pineal glands is usually reported as localized to blood vessel or capillary walls,[40,92,593,938,979] but mild to moderate cytoplasmic activity has been reported sometimes within pinealocytes[593,634,938] and strong activity within neuron cell bodies in squirrel monkey pineal glands.[593] Thyroxine was reported by Milcu *et al.* to increase ATPase activity of infant rat pineal glands in culture.[634] Electron microscopic cytochemistry of ATPase localizations in rat pineals and brain regions has shown that in pineal, choroid plexus and area postrema the enzyme is largely confined to pinocytotic invaginations and vesicles within endothelial cells and adjacent pericytes. There was no activity in the basement membranes of these tissues, in contrast with the localization here characterizing cerebral capillaries. Electron microscopic study reveals in addition ATPase activity (substrate = cytidine triphosphate) at the cellular interface between pinealocytes and neuroglia. Since this resembles the ultrastructural localization observed between Sertoli cells and spermatozoa a nutritive rather than a merely supportive function has been suggested by Torack and Barrnett for the pineal glia.[979]

3.6.1.6 *Nucleosidediphosphate phosphohydrolase* (Nucleoside diphosphatase).

A nucleoside phosphatase activity acting on inosine diphosphate (IDP) was apparently found by Torack and Barrnett to have a localization within rat pineal vessel walls similar to that described above for ATPase.[979]

3.6.1.a (Adenyl cyclase).

Adenyl cyclase catalyzes the conversion of ATP to cyclic 3′,5-AMP and inorganic pyrophosphate (Fig. 52). The only cofactor known to be required for this reaction in metazoan tissues is a divalent cation. Magnesium has been used most frequently as this ion since it is thought to be the natural cofactor.[851,852] Most of the adenyl cyclase in bovine pineal glands occurs in material sedimenting with mitochondria and heavy microsomes, in contrast with bovine pineal phosphodisterase (Table LXXXI). Adenyl cyclase activity of pineal homogenates declines rapidly during standing. The best tissue comparisons of adenyl cyclase activity have been obtained with rats, where postmortem time was minimal (within 30 seconds). Here, pineal adenyl cyclase activity has an intermediate rank in relation to that of various brain regions (Table LXXXII).

Recent research, especially by Weiss, Costa, and Crayton, on rats revealed for pineal adenyl cyclase an important role in the mechanism by which sympathetic fibers and norepinephrine (NE) regulate the biosynthesis of indoleamines. This has been discussed in the chapters on indole- and catecholamines. The factors that regulate pineal adenyl cyclase, and consequently the dependent metabolic and endocrine events, can be summarized. Pharmacologically active catecholamines can stimulate pineal adenyl cyclase activity acutely.[1040] This effect can be blocked by β-adrenergic blocking agents. Both neural and hormonal factors can produce chronic changes in the NE-activatable pineal adenyl cyclase system. This has been demonstrated in relation to three experimental situations. (a) NE-induced activation of pineal adenyl cyclase increases in strength during ontogeny, but the basal level of enzyme activity is unaltered. This increasing sensitivity to NE develops even when the sympathetic innervation has been abolished since the time of birth. (b) In adults, either chronic sympathectomy or long-term exposure to continuous light increases the responsiveness of the pineal adenyl cyclase system to NE. However, here too there is no change in the basal level of enzyme activity. (c) Estrogen administration to ovariectomized rats leads to inhibition of the NE-induced activation or stimulation of the pineal adenyl cyclase system. This leads to the proposal of a general endocrine model in which a hormone (estradiol) secreted by a peripheral and perhaps indirect pineal target organ (the ovary) has a feedback action on the adenyl cyclase and dependent biosynthetic activities of a more centrally located neuroendocrine organ, the pineal gland.[1035,1036,1039,1042-1044]

4. LYASES

4.1 Carbon-carbon lyases

4.1.1.15 *L-Glutamate 1-carboxy-lyase* (Glutamate decarboxylase).

This pyridoxal-dependent enzyme together with γ-aminobutyric acid (GABA) is in notable concentration in gray matter of the brain. The enzyme is lacking in pineal tissue, in keeping with the negligible pineal content of GABA.[14]

4.1.1.26 *3,4-Dihydroxy-L-phenylalanine carboxy-lase* (DOPA decarboxylase)

In the case of many tissue sources the substrate specificities and other characteristics of this enzyme overlap or are identical with those of the following enzyme (E.C. 4.1.1.28). They are, therefore, often lumped as "aromatic-L-amine acid decarboxylase". Inasmuch as these enzyme activities are not identical in some animals, and as there are some suggestions of differences within pineal samples, we will retain separate designations based on the use of DOPA as opposed to 5-HTP as substrate.

This enzyme is of a particular significance in the biosynthesis of various catecholamines as discussed and diagrammed (Fig. 46) in Chapter Eight. In comparison with thirty brain regions human pineal enzyme concentration was found to be exceeded only by that of putamen, caudate nucleus and mesencephalic reticular tegmentum, regions having relatively greater contents and presumed productivity of catecholamines.[568] However, human pineal content of DOPA-decarboxylase is reputedly much less than that found in pineal glands of some other species (Table LXXXIII). Variable reduction of pineal enzyme activity was found 2 to 3 weeks after bilateral superior cervical ganglionectomy. The species differences in the postsympathectomy decline in pineal enzyme activity suggested that in rat and rabbit the enzyme is mostly parenchymal in localization while in the cat it is mostly in pineal sympathetic fibers (Table LXXXI).[357]

TABLE LXXXIII

Pineal dopa decarboxylase activity according to species and the effects of bilateral superior cervical ganglionectomy.*

Species	Normal Mean ± Se	(N)	Ganglionectomized Mean ± Se	(N)
Rabbit	6460 ± 990	(14)	4610 ± 300	(5)
Rat	3790 ± 580	(11)	5240 ± 1150	(4)
Cat	580 ± 110	(8)	†140 ± 40	(6)
Pig	1990 ± 480	(8)	—	
Cow	1610 ± 380	(8)	—	
Man	30 ± 10	(6)	—	

* Results of Håkanson and Owman[357], expressed as CPM (1μg of ^{14}C-dopamine produced/hr = about 10,000 CPM).
† P for ganglionectomized vs normal < 0.001.

4.1.1.28   *5-Hydroxyl-L-tryptophan   carboxy-lyase*   (5-

Hydroxytryptophan decarboxylase, 5-HTPD) (see also
E.C. 4.1.1.26).

This enzyme activity figures prominently in pineal
biochemistry as that responsible for the synthesis of 5-HT
from 5-HTP (Fig. 31). It is, however, apparently not usually
rate-limiting since pineal 5-HT content can be markedly
increased in the presence of added 5-HTP, but not with added
tryptophan.[899] In rat tissues the highest recorded enzyme activity occurs in the pineal gland (12.96 μmoles 5-HT formed/
g/hr), with the next highest levels in liver (3.95 μmoles
5-HT/g/hr) and ileum (1.67 μmoles 5-HT/g/hr).[924] High
activities occur also in bovine and japanese quail pineal
glands, but at levels a little less than half of that in rat glands.[924]
Enzyme activity is not detectable in rat pineal glands within
12 hours after birth and is relatively low for the first 6 days.
It then rapidly increases with the attainment of adult concentrations by 20 or 40 days after birth.[425,1102] In thirty-three adult
human pineal glands 5-HTPD activity ranged from .0016 to
.328 μmoles 5-HT formed/g/hr (or 1.3 to 476.0 μmoles/pineal
gland/hr). This great individual variability could not be
explained, and it correlated neither with postmortem time
before tissue analysis nor with age of the subject (25–78
years).[705]

4.1.2.13 *Fructose-1,6-diphosphate   D-glyceraldehyde-3-phosphate lyase* (Fructose diphosphate aldolase).

This enzyme activity has been reported in lambs to be
present in pineal glands at the same level as in the
epithalamus and at a slightly lower level than in cerebral
cortex.[967,968]

4.2 Carbon-oxygen lyases

4.2.1.1 *Carbonate hydro-lyase* (Carbonic anhydrase CA).

Carbonic anhydrase has been measured in rat and human
pineal organs. In the former the very low enzyme content
and its circadian changes can be explained largely if not
entirely on the basis of the enzyme content of red blood cells
remaining in the tissue.[817-819] In the two human pineal glands
studied, carbonic anhydrase activity was less than that found

in all brain regions with the possible exception of those consisting of heavily myelinated white matter (corpus callosum and pyramid of the medulla).[689] The extremely low pineal activity is consistent with the endocrine function of the organ.[598,819]

4.2.1.2 *L-Malate hydro-lyase* (Fumarate hydratase, fumarase).

This enzyme was found in lamb pineal tissue at levels greater than those in cerebral cortex and epithalamus (approximate ratio of activity, respectively, 10:5:0).[967,968]

4.2.1.3 *Citrate (isocitrate) hydro-lyase* (Aconitate hydratase, aconitase).

Low concentrations of this enzyme activity were found in lamb pineal gland and cerebral cortex but not in the epithalamus.[968]

5. ISOMERASES

5.3 Intramolecular oxidoreductases

5.3.1.9 *D-Glucose-6-phosphate ketol-isomerase* (Glucose phosphate isomerase, phospho-hexose isomerase).

The lamb pineal is a rich source of this enzyme. The ratio of pineal : cerebral cortical : epithalamic tissue concentrations approximates 12:10:9.[967,968]

CONCLUSIONS

1. The very high relative levels of particular enzymes within pineal tissue from adult man and other mammals and the near pineal specificity of the melatonin-forming enzyme, hydroxyindole-*O*-methyltransferase, suggest that this organ has biochemical individuality and probably significant functional activity.

2. The primarily postnatal development and increase in at least several of the more important pineal enzymes in laboratory species and the slight if any decreases detectable in these with aging and calcification of the human pineal, suggest that pineal biochemical and probable functional activity, in whole or in part, extend from the time of maturation through

adulthood and possibly old age. There is no enzymatic evidence for a primarily fetal or juvenile period of pineal activity followed by waning or degeneration.

3. A number of different pineal enzymes follow circadian (24-hour) rhythms of remarkable amplitude. In the case of at least several of these the amplitudes, rapidity of response, and precision of timing are greater in the pineal gland than in other organs. Although metabolic interrelations and controls of these rhythms are in many cases still to be investigated, two or more are markedly and acutely influenced through cyclic 3′,5′-AMP, the production of the latter by adenyl cyclase, and the potent induction on stimulation of this enzyme by norepinephrine.

4. It is likely that eventually pineal cytochemical enzymology will provide important evidence concerning the derivation and phylogeny of the pineal-specific secretory cells, the pinealocytes. However, at the present time the evidence is still weak and ambiguous. Mammalian pinealocytes in their enzyme activities, particularly those active in monoamine biosynthesis, resemble neuronal and retinal cells more than neuroglia, ependyma or various cells of the mesodermal series, on the basis of available information. The enzymatic evidence for a nutritive relation of pineal neuroglial cell processes impinging on pinealocytes is consistent with either neuronal or photoreceptor evolutionary derivations for the mammalian pinealocytes.

5. Although great advances have been made in recent years in our knowledge of many pineal biosynthetic and metabolic acitvities, little is known about how these relate to the release of a secretory material, aside from the apparent release of melatonin. Enzymes involved in pineal protein synthesis and the control of such synthesis have been neglected.

Chapter Eleven

MITOCHONDRIA AND OXIDATIVE METABOLISM

MITOCHONDRIA

THE FOREGOING CHAPTERS concerned with pineal metabolites and enzymes serve to describe many of the components and detailed characteristics of pineal metabolic activities. Remaining to be described are some more general characteristics of pineal metabolism, which relate primarily to oxidative metabolic systems, but through less direct and less specific lines of evidence than we have been considering. Although chemically less specific and more difficult of interpretation these more general characteristics aid in a preliminary way in filling some gaps in our knowledge of pineal oxidative metabolism, particularly its peculiarities related to cell type and its changes with age and experimental manipulations.

Mitochondria are the cytoplasmic organelles which are the sites of energy production and transduction. The mitochondrial outer membrane controls the permeability of the organelle and has localized on it most of the enzymes of the citric acid cycle and some of the accessory oxidative enzymes, including the pyruvic dehydrogenase complex and the β-oxidation system for fatty acids. The mitochondrial inner membrane, and its attached particles, is the site of the enzymes in the electron transport series from NADH and succinate to molecular oxygen, and of oxidative phosphorylation. The elementary and attached particles are believed by some investigators to be concerned exclusively with electron transport, while the inner membrane proper

281

contains the dehydrogenases and enzymes involved in oxidative phosphorylation. The inner membrane along with its attached materials is involved with the generation of oxidative energy and its transduction into: (a) chemical energy, as in the form of ATP; (b) mechanical energy as demonstrated by mitochondrial contractions; or (c) osmotic energy, such as that responsible for the uptake into the mitochondrial matrix of various ions.

Pinealocytes typically contain numerous and structurally distinctive mitochondria. Even with the aid only of the light microscope early pineal cytologists generally recognized an abundance of rod-shaped to filamentous mitochondria within the perikaryal cytoplasm of pinealocytes.[146,201,416,432,446] Our knowledge of these has been greatly extended and made more precise by electron microscopy. However, caution must be maintained since among other peculiarities of pinealocyte mitochondria is a greater than usual osmotic sensitivity and tendency for artifactual changes with suboptimal fixation.[223] Nevertheless, all recent investigators agree that in diverse mammalian species, pinealocyte mitochondria are distinctive for their great size (to 4 μ in length in the rat),[206,347] polymorphism, variability in number and arrangement of cristae, and electron density or relative "staining" of the matrix and the (intracristal) spaces between the lamellae of the cristae.[24,37,223,345,471,575,638,730,1028,1056] Among mitochondrial shapes observed in pinealocytes of some species are: saccular, tubular, branched or ramified,[471] giant ("riesen-") and club-shaped ("keulenformiges").[346] Within the larger types the cristae are sometimes few and peripheral in location, numerous and transversely densely packed through the interior, or variable in number, arrangement and interlamellar distance within the cristae. Various mitochondrial inclusions have been described in pinealocytes, most often from adult or old rats. These include concentrically lamellated bodies,[524,638] clusters of osmiophilic granules within the matrix,[638] dense intracristal layers,[1056] and dense-cored microcylinders 270–330 Å wide and of indeterminate length.[562] Present evidence does not allow any chemical or metabolic correlations to be made with these variations in pinealocyte mitochondrial structure and content. However, on the basis of correlative structural and chemical studies made on mitochondria of other organs and cell types such correlations should be demonstrable in pinealocytes. The abundance, variety and morphological lability of pinealocyte mitochondria suggest that they may be especially informative in experimental studies on the relations of mitochondrial morphology and subunits to particular transport and enzymatic activities.

The relative volume of the rat pinealocytes' perikaryal cytoplasm occupied by mitochondria increases postnatally to attain a maximum at about four weeks (Fig. 57). The total mitochondrial mass per pinealocyte must continue to increase beyond this time since pinealocyte cell volume continues to increase

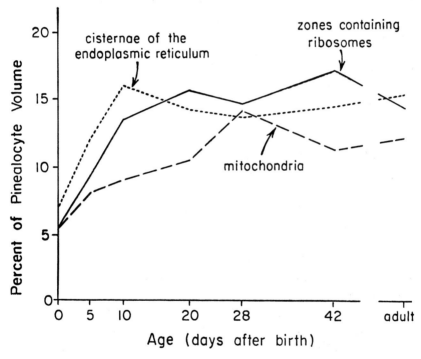

Figure 57. Postnatal changes in percent of rat pinealocyte perikaryal volume occupied by particular organelles, determined from electron photomicrographs by a stereological morphometric method. Volumes represented by Golgi apparatus and smooth vesicles in the cell bodies were generally represented as less than 5 percent and did not show a consistent change with age. (Modified from Bayerová and Malínský.[95])

greatly[825] while the relative mitochondrial volume remains about the same or decreases slightly. Succinic dehydrogenase, a mitochondrial enzyme, has been shown to increase in concentration or activity in rat pineal glands from one day to about 6 weeks after birth.[773]

Experimentally produced changes in pinealocyte mitochondrial numbers and characteristics have been reported for many decades,[873] but only since the use of electron microscopy do these reports seem worthy of attention. The more marked and frequent changes are described for the so-called light ("hellen") pinealocytes in contrast to the less numerous dark ("dunklen") pinealocytes which are variably interpreted as either a different cell type or as a different physiological phase of the former. The light pinealocytes differ from the dark ones not only in having a less electron dense cytoplasm but also in having commonly mitochondria of the long tubular type and endoplasmic reticula of the smooth variety. The dark cells have tubular mitochondria rarely and show richly granular endoplasmic reticula.[575] The mitochondrial volume fraction of rat pinealocyte perikarya measured from electron micrographs (Fig. 57) is similar to, or slightly greater than, that of the epithelial cells of the choroid plexus of the fourth ventricle. In a study of mitochondrial volume of fractions of diverse rat brain cells, Pysh and Khan have demonstrated a maximal mitochondrial volume in the latter cells and significantly lower (to 2–3% of perikaryal volume) volumes in neurons, neuroglia and ependyma from diverse brain regions.[757]

Numerical and structural changes in pinealocyte mitochondria have been described after various conditions or experimental treatments (Table LXXXIV). Increase in apparent or relative numbers of mitochondria is often associated with mitochondrial hypertrophy and increased polymorphism, possibly suggesting increased mitochondrial activity. However, in some conditions, when the treatment is prolonged or the dose extreme, as with norepinephrine or Niamid (20 mg/day, 8 days), the hypertrophy is accompanied by vacuolation and loss of cristae and swelling of the matrix. Regressive changes in pineal mitochondria are most clearly evident following

TABLE LXXXIV

Modifications *in vivo* of rodent* pinealocyte mitochondria as revealed by electron microscopy†.

Conditions or treatments	Structural changes†	References
Conditions increasing numbers of mitochondria:		
1. Pregnancy (guinea pigs at thirty days of gestation).	↑ Polymorphism, ↑ frequency of longitudinal cristae	575
2. Bilateral adrenal enucleation (one to sixty days).	↑ Size (to 5 μ long).	470
3. Estradiol implanted in median eminence (with ↑ in pituitary LH content).	↑ Polymorphism.	166
4. Norepinephrine, 50 mg/day, 5 days.	Lightening and dilation of	143
5. Niamid‡, 5 mg, twenty hours.	osmiophobic intracristal material.	143
Conditions causing structural but not (?) numerical changes:		
1. Immobilization stress + food and water deprivation, twenty-four hours.	Hypertrophy.	638
2. Hypophysectomy, ♂ s, fourteen days.	↑ Polymorphism and hypertrophy (to 1.5 × 5 μ) of mitochondria with clear matrix; ↑ relative number of mitochondria with dense (osmiophilic) matrix and clear intracristal compartment.	471
3. Ovariectomy, thirty to sixty days.	Possible hyper↑rophy.	166
4. Testosterone-induced (1.25 mg at four days) constant estrus.	Hypertrophy of some.	166
Conditions decreasing numbers of mitochondria:		
1. Continuous light.	Swelling + rarification and reduction in cristae.	165,358,359,575
guinea pigs, twenty-six to thirty-three days. rats, eighty days.		
2. Estradiol, systemic injections. 800 μg/kg/day, seven days.	↓ In size, with wrinkling of outer membrane and ↓ in matrix.	165,166

* = Rats except as noted otherwise.

† ↑ = Increase, ↓ = decrease.

‡ = A monoamine oxidase inhibitor, *N′isonicotinoyl-N²-[β(N-benzylcarbamoyl)-ethyl]-hydrazine.*

continuous light, a treatment that leads to marked decrease in pineal content of succinic dehydrogenase and some other mitochondrial enzyme systems.[131,781] The two other major categories of conditions studied, modification of the sympathetic system by stress, surgery or drugs, and modification of the endocrine-reproductive systems by pregnancy, surgery or hormones, give variable or contradictory results (Table LXXXIV). This is probably due to the variable and often extreme doses or conditions imposed and to variations in length of treatment and timing of the killing of the animal. In any case the available observations do not allow any sure or simple correlation between activity of either the sympathetico-adrenal system or the endocrine-reproductive system and pinealocyte mitochondrial activity.

OXIDATIVE METABOLISM

Oxygen uptake and oxidative metabolism of rat, goat and bovine pineal tissue has been studied in different ways and with often different objectives. The study on rat pineal respiration was concerned primarily with comparisons of pineal and choroid plexus in their O_2 uptake in the presence of particular metabolites and concentrations of inorganic ions.[780] Goat pineal respiration was investigated with a view toward revealing age changes in pineal metabolism of glucose and its conversion to various amino acids.[380] Bovine pineal respiration was examined in regard to relative oxidation of the C-1 and C-6 positions of glucose as an indicator of the relative activity of the hexose monophosphate pathway and of metabolism characteristic of endocrine glands.[520] Warburg respirometry of minced adult rat pineals by Quay showed succinate and glutamate to be the best substrates for pineal tissue and a quite different pattern for pineal and choroid plexus samples (Fig. 58). With glucose as exogenous substrate maximal respiration by both tissues was obtained with a Na:K ratio of 125 mmole: 19 mmole. In contrast with that of choroid plexus, pineal respiration was not modified by changes in concentrations of Ca, Mg, PO_4 or Cu^{++}.[777,780] It is not clear to what extent these latter differences are due to differences in rupture or permeability of plasma or other membrane systems. Hell-

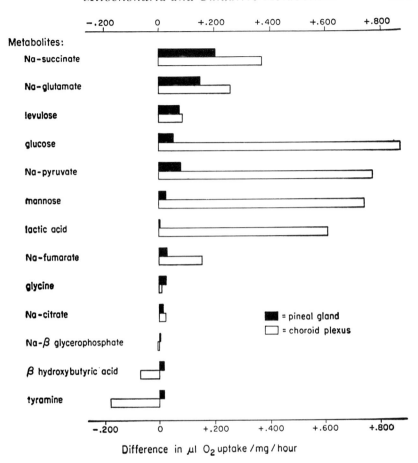

Figure 58. Respiration of rat pineal and choroid plexus (of ventricle IV) tissues in the presence of selected substrates and other metabolites. Results are given as the difference in O_2 uptake in comparison with simultaneous incubations in medium without added metabolite. (Modified from Quay.[780])

man and Larsson found relatively very high pineal O2 consumption as well as CO_2 and lactic acid formation from glucose in glands from young animals, and a gradual decline in these activities with age.[380] Marked age differences of the same nature were found in the pineal conversion of glucose to amino acids. These results have been discussed in detail in Chapter V. Bovine pineal conversion of 1-^{14}C label from glucose to [14]CO_2 *in vitro* was found by Krass and LaBella to be seven to twenty-four times as great as that of [6-^{14}C].

This high C-1:C-6 oxidation ratio of pineal tissue is similar to that found for all known endocrine glands and differs from that (1.0–1.4) characterizing brain. Total pineal glucose oxidation, both C-1 and C-6, and their ratios were lower in samples from adults (3–8 years) than in those from young (5–10 months) animals.[520]

Two kinds of experimental treatments have been described which modify pineal respiration. Both of these are matched by results discussed in the previous chapter concerning particular pineal enzymes and especially succinic dehydrogenase. Epinephrine (10^{-4} M *in vitro*) has been shown to increase pineal glucose oxidation at the C-1 position by 170 percent and at the C-6 position by 46 percent. Similar increases were obtained using glands from young and adult animals. Continuous light has been shown to suppress pineal oxidative metabolism. This is clear from the increase in pineal lactate noted by Nir *et al.*[684] and the decrease in pineal succinic dehydrogenase and other related enzymes studied by Quay[773,781] and Bostelmann.[131] Remaining less certain is whether continuous darkness has the opposite effect on pineal oxidative metabolism (cf. Bostelmann).[131] Fewer studies have been made following this procedure and the conditions (time of day, lighting, etc.) under which the control animals were maintained are often obscure. Comparisons of animals killed following continuous darkness with those killed during the morning of a normal daily photoperiod may be misleading, since pineal succinic dehydrogenase (Fig. 55) and perhaps related oxidative systems are maximal at night and low during the morning.

CONCLUSIONS

1. Mammalian pinealocyte mitochondria are notable for their relatively great number or concentration in the cytoplasm of the perikaryon, and for their polymorphism and frequently great size.

2. Sympathetic activation or sympathetomimetic treatments *in vivo* on a short term basis increase pinealocyte

mitochondrial numbers and/or size and epinephrine *in vitro* stimulates pineal glucose oxidation.

3. Pinealocyte mitochondrial volume and succinic dehydrogenase activity in the rat increase progressively from shortly after birth until four to six weeks later. In adulthood an appreciable decline in bovine and goat pineal oxidative metabolism occurs.

4. Continuous light decreases rodent pinealocyte mitochondrial numbers and cristae, and suppresses pineal oxidative metabolism as revealed by increased lactate and decreased succinic dehydrogenase and related enzymes.

5. Endocrine manipulations relating to regulation of the reproductive system have been reported to cause modifications in number and structure of pinealocyte mitochondria. However, the results are equivocal and inconsistent in terms of suggesting either stimulatory or inhibitory actions.

6. Possible stimulation of pineal oxidative enzymes by continuous darkness *in vivo* remains uncertain, since the control animals used for comparison were killed during the time of day when succinic dehydrogenase and probably related enzymes are normally near their daily minima in activity.

□ □

Chapter Twelve

SOLUBLE PROTEINS AND PEPTIDES

PROTEIN CONTENTS AND CELLULAR LOCALIZATIONS

AMONG A SMALL number of endocrinologists there has
been maintained over several decades an interest in
pineal peptides and soluble proteins as possible pineal
hormones.[108,109,246,247,274,623,970] Within the current decade
there is increasing interest in, and improving evidence for,
such pineal protein hormonal activity. Although the occurrence of pineal-specific proteins has been demonstrated, especially by electrophoresis, the correlation of any of these
with pineal-specific biological activities remains to be established. Biologically active pineal peptides and proteins are
on one hand not yet shown to be specific or peculiar to pineal
tissue. On the other hand, pineal peptide and protein fractions having distinctive activity are very imperfectly known
chemically. Despite these circumstances pineal homogenate
supernatant fractions and suspensions have been used
therapeutically for many years by a small number of physicians in Europe and the Americas. However, since the chemical composition of these agents is uncertain at best and since
their alleged clinical effects have not been sufficiently tested
to be accepted, we will not review all of the named pineal
therapeutic preparations. Nearly all of these have been prepared from bovine, ovine or porcine pineal glands. Available
published evidence suggests that in most cases they are
unstandardized mixtures of pineal materials including proteins, and that the methods used for their separation and
purification must in many cases have led to appreciable protein denaturation and hydrolysis.[274,472,820]

We are concerned in this chapter with the dynamic aspects of pineal protein synthesis and rhythmicity and with soluble pineal protein fractions and peptides that may possibly have hormonal or humoral activities or be precursors of molecules having such activities. Little will be presented on structural proteins. Light and electron microscopy suggest that mammalian pineal glands contain many of the structural proteins found in other organs, such as collagen and elastin, and the components of cytoplasmic membranes, microtubules, fibrils and filaments. Neither quantitative nor qualitative chemical studies are available concerning pineal structural and fibrous proteins.

Protein Content

Total protein contents of ungulate pineal glands have been estimated by Fenger[270] (Table LXXXV) and by Roux.[868] A protein content of 13.1 percent/wet weight given by the latter author for cattle pineal glands is probably not significantly different from Fenger's estimate for glands of the same species (Table LXXXV). Pineal total protein content thus derived from total nitrogen, and as reported in ungulates is at, or within the upper limit of protein content found for both gray and white matter of mammalian brain tissue.[864] However, recent and probably more accurate measurements of pineal protein in man and rat indicate that the pineal is at the other end of the scale. Comparative measurements of protein contents of human pineal glands and brain regions show the pineal gland

TABLE LXXXV

Total nitrogen and estimated protein contents (6.25 × N) of pineal glands.*

Species Months	Number of Glands	Total Nitrogen		Total Protein	
		/ Wet Wgt.	/ Dry Wgt.	/ Wet Wgt.	/ Dry Wgt.
Lambs					
Dec.-Jan.	5,062	1.80	13.7	11.2	85.6
Sheep					
Dec.-Jan.	1,348	1.88	13.4	11.7	84.0
Cattle					
Dec.-Jan.	1,458	1.98	13.3	12.3	83.2
March	886	1.77	13.2	11.0	82.6

* Data of Fenger[270]; results expressed as g/100g.

to be consistently the lowest, averaging 54.5 ± 3.2 mg/g fresh tissue. The range in mean protein concentrations in human brain regions was reported to be 67.7 ± 3.3 (frontal gray matter) to 103.0 ± 1.3 mg/g (putamen).[900] The daily range in rat pineal protein content (Fig. 59) lies within the order of magnitude found for human pineal protein content.

Pineal glands and many brain regions from human necropsies and biopsies contain α-albumin.[153] This protein shares antigenic properties with human serum albumin but has a lower mobility in agar gel electrophoresis. It has been proposed as an example of an easily diffusible protein, since it occurs in the leptomeninges surrounding structures rich in α-albumin, namely the olfactory bulbs and tracts and the pineal body. Its possible functional or pathological meaning is obscure. Roux has reported that albuminoid material has about the same concentration in pineal as in cerebral tissue.[868]

Cellular Localizations

Endocrine cells secreting a proteinaceous hormone usually contain microscopically visible secretion granules which are distinctive in structure as well as chemical composition. Mammalian pinealocytes contain cytoplasmic granules which may be of this nature. But their occurrence is variable, probably for technical reasons, and their significance and chemistry have not been elucidated.

Light microscopy of pineal tissue sections stained according to various histological procedures frequently shows many of the pinealocytes to have cytoplasmic chromophilia and others to be chromophobic and relatively empty appearing. It is probable that much of the pinealocyte's cytoplasmic protein is lost during treatment with many aqueous fixatives, subsequent washing and first steps of dehydration. Pinealocytes having cytoplasmic regions staining with acidic dyes such as orange G and aniline blue, have been observed by many authors.[304,375,766] However, the cloudy and finely granular character of the chromophilia of these acidophils is not readily correlated with any particular granules or intact cytoplasmic structures revealed by electron microscopy. Other pinealocytes having basophilic cytoplasmic granules

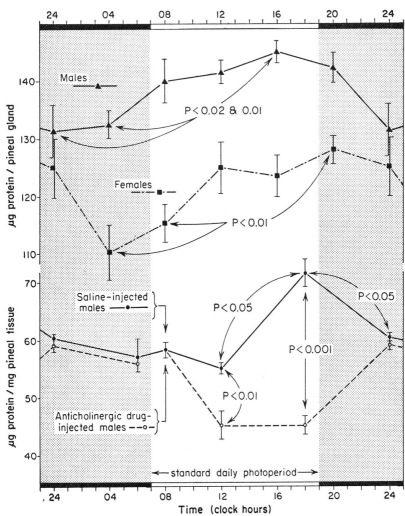

Figure 59. Circadian rhythms in protein content of adult rat pineal glands, as reported from two laboratories, animal strains and sets of circumstances. The upper two graphs, from Nir *et al.*[685], suggest a possible sexual difference in time of peak. The lower graphs, from Merritt and Sulkowski[618], demonstrate the inhibition of the daily peak by injection of an anticholinergic drug (N-methyl-3-piperidyl benzilate). Means ± standard errors are plotted.

are more easily pictured as secretory cells and their distinct cytoplasmic granules of larger size may possibly correspond to some of the larger dense—or variably cored vesicles or granules seen by electron microscopy. Pineal basophils have been known for many years,[173,189] but are most often observed, or are most heavily granular, in pineal organ and tissue cultures.[110,416,634] The distinctive cytoplasmic granules of these cells stain with the azure dyes and their relatives, as in May-Grünwald-Giemsa techniques, and with del Rio Hortega's silver carbonate and the aldehyde fuchsin methods.[786,810] Milcu and coworkers have reported that these cells in cultured rat pineal glands are the most active enzymatically.[634] Review of the light and electron microscopy of pineal basophils and similarly granular cells still leaves unanswered the question concerning the relation of some of these cells to granular neuroglial cells, such as observed by del Rio Hortega and more recent authors.[766,786] Nevertheless, electron microscopy of pineal glands of several mammalian species[429,636,730,903] and of a human pinealoma[644] usually show some of the pinealocytes to be characterized by the presence of large (1,100–10,000Å) dense granules in perikaryon and in pericapillary processes. The usual diameter of these granules apparently varies with species. They are larger and more variable than the dense-cored vesicles believed to contain NE and possibly other amines (see Chapter Eight). The best description of the probable secretion of material in these large granules into the perivascular space has been provided by Leonhardt[544] on the basis of reconstruction of the process as seen in electron micrographs of the rabbit pineal gland. In hamsters blinding leads eventually to an increase in the concentration of these large (1,000–1,200Å) granular vesicles in the pinealocytes.[901] This can probably be interpreted as representing a storage phase of pinealocyte secretory activity, since hamsters blind for 24 weeks or more have a rebound of the gonads to an apparently normal state after alleged suppression by the pineal gland during the early weeks of blindness.[160]

Smith *et al.* have shown in some rabbit pinealocytes granules about 1μ (10,000Å) in diameter which are autofluorescent.[915,916] They are increased in number under chronic treatment with *p*-chlorophenylalanine, thus presenting an opposite trend to that shown by the 5-HT-containing fluorescent cells in the same animals. The autofluorescent granules may possibly correspond to the large ones seen by electron microscopy. Smith has presented evidence that the autofluorescent pinealocyte granules may contain a pineal-specific and tryptophan-containing protein whose pineal concentration also increases under chronic treatment with *p*-chlorophenylalanine.[915]

PINEAL PROTEIN SYNTHESIS

Pineal synthesis of proteins has been studied by following changes *in vivo* and *in vitro* of particular enzymatic (protein) activities and *in vitro* of proteins labeled with radioactive precursor compounds. Only the second of these kinds of studies will be reviewed here, since the first has been covered in earlier Chapters (Seven, Eight and especially Ten). In both kinds of studies as applied to pineal tissue, protein breakdown and turnover rates have not been calculated.

Adult female rat pineal glands in organ culture have been shown to incorporate ^{14}C-tryptophan into proteins at an approximately constant rate for at least 48 hours. Large amounts of ^{14}C-methionine and ^{14}C-leucine were also incorporated with pineal protein during similar incubations. Total protein content of the pineal organs decreased during the incubations and any protein that might have been released into the culture medium was in too low a concentration for measurement. Nevertheless, Wurtman *et al.*[1090] in these studies were able to arrive at the tentative conclusion that rat pineal protein synthesis occurs at a relatively high rate; at least 0.1 μmole of ^{14}C-tryptophan per gram of tissue was incorporated into pineal protein per day. Moreover, the true rate of incorporation may have been considerably greater since their procedures did not include measurement of ^{14}C-labeled protein released or secreted into the culture medium. However, the relative amount of ^{14}C-tryptophan taken up into tissue proteins *in vitro* was about 1/40th of that converted to ^{14}C-5-HT, ^{14}C-melatonin and ^{14}C-5-HIAA.[1090]

Wurtman and colleagues also showed that norepinephrine (NE) stimulates the *in vitro* pineal synthesis of ^{14}C-protein from ^{14}C-tryptophan. It was believed that this stimulation involved an increased uptake of ^{14}C-tryptophan by the pinealocytes, because: (1) NE increased the intracellular content of ^{14}C-tryptophan as well as its conversion to protein and indoleamine derivatives; (2) NE did not enhance ^{14}C-protein synthesis in pineal glands which contained a previously established content of ^{14}C-tryptophan; and (3) NE did not stimulate ^{14}C-protein synthesis from ^{14}C-methionine or ^{14}C-leucine (Table LXXXVI). The possibility of there being a stimulatory effect of cyclic 3',5'-adenosine monophosphate (c-AMP) on this kind of pineal protein synthesis has not yet been explored. Comparisons with endocrine glands are suggestive of such a relationship. For example, c-AMP stimulates protein synthesis by adenohypophyseal polyribosomes.[10] However, it may be recalled from Chapter Seven and Figure 36, that NE's stimulation of pineal indoleamine synthesis is apparently not mediated by c-AMP in regard to stimulated tryptophan uptake, but is mediated by c-AMP in regard to

LXXXVI

Effects of catecholamines and indoles on synthesis of ^{14}C-protein from ^{14}C-tryptophan by adult female rat pineal glands in organ culture for 48 hours.[°]

Compounds	Concentrations Tested (Molarity)	Percent Difference From Controls	P[†]
Catecholamines:			
L-Norepinephrine	3×10^{-6}	+10	n.s.
	3×10^{-5}	+22	<0.05
	3×10^{-4}	+46→+123[‡]	<0.001
D-Norepinephrine	3×10^{-4}	+122[‡]	<0.001
L-Epinephrine	3×10^{-4}	+74	<0.05
Dopamine	3×10^{-4}	+208[‡]	<0.001
Indoles:			
5-Hydroxytryptamine	1×10^{-5}	+26	n.s.
	3×10^{-5}	−18	n.s.
	1×10^{-4}	−15	n.s.
Melatonin	3×10^{-5}	−13	n.s.
	1×10^{-4}	−30	n.s.
	3×10^{-4}	−10	n.s.
5-Hydroxyindole-3-acetic acid	3×10^{-4}	−12	n.s.

[°] Calculated from the data of Wurtman *et al.*[1090]

[†] Probability of significance of difference between means of experimental and control cultures within the same experiment; n.s. = not statistically significant.

[‡] P<0.05 in comparisons of dopamine mean with those of L- and D-norepinephrine.

increased levels or activities of tryptophan hydroxylase and N-acetyltransferase.

Pineal synthesis of glycoproteins has been studied also, using incubations 68 hours in length and protein incorporation of ^{3}H-L-fucose. This precursor is advantageous in such studies, since, unlike some other sugars, fucose is not transformed significantly into compounds other than glycoproteins. Polyacrylamide gel electrophoresis of pineal glycoproteins shows, as in brain, a heterogeneous array of compounds. The same is true of solubilized pineals which had been incubated with radioactive fucose.[570] The labeled glycoproteins in the glands were in the molecular weight range of 20,000–200,000. In contrast about 50 percent of the TCA-insoluble material in the media formed a single peak in electrophoretic separation and had a molecular weight of 30,000–50,000. The labeled material in both glands and culture medium could be degraded by pronase, but not by hyaluronidase, DNAase or RNAase; the lipid fraction was without radioactivity.[570]

Treatment of such cultures with NE had no effect on ^{3}H-L-fucose incorporation by glycoprotein fractions. However, when labeled N-acetylglucoseamine was used in other experiments, NE did increase the incorporation of this precursor into macromolecules (P < 0.001). In this case, no one glycoprotein product was involved. The stimulated increase in precursor uptake and incorporation was general among the group of glycoproteins.[758]

CIRCADIAN AND PHYSIOLOGICAL CHANGES

A circadian rhythm in adult male rat pineal protein content was demonstrated by Merritt and Sulkowski[618] and confirmed by Nir *et al.*[685] (Fig. 59). The latter workers showed also a similar rhythm in adult females, but with the peak shifted about four hours later in the evening. They also discovered that the rhythm in pineal protein was not detectable in young (21-day-old) females. In adults pineal protein content increased during the daily period of light to reach a peak in the late afternoon, or near the time of the start of darkness.

As noted in Chapter Nine (and Fig. 54), the peak in rat pineal protein content follows by two to four hours those in RNA content and nuclear and nucleolar size. This temporal relationship is what might be predicted on the basis of the relations of cytological changes and synthetic processes observed in other tissues and in other cell types active in protein synthesis. Circadian rhythms in rabbit pineal total protein, tryptophan-containing protein and relative fluorescence of tryptophan-containing protein have been demonstrated by Smith.[915] Two times were compared, 09:00 and 23:00 (photoperiod = 07:00–19:00. Significantly higher values for all three variables occurred in the samples taken at 23:00. In the absence of data for intermediate times, it is not clear whether or not the rabbit pineal's protein rhythms match those described in rats.

Three chemical agents have been shown to be able to modify pineal protein content or circadian rhythmicity. N-methyl-3-piperidyl benzilate (1 mg/kg ip) can block the rise in rat pineal protein content that normally occurs during the daily period of light (Fig. 59).[618] This drug has anticholinergic and psychogenic activity and has been interpreted as blocking central cholinergic synapses involved in EEG arousal. Inasmuch as the drug's blockade of pineal protein content occurs during the behaviorally relatively quiescent phase of the rat's daily rhythm, it is not all clear how the generalization of the drug's central mechanism of action is related to the pineal effect. Either acute or chronic administration of p-chlorophenylalanine (pCPA) to rabbits has been shown by Smith (1972) to lead to an increase in pineal morning content and relative fluorescence of tryptophan-containing protein (Fig. 60):[915] A single injection of 17 β-estradiol (10 μg) to 31-day-old female rats also caused an increase in pineal morning protein content (Table LXIV).[688] But clearly significant changes in pineal protein content have not yet been found in association with the phases of the rat's estrous cycle.[686] In the absence of information on the daily time course of changes in pineal protein content after either pCPA or estradiol, it is impossible to decide whether the morning difference observed is due to a shift in the timing of the circadian

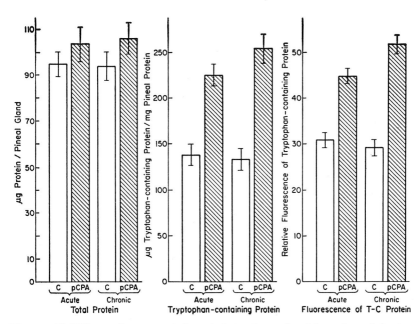

Figure 60. Effects of acute and chronic injections of p-chlorophenylalanine (pCPA) on adult male rabbit pineal total protein, tryptophan-containing protein and relative fluorescence of tryptophan-containing protein (adapted from Smith[915]).

Control (=C; Ringer saline) and pCPA (316 mg/kg) animals were injected i.p. at 09:00 either on one day (= acute) or daily for one to five days. All animals were killed 24 hours after the last injection (lights on 07:00–19:00).

peak or due instead, or as well, to a general increase in the pineal's basal or average content.

Light and heat are environmental factors that have been shown in chronic or extreme experiments to be capable of influencing pineal protein content. Both decreased it, possibly through actions as chronic stressers. Table LXXXVII shows that continuous (40 watt, "daylight" fluorescent) light led to a significant lessening of the increase in pineal RNA and protein concentrations during the post weaning growth of the organ. This deficit in pineal protein concentration is in addition to the deficit in pineal growth caused by continuous light and shown by earlier investigators.[276,775,776] Since the DNA concentration/pineal gland was not changed by continuous light in these experiments, the changes in RNA and

TABLE LXXXVII

Effects of continuous light (LL) and darkness (DD) on pineal RNA and protein contents of female rats starting at weaning (twenty-one days old).[*]

Constituent Treatment	Days of Exposure After Weaning			
	0	10	20	30
RNA				
LD (controls)	6.01 ± 0.27	9.27 ± 0.29	10.93 ± 0.34	11.93 ± 0.29
		$P<0.001$	$P<0.001$	$P<0.001$
LL	— —	7.53 ± 0.26	8.59 ± 0.26	9.43 ± 0.24
DD	— —	9.66 ± 0.33	11.17 ± 0.32	11.39 ± 0.43
Protein				
LD (controls)	68.4 ± 1.5	88.0 ± 2.3	112.7 ± 5.3	115.4 ± 3.2
		$P<0.001$	$P<0.01$	$P<0.01$
LL	— —	72.2 ± 2.5	92.3 ± 5.7	97.6 ± 2.6
DD	—٠—	90.8 ± 3.6	112.6 ± 3.0	107.8 ± 3.1

[*] Data of Nir *et al.*[983]; results expressed as mean $\pm$ standard error μg/pineal gland; $N = 20$ samples/group and with 6 pineals/sample.

protein concentration are attributable to changes in average concentration per pinealocyte. This is supported by cytophotometric results reviewed in Chapter Nine (cf. Table LXIII). On the other hand, continuous darkness did not affect significantly the DNA, RNA or protein contents of growing rat pineal glands (Table LXXXVII). In adult rabbit pineal glands, continuous darkness abolished the day-night difference in concentrations of total protein, tryptophan-containing protein and of the relative fluorescence of the tryptophan-containing protein.[915] After two weeks in continuous darkness, pineal total protein concentration remained within the confidence limits of the normal (LD) morning trough values, and the tryptophan-containing protein and its relative fluorescence remained within the limits of the normal (LD) nocuturnal peak values (Fig. 61). The desirability is apparent of more extensive and detailed investigation of the effects of light and darkness on different pineal soluble proteins or protein fractions.

Continuous exposure of maturing female rats to environmental temperatures of 32–34°C has been reported to cause a decrease in pineal RNA content by 20 days and then subsequently a decrease in pineal protein content by 30 days. Pineal weight and DNA content were not affected significantly.

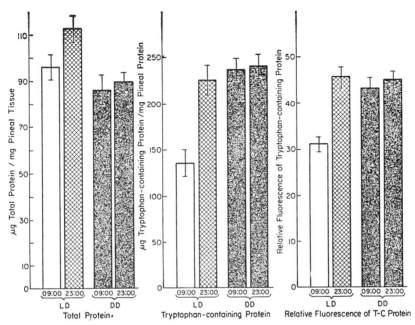

Figure 61. Day-night differences and the effects of continuous darkness (DD) for two weeks on adult male rabbit pineal concentrations of total protein, tryptophan-containing protein and relative fluorescence of tryptophan-containing protein (adapted from Smith[915]). The daily photoperiod for LD animals was 07:00–19:00.

PINEAL-SPECIFIC PROTEINS

The first experimental evidence of pineal-specific protein is probably that of Witebsky and Reichner (1933).[1055] Their comparative serological studies indicated that among bovine organs tested the pineal gland contained a serologically specific, heat labile and alcohol insoluble protein constituent. Additional serological or immunochemical studies on pineal components have not been made but would appear to pose important opportunities for future investigators, especially since the state, applications, sensitivity and significance of immunochemistry have been so greatly extended within the last twenty years.

Recent evidence for pineal-specific proteins is based largely on gel electrophoresis of supernatant or water soluble fractions from pineal homogenates. Microelectrophoresis of the supernatant from 1–1.5 mg tissue homogenates in 0.25M sucrose was employed by Pun and Lombrozo to separate stainable protein bands on polyacrylamide gel columns.[756] Seventeen bands stainable with Amido Black (Allied Chemicals) in 7.5 percent acetic acid were demonstrated from homogenates of twelve week old female rat pineal glands. Several of these (regions 4–7, Fig. 62) were not detectable in parallel simultaneously run columns containing supernatant fractions from whole brain and several brain regions. Separations of pineal proteins were reported by other laboratories at about the same time but without evidence for pineal specificity.[255,449]

In recent studies using rabbit pineal glands and brain regions, Smith has found apparently the same four pineal-specific bands (regions 4–7, Fig. 62) as described by Pun and Lombrozo.[915] He has furthermore discovered band 6 to be unique among the pineal protein bands and not to be duplicated in characteristics by bands electrophoretically

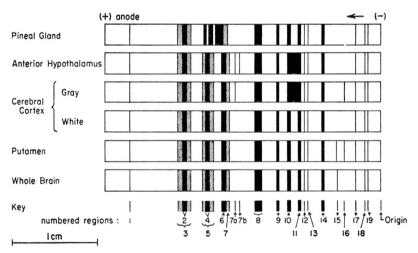

Figure 62. Diagrammatic map of protein bands separated by microelectrophoresis on polyacrylamide gel columns and stained with Amido Black (adapted from Pun and Lombrozo[756]). Pineal and brain fractions from twelve week old female rats were run in parallel with a constant current (0.5 ma). Pineal-specific protein bands occur in regions 4 through 7.

separated from pons, medulla oblongata, cerebral cortex, whole brain and blood plasma. Only band 6 reacted with staining methods for tryptophan and had autofluorescence (excitation maximum at 425 nm, emission maximum at 520 nm). This autofluorescence was believed to originate from the high tryptophan protein and to be the same as that observed in pinealocyte cytoplasmic granules measuring about 1 μ in diameter. It has not been ascertained whether this high tryptophan and autoflourescent band or fraction contains only one or whether it contains more than one protein. It will be recalled from the previous section that the rabbit pineal's content of this tryptophan-containing and auto-fluorescent protein is greater at night than during the day and is increased in relative amount by injections of *p*-chlorophenylalanine (pCPA). Three possible mechanisms can be suggested for the increased pineal-specific, tryptophan-containing protein following pCPA; other and less direct mechanisms are also possible. (1) By its inhibition of tryptophan hydroxylase and hence pineal synthesis of indoleamines, pCPA may allow a metabolic shunting of more tryptophan into protein synthesis. (2) Through a possible shifting of the circadian peak in pineal protein synthesis pCPA may give rise to the impression that increased tryptophan-containing protein is present during the morning or the usual time of analysis. (3) By means of causing changes in pineal contents and kinetics of 5-HT and NE and secondarily of c-AMP, pCPA may affect tryptophan uptake, synthesis or other processes (cf. Fig. 36) favoring either increased content of the tryptophan-containing protein or a temporal expansion of the circadian peak in the pineal's content of this protein.

PHYSIOLOGICALLY ACTIVE PINEAL PEPTIDES AND PROTEIN FRACTIONS

We are concerned here with evidence that particular biological or physiological effects obtained by administering pineal extracts or fractions to man and other mammals are due to pineal peptides or protein fractions. These physiologically active pineal peptides and proteins can be postulated to have

one or more of the following origins and tissue relationships:
(1) Biosynthesis in other organs in addition to the pineal gland
and with either true hormonal activity or pharmacological
effects when administered. (2) Biosynthesis in other organs
than the pineal gland with secondary uptake, modification
and/or storage in pineal tissue and with probable humoral
or hormonal activity. (3) Biosynthesis only in the pineal gland
and possession of a unique hormonal role or effect. Of these
three categories, the first still cannot be excluded for most
of the pineal's biologically active materials as studied by not-
ing effects of injections of homogenates, extracts, or partially
purified fractions of pineal tissue. The second category is
suggested here as a real possibility on the basis of the confus-
ing and conflicting reports of pineal contents of neurohypophyseal hormonal principles or peptides and biological activities. The third possibility, which alone would confer
credibility on hypotheses for a true pineal peptide or protein
hormone, remains open for necessarily rigorous research and
evaluation.

Antigonadotropic Pineal Constituents

The most frequently studied type of biological action of
pineal extracts and chemical constituents is that which is often characterized as being *antigonadotropic*. However,
opposite, or progonadotropic effects are sometimes claimed
for administered pineal materials. Moreover, the tissue target
of presumptive hormonal activity is variously interpreted as
being higher brain centers, hypothalamus, pituitary gland,
gonads, and, possibly as well, regulators of circulating levels
of gonadal hormones, such as the liver.

Two chemical categories of pineal compounds have been
shown to affect the reproductive organs, 5-methoxyindoles
(see Chapter Seven) and peptides or protein fractions. Table
LXXXVIII summarizes the pineal tissue preparations and constituents that affect in assay systems the reproductive organs.
Within the category of antigonadotropic materials, there are
two or more pineal peptidic compounds. These have been
partially purified and are free of methoxyindoles. At least
one of them has antigonadotropic potency greater than that

TABLE LXXXVIII

Characteristics of anti- and progonadotropic pineal extracts, protein fractions and peptides tested in mammals.

Action Type of preparation or constituent	Characterization	References
I. Antigonadotropic (usually in adults)		
A. Aqueous extracts, usually of acetone-dried or lyophilized pineals.	?	88,114,115,174,248,439,491, 621,660,663,679,884,933, 1004,1005,1017,1070.
B. Supernatant from TCA ppt extract.	?	839.

C. Fraction "F₃" in Sephadex G25
(0.2 M pyridine, 0.05 M acetic acid, pH 5.9)
  1. Paper chromatography gives 2 active materials.
  2. Paper chromatography and electrophoresis at 2 pHs.
	? Peptide(s)
	(≠ D).
	Peptides.
	Peptide(s).
		231,232,970–972.
		229,662.
		966.

D. Isolated and identified compound.	Arginine vasotocin (Fig. 63).	155,156,633,721.
E. Separation in Sephadex G25 and partially purified from bovine and human pineal glands.	Fraction or peptide (?) of MW 500–1000; activity > melatonin.	101,103,115,918,919.
II. Progonadotropic (usually in young)		
A. Aqueous extracts usually of acetone-dried or lyophilized bovine pineals.	?	115,543,679
B. TCA insoluble ppt from extracts.	?	839.
C. Fraction "F₂" in Sephadex G25 (0.2 M pyridine, 0.05 M acetic acid, pH 5.9).	Peptide(s).	229,231,232,662.

of melatonin. According to Moszkowska and Ebels, their fraction F_3 peptide (I.C.-Table LXXXVIII) is not arginine vasotocin (I.D.-Table LXXXVIII), since it acts on anterior hypophyseal secretory activity whereas arginine vasotocin apparently does not and acts instead on the gonads or on the gonadotropic hormone(s).[664] It may be noted too that there is no evidence as yet that differentiates the antigonadotropic peptide fraction (I.E.-Table LXXXVIII) of Benson and co-workers from arginine vasotocin (I.D.-Table LXXXVIII). The occurrence of arginine vasotocin (Fig. 63) in bovine pineal glands and demonstration of its antigonadotropic activity were first reported by Milcu and Pavel and their co-workers at Bucharest.[633,721,722] Although the occurrence of this compound in bovine pineal glands has been disputed,[234] it has been convincingly confirmed by Chessman's analytical chemical studies.[155] However, the compound is present in bovine pineal tissue at only extremely low concentrations and the ability of pineal glands to synthesize it has not yet been shown. Arginine vasotocin has been identified in human cerebrospinal fluid,[720] and it is conceivable that the pineal's content of this compound may be secondary, by means of uptake from either or both cerebrospinal fluid and blood. However, arginine vasotocin is generally considered to be a neurohypophyseal product only in submammalian vertebrates and to be evolutionarily replaced here in mammals by arginine vasopressin.[888,889] Indirect evidence for the possibility of pineal uptake of this compound can include the recently described pineal uptake *in vivo* of the related hypothalamic MSH-release-inhibiting peptides (Fig. 63).[673] Neither the primary nor secondary occurrences of arginine vasotocin and related compounds in pineal tissue improve the confused state of knowledge concerning the specificity and chemical sources of the biological or pharmacological activities reported for pineal extracts. Arginine vasotocin and related compounds have significant actions in a wide variety of bioassay systems (Table LXXXIX).

Comparatively little is known about the chemical nature of pineal progonadotropic materials. While a peptide or proteinaceous nature is likely, there are no analytical studies

A. VASOPRESSOR – ANTIDIURETIC PEPTIDES

I. Arginine Vasotocin (Bovine Pineal and Submammalian Neurohypophysis)

CyS – Tyr – *Ileu* – Glu(NH$_2$) – Asp(NH$_2$) – CyS – Pro – *Arg* – Gly(NH$_2$)

   I   2   3   4   5   6   7   8   9

2. Lysine Vasotocin (Pig Pineal)

CyS – Tyr – *Ileu* – Glu(NH$_2$) – Asp(NH$_2$) – CyS – Pro – *Lys* – Gly(NH$_2$)

3. Arginine Vasopressin (or Antidiuretic Hormone, ADH, of Human and Most Mammalian Neurohypophyses)

CyS – Tyr – *Phe* – Glu(NH$_2$) – Asp(NH$_2$) – CyS – Pro – *Arg* – Gly(NH$_2$)

4. Lysine Vasopressin (Pig Neurohypophysial Vasopressin)

CyS – Tyr – *Phe* – Glu(NH$_2$) – Asp(NH$_2$) – CyS – Pro – *Lys* – Gly(NH$_2$)

B. OXYTOCIN – LIKE PEPTIDES

I. Oxytocin (Neurohypophysis from Fish to Man)

CyS – Tyr – *Ileu* – Glu(NH$_2$) – Asp(NH$_2$) – CyS – Pro – *Leu* – Gly(NH$_2$)

C. MSH – RELEASE – INHIBITING PEPTIDES (of Bovine Hypothalamus and Taken Up *in Vivo* by Rat Pineal Glands)

I. MIF – I

H – Pro – *Leu* – Gly(NH$_2$)

2. MIF – II

H – Pro – *His* – *Phe* – *Arg* – Gly(NH$_2$)

Figure 63. Amino acid structures of peptides found in, or taken up by, mammalian pineal glands, and comparisons with related hypothalamo-neurohypophyseal hormones. Italicized amino acids are the ones differing within this series of closely related compounds. Adapted from references 155, 673, 718, 888 and 889.

extending the preliminary findings of Ebels and Moszkowska (Table LXXXVIII).

Antidiuretic Activity

Antidiuretic and sodium-retaining activities have been reported for pineal extracts and chemical constituents at various times. In Chapter Seven we reviewed indole derivatives that have been claimed to have the latter activity, reputedly or possibly through adrenoglomerulotropic or related actions.

TABLE LXXXIX

Structure-activity relationships of pineal and neurohypophyseal peptides in some standard bioassay systems.*

Compound†	Potency (units/mg peptide)	Potency Relative to Oxytocic Activity						
		Rat Uterus (0.5mM Mg)	Milk Ejection	Avian Depressor	Rat Blood Pressure	Rat Antidiuresis	Frog Bladder	Frog Natriferic
Oxytocin	360	86	100	100	1.9	1.1	100	100
Arginine Vasotocin	37	192	297	—	177	177	19500	1470
Lysine Vasotocin	20	—	275	269	196	91	1250	1300
Arginine Vasopressin	9	165	566	466	3330	3330	780	100
Lysine Vasopressin	5	255	680	560	4000	—	<100	160

* Extracted from Heller.[379]

† Amino acid structures shown in **Figure 63.**

In the present section we wish to consider pineal antidiuretic activity of a possibly peptidic origin. The tentative suggestion here of a peptide as the agent bearing this activity is based on the demonstration of both lysine vasotocin[718] and arginine vasotocin (Table LXXXVIII) in mammalian pineal glands, and the well known antidiuretic activity of these compounds (Table LXXXIX). König and Meyer have found an antidiuretic activity in adult male rat pineal glands which follows a circadian rhythm and which is abolished by four weeks of continuous light (Fig. 64).[511,512] Antidiuretic activity of pineal extracts was tested on rats under alcohol narcosis and satiated with water. Synthetic lysine vasopressin (Sandoz) served as a reference standard. But it is not known which if any of the peptides of this series (Fig. 63) were responsible for the pineal activity. It should be recognized also that antidiuretic activity can be found in mammalian brain regions well separated from the pineal and from the usually considered hypothalamo-neurohypophyseal centers containing antidiuretic hormone and related compounds.[981]

Natriuretic Activity

Pavel has reported that a purified bovine pineal peptide and synthetic arginine vasotocin (Fig. 63) similarly caused in mice cytological changes in the adrenal zona glomerulosa suggesting decreased activity along with natriuresis.[719] There is no evidence as yet that this represents a normal physiological action of a pineal peptide such as arginine vasotocin, but there have been diverse experimental attempts to show the presence in the pineal region of both stimulatory and inhibitory activities on the zona glomerulosa and sodium retention.[140,265,516,712]

Lipolytic and Melanotropic Activities

Rudman and co-workers have purified and studied from ovine and bovine pineal glands and other tissues peptides having lipolytic and melanotropic activities.[870] Lipolytic (fat mobilizing) activity was assayed *in vitro* with rabbit perirenal adipose tissue, and melanotropic (melanocyte-expanding, skin-darkening) activity was measured *in vitro*

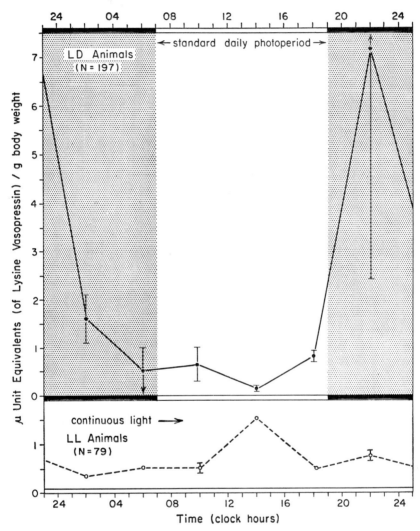

Figure 64. Circadian rhythm in the antidiuretic activity of male rat pineal glands and the effects of continuous light for four weeks. (Modified from König and Meyer.[512])

with frog (*Rana pipiens*) skin samples according to the method of Lerner and Wright.[552] From ovine and bovine pineals, peptides having both activities and similar or identical properties were obtained.[871] The similarities pertained to electropho-

TABLE XC

Amino acid compositions of pineal peptide fractions
having lipolytic and melanotropic activities.[*]

Amino Acid[†]	Ovine Pineal Fractions		Bovine Pineal	
	"21"	"24"	"15-A"	"15-B"
Glycine	101	112	110	93
Arginine	62	71	50	54
Lysine	141	152	127	131
Proline	70	76	50	55
Aspartic Acid	76	70	98	88
Glutamic Acid	138	121	135	141
Isoleucine	18	13	21	23
Tyrosine	13	9	10	10
Half-cystine	48	53	31	36
Threonine	33	42	42	38
Serine	67	62	83	89
Alanine	81	91	83	86
Valine	29	31	46	50
Methionine	10	11	8	9
Leucine	68	51	64	54
Phenylalanine	22	19	20	24
Histidine	23	16	22	19
Tryptophan	0	0	0	0

[*] From Rudman *et al.*[871] Data expressed as moles/1000 moles amino acid.
[†] Amino acids above the dashed line are those found also in arginine or lysine vasotocins.

retic mobility, molecular weight (1000–3500), lipolytic and melanotropic potencies (10–80 percent of those of ACTH) and amino acid composition (Table XC). From their most recent study these investigators report the presence of at least two different lipolytic-melanotropic peptides in bovine pineal glands on the basis of species differences in the lipolytic response to the peptides. One of these pineal peptides has a similar or identical counterpart in the choroid plexus. It has a molecular weight of about two thousand and has about nineteen amino acid residues.[872] The size and composition of these pineal peptides suggest that they are not identical with other pineal peptides that we have discussed and for which we have information either on molecular weight or on amino acid composition. There is no reason to believe at this time that the pineal peptides having lipolytic and melanotropic activities are necessarily hormonal in nature. Tissue specificity in origin and chemical specificity of action are apparently low, or at least shared by other brain structures and hypothalamo-hypophyseal compounds respectively.

Hepatic and Metabolic Effects

Milcou and colleagues in Bucharest have proposed that the mammalian pineal gland secretes a polypeptide ("pinealin"), which is a potent and specific hypoglycemic agent or hormone.[623-625] Melatonin tested in the same way (0.6 µg subcutaneously to rabbits) had no such effect.[630] The pineal polypeptide was thought to act synergistically with insulin and to be able to provide protection to the pancreatic β-cells of animals treated with alloxan. The interested reader can refer either to a brief review of this work[807] or to a bibliography of Milcu's papers[28] for further information. There is apparently very little information available concerning the chemical nature of this pineal fraction or polypeptide.

Neurological and Behavioral Effects

Pineal extracts of poorly known composition, and variously named "epiphysormone", "epiglandol" and "epiphysan", have been used in attempted therapy of diverse mental diseases, and most frequently of schizophrenia. Kitay and Altschule have provided a concise tabulation of the reports concerning these early, and generally inconclusive, experiences.[490] Recent investigations on possible neurological and behavioral effects of the pineal gland have been concerned more with either the changes following pinealectomy in laboratory species or those attending administration of pineal indole derivatives (see Chapter Seven) to man as well as other species.

However, in former years Altschule studied the short-term results of bovine pineal extracts and extract fractions of various sorts administered to psychotic patients.[19,21] Preliminary evidence suggested the possibility of improvement in cases of schizophrenia and affective disorders. The active agent in the extracts was found to be not related to pineal constituents inducing blanching in amphibian skin. It was believed to be a peptide having a molecular weight of about 1000. Regrettably, little has been published concerning its chemistry. Some of the clinical effects of the bovine pineal extracts could be elicited also by extracts of whole brain without the pineal gland, but at one tenth to one fifth of the concentration or activity level found in pineal preparations.[20] A further and very carefully designed study, also at McLean Hospital, compared over a period of eight weeks the effects of Altschule's pineal extract and a placebo in eight chronic schizophrenic women (4 per group). One measure, the Lorr Psychiatric Scale score, was thought to suggest a small but statistically significant ($P \leq 0.05$) improvement associated with injections of pineal extract. However, the results are far from conclusive and their marginal statistical significance is weakened if probability evaluations encompass group comparisons at various test intervals and not just those showing the greatest mean differences.[240]

CONCLUSIONS

1. Pineal tissue protein concentration in man and other mammals is lower than that of brain regions but recent studies suggest that adult pineal protein synthesis is active and involves compounds that are pineal-specific and others that have demonstrable actions *in vitro* or *in vivo*.

2. *In vitro* synthesis of protein by rat pineal glands has been demonstrated by the incorporation into pineal proteins of radioactively labeled tryptophan, methionine and leucine, and into pineal glycoproteins of labeled fucose. Norepinephrine stimulates pineal synthesis of ^{14}C-protein from ^{14}C-tryptophan *in vitro* through stimulation of pinealocyte uptake of tryptophan.

3. Pineal total protein concentration follows a circadian rhythm in the adult laboratory rat, the level rising during the period of light and falling during the early or mid portions of the period of darkness. The daily rise in pineal protein can be blocked by an anticholinergic drug.

4. At least four pineal specific proteins or protein fractions

are demonstrable in rat and rabbit glands by electrophoresis. One of these bands, as studied in rabbits, is unique among pineal and brain proteins for its high tryptophan content and its autofluorescence. It also appears to be localized in large (near 1 μ diameter) cytoplasmic granules of certain of the pinealocytes, to follow a circadian rhythm dependent on environmental light-dark cycling, and to be increased by administration of p-chlorophenylalanine.

5. Effects of administered pineal protein fractions and peptides have been studied most frequently in relation to an often proposed pineal hormonal regulation of the activity of the reproductive organs. Two or more antigonadotropic peptides and perhaps one or more progonadotropic peptides can be identified in pineal tissue, but the pineal-specificity of these, as well as their potency, is low or open to critical evaluation.

6. Antigonadotropic, antidiuretic and perhaps certain other biological activities of bovine pineal extracts can be attributed to the proven but low pineal concentration of 8-arginine vasotocin. Porcine pineal glands contain the related peptide, 8-lysine vasotocin. A circadian rhythm in rat pineal content of antidiuretic materials has been shown and presumably depends on daily changes in pineal uptake and/or synthesis of these and perhaps related peptides. The nocturnal rise in pineal antidiuretic activity is abolished by continuous light.

7. Experimental evidence of varying quality suggests that pineal peptides or polypeptides may have lipolytic, melanotropic, hepatic, metabolic, neurologic and behavioral effects. But evidence for either pineal-specificity or hormonal action being involved in any of these actions is in part incomplete and in part negative.

8. The incompleteness, and often discouraging status, of evidence for pineal peptide or protein hormones should not dissuade further investigation. The evidence for pineal-specific peptides or proteins and an active protein synthesis, coupled with greatly improved methods of analysis both of chemical compositions and biological activities, provides a basis for rational encouragement of research on this subject.

Chapter Thirteen

MISCELLANEOUS COMPOUNDS AND PIGMENTS

MISCELLANEOUS COMPOUNDS

Ubiquinone

UBIQUINONE OR COENZYME Q (Fig. 65) is a member of a family of terpenoid quinones associated with the energy-transducing system of cells, especially in chloroplasts and mitochondria.[181] It is not surprising, therefore, that it is widely distributed among metabolically active tissues. Ubiquinone 10 (coenzyme Q_{10}) is the member compound found in diverse cell types of man and other investigated mammalian species. But in tissues of the laboratory rat, ubiquinone 9 (coenzyme Q_9) is found as well.[180] These and other ubiquinones differ only in the number of replicated segments in the side chain (Fig. 65).

Pineal content of ubiquinone was appreciated first in relation to its inhibitory effect on biosynthesis of aldosterone.[1095] This pineal lipid-soluble constituent which had been found to inhibit aldosterone secretion was thought by Fabre and co-workers to be largely responsible for this effect. They also succeeded in isolating ubiquinone from beef pineal glands (1 mg/5 kg tissue).[253] The comparatively moderate pineal level of ubiquinone has been confirmed by a histochemical study, which showed a uniform distribution of the compound through the mouse pineal gland.[382]

Some interesting but enigmatic studies on photoperiodic control of activities of a malaria parasite (*Plasmodium berghei*) in mouse blood suggest that the pineal organ may have an effect, perhaps indirectly, on blood values of ubiquinone and

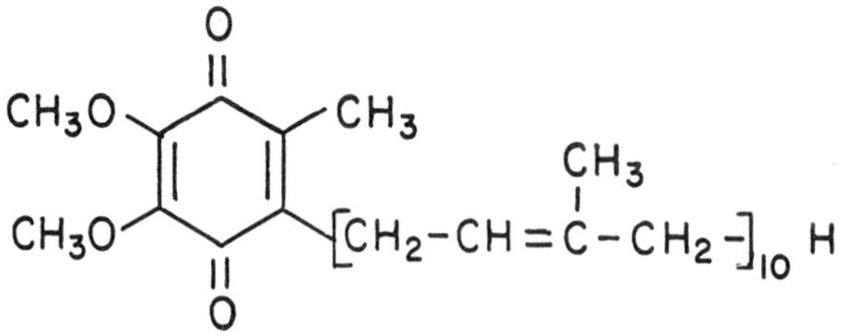

$$CH_3O \quad \overset{O}{\underset{\|}{C}} \quad CH_3$$

$$CH_3O \quad \overset{\|}{\underset{O}{C}} \quad \overset{CH_3}{\underset{|}{[CH_2-CH=C-CH_2-]_{10}}} H$$

Figure 65. Structure of ubiquinone 10 (= coenzyme Q_{10}).

related compounds. Such an effect seems unlikely to be due to a release of ubiquinone by the pineal gland, but it may possibly be due to a pineal action eventually affecting liver and blood chemistry. Arnold and co-workers have shown that pinealectomy abolishes the photoperiodic synchronous behavior of the malaria parasites.[35] The augmented synchrony typical of intact animals could be restored in pinealectomized animals by administration of ubiquinone, or of members of the chemically related vitamin K series, or partly of α-tocopherol. This chemical restoration of the parasites' synchronous behavior required the continued exposure of the pinealectomized host mice to an appropriate environmental photoperiodic rhythm.[36] Diets deficient in vitamins K or E had the same result as pinealectomy. Investigation of possible pineal effects on uptake, transport and storage of ubiquinone seems desirable. Orally administered ubiquinone is transported by lymphatics to the liver where it is primarily stored. Excretion of the mostly unaltered compound in feces is largely by way of the liver's biliary secretion.[303]

Other Compounds and Substances

The presence of vitamins or closely related compounds in pineal tissue has been discussed already in connection with evidence for ascorbic acid (vitamin C, Chapter Five) and ubiquinone (vitamins E and K, preceding paragraph). Remaining to be mentioned is an early reference to pineal thiamine (vitamin B_1) content. Extraction of cow pineal glands and assay with yeast suggested a pineal potency or concentration somewhat higher than that of the pituitary gland.[954] This is to be expected since thiamine pyrophosphate is a nearly ubiquitous coenzyme in living systems.

Porphyrins are probably not present at appreciable levels in pineal tissue of adult mammals since the characteristic fluorescence of these compounds could not be detected.[507]

Amyloid bodies and amyloid-like plaques have been described and figured in human pineal glands of advanced age.[560,748] In some instances the formations microscopically resemble corpora amylacea, but in the absence of chemical or ultrastructural descriptions, little of significance can be said about them. These materials have been reported rarely in laboratory or domestic animals. A microscopic and histochemical study has been made of them in an orangutan (*Pongo pygmaeus*) pineal gland and associated cerebral structures.[813]

PIGMENTS

Three classes of pigments have been noted in human and mammalian pineal glands, melanin, iron-containing pigment (probably mostly hemosiderin) and lipoprotein (lipofuscin) pigment (Table XCI). The occurrences of all of these vary greatly on an individual basis as well as by species. There is little if any reason to believe that these variations have any pineal-specific functional significance in mammals.

Melanins

Melanin pigments are variably present in the connective tissue and leptomeningeal tissues of the pineal capsule and interlobular septa. Microscopic cytochemical studies have been published concerning them in man[94,408,694,763] and other mammalian species.[622,804,810,882] In addition to cytochemical tests (Table XCI) there are available chemical tests appropriate for identifying these pigments.[349] With electron microscopy the characteristic structures, melanosomes, usually containing the pigment, can be identified. This has been done in an ultrastructural study of the developing human pineal gland.[413] Melanosomes were found in the periphery of the pineal organ

Pineal Chemistry

TABLE XCI

Comparisons of cytochemical reactions of yellowish brown to black pigments sometimes found in mammalian pineal glands*

Test*	Pigment Class		
	Melanins	Hemosiderin	Lipofuscins
Blackening in acidic silver nitrate solution	++	0	0
Blackening in ammoniacal silver solution	++	0	0→(+)v
Staining for iron (Perl's prussian blue reaction)	0	+	0
Schmorl reaction	+++	0	(+)→+v
Basophilia	++	0→(+)	0→+
Bleaching (H$_2$O$_2$)		0	0→+
Periodic acid-Schiff	(+)→+v	0	0→++v
Lipid staining	0	0	(+)→+v
Fluorescence	0	0	++
Chrome alum hematoxylin	0	0	0→++

* For further information see references 724 and 1059.
Reaction results are characterized as: 0 = negative, (+) = weakly positive, + = moderately to strongly positive, v = variability in reaction within the same pigment deposit.

of an embryo of 150 days, confirming an earlier but equivalent finding from light microscopy.[993]

Attempts have been made to correlate pineal melanization in domestic mammals and in man with age, sex and reproductive state.[761,763,881] However, none of these is convincing. There are no quantitative treatments of the data and the latter are drawn from heterogeneous populations of unknown composition in terms of melanization in other parts of the body as well as other characteristics. In the course of examining thousands of rat pineal glands over the last two decades, I have found pineal melanization to be erratic in individuals from various pigmented strains. This is probably no different from what has been described for the occasional pigmentation of other endocrine glands in the same species.[9] Furthermore, there is no evidence of functional or metabolic differences in the rat pineal gland correlated with either pineal or general body pigmentation. For many years personal studies on pineal composition and physiology purposely employed a strain of rats in which different degrees of pigmentation were maintained by selective breeding, from albino to hooded and solidly colored (agouti brown and black) types. In various studies results from selected or matched groups differing in pigmentation failed to suggest any correlated differences in pineal composition or level of activity. The only conceivable difference of this sort that can be supported at this time is related to the greater photosensitivity or photophobia of albino as compared with pigmented animals. This can be a source of interference or variation in experiments on the effects of the pineal gland on behavioral responses to light.[795a]

The region of the pineal complex of organs in some lower vertebrate animals, from lampreys to reptiles, occasionally shows a distinctive distribution of melanin pigment, suggesting selective interference or transmission of environmental light. These distinctive patterns of melanization in and about the pineal complex are usually consistent within a species or larger group of related animals. In no avian or mammalian species, however, has any such consistent pattern of pigmentation been observed in the pineal region. Personal experience with variable pigmentation in and around human, ungulate and rodent pineal organs supports this negative conclusion. Pineal-related patterns of modified pigmentation in lower vertebrates can probably be attributed to adaptations enhancing control of incident irradiation on the photosensory cells of the organ. As noted earlier, mammalian pineal glands lack photosensory cells.

Hemosiderin

Human pineal glands of adult or older age sometimes have iron-rich interlobular pigmented cells.[134,941] These are probably macrophages and their pigment is probably mostly hemosiderin, resulting from the phagocytosis and destruction of extravasated red blood cells. Increased iron pigment deposits occur in the human pineal gland as well as in a wide variety of other organs in cases of hemochromatosis.[941] There is no reason to believe at this time that pineal occurrences of hemosiderin-laden cells relate to any specifically pineal peculiarity or pathology. Nevertheless, in the central nervous system regional differences and pathological correlations have been observed or suggested.[351,362,579,941,944] Comparisons with pineal involvement are essentially nonexistent.

Lipofuscins

Lipofuscins are complex products from the peroxidation of unsaturated lipid, usually combined with protein. Darkness of color and characteristics of solubility and of chemical and staining reactions change with the aging and progressive oxidation of the material.[724,749] Granules of yellow to brown lipofuscin pigment have been found in almost all organs and tissues of man and other mammals. In most of these, there is an increasing prevalence and amount with age. In some instances, altered nutrition (vitamin E deficiency) or pathological conditions are suggested inducing or contributing factors[749] Pineal lipofuscin has been described most frequently among mammals in ungulates and primates, especially by pathologists writing during the first third of this century. Bargmann's monograph on pineal structure and pathology can serve as entrance to this early descriptive and fragmentary literature.[84]

Lipofuscin in human pineal glands is found in two tissue compartments, pinealocytes (intralobular) and interlobular cells.[93,769] The cells of the second category containing lipofuscin probably include neuroglia and connective tissue macrophages. Within the cells of both compartments the lipofuscin appears to be preceded by lipid. However, the relative sizes and reactions to cytochemical procedures differ for the lipids in the two compartments (cf. Chapter Four).[769] Human pineal lipofuscin makes its major appearance in the vicinity of, and following, the age of puberty (Table XVII).[762] It is generally agreed that it increases with age, but with great individual variation.[93,408,560,635,700,761,769] No correlations have been proposed between pineal contents of lipofuscin and particular diseases or antecedent conditions.

There also have been no experimental studies attempting to induce or modify lipofuscin contents of pineal glands *in vivo*. Results of investigations of this kind focused on other organs[749] suggest that examination of the pineal gland in these circumstances may be informative. Although some electron microscopists have described a lipoidal or lipofuscin pigment in rat pineal cells,[130,346,347] I have never found pineal lipofuscin in this species. It is possible that differences in dietary treatment are responsible. Whatever the explanation turns out to be, the rat pineal gland might be an advantageous target organ for experimental studies on induction and cytogenesis of lipofuscin pigment.

The metabolic implications of intracellular lipofuscin are not agreed upon. But occurrences do not usually at least signify any broadly degenerative process. In the aging human brain Friede reported a positive association of occurrences of lipofuscin in neuronal perikarya with those particular neuron groups (brain nuclei) that have in general stronger oxidative enzyme activities.[298] Microchemical comparisons by Hirsch of enzyme activities of individual human spinal cord ventral horn neurons with high and low lipofuscin contents failed to show significant differences in enzyme activity.

However, when she subdivided single neurons into pigmented and unpigmented portions, she found lysosomal enzymes (acid phosphatase, β-galactosidase) more active in the former and oxidative enzymes (malate and lactate dehydrogenases) more active in the latter.[391]

CONCLUSIONS

1. Moderate concentrations of ubiquinone and thiamine have been reported in pineal tissue, where, as in other organs, they represent coenzymes of general metabolic significance.

2. The abolishment by pinealectomy of a photoperiodic and ubiquinone-dependent synchronous behavior of a protozoan parasite in mouse blood, lends support to belief in a pineal action on liver and blood chemistry.

3. Melanins, hemosiderin and lipofuscins are yellowish brown to dark brown or black intracellular pigments found variably in human and mammalian pineal glands. Neither their topographical patterns in or around the gland nor their quantitative or other characteristics suggest any necessarily pineal-specific functional or degenerative processes.

4. Human pinealocytes containing lipofuscin are rare until about the time of puberty, or later, depending on the individual. An age increase in the percent of cells containing lipofuscin occurs as well in the stromal and interlobular compartment. There is no convincing evidence from pathology for correlations of pineal lipofuscin with particular diseases or circumstances of life before death. Nevertheless, the advent of means for experimental induction *in vivo* of lipofuscin suggests that a rationale for attempting such correlations may not be far off.

Chapter Fourteen

INTEGRATION AND CONCLUSIONS

THE PURPOSE OF this final chapter is to integrate the more important findings from our review of pineal composition and activities and thence to arrive at general conclusions and hypotheses about the organ's functional significance and operational mechanisms. The resulting concepts concerning pineal mechanisms attempt to accommodate, in so far as is reasonable, along with different kinds of evidence, different points of view or schools of thought among recent investigators. However, the input is eclectic and the results are surely incomplete and oversimplified. A substantive and coherent basis, nevertheless, emerges, supporting recognition of pineal endocrine and distinctive functional activity. It is hoped that this fitting together of disparate findings into generalizing and provisional schemata will facilitate understanding of pineal activities and relationships and foster more effective pineal research.

STRUCTURAL-FUNCTIONAL RELATIONS

The structure and histology of mammalian pineal organs exclude the likelihood of most of the kinds of functions seen in other and diverse body cells and tissues, such as sensory exteroception, fluid transport, filtration, contraction, physical support, antibody formation, exocrine secretion and many others. Internal cellular composition and organization, now known in detail for pineal organs of man and many other mammalian species, are most clearly consonant with an endocrine activity. The only available pathway for transmittal of information from the pineal organ is the bloodstream.

323

Cerebrospinal fluid in the brain's ventricular and sub-arachnoid compartments is a partially possible route in a few mammalian species. But afferent neurons are possibilities in none, since pineal nerve fibers consist only of efferent (autonomic to the pineal) and commissural (in transit) types. The numerically dominant and metabolically most active pineal cell type, the pinealocyte, is structurally and chemically unique. Its primary activities are synthesis and secretion of specific indole derivatives and peptides or proteins. The secretions are released into the pericapillary space. There is evidence that at least one of the pineal's secreted products (melatonin) reaches the bloodstream, where its occurrence depends upon the presence of the pineal gland.

Pinealocyte and intercellular pineal control mechanisms as understood concurrently can be summarized by means of a diagram (Fig. 66). Six major categories of cellular and intercellular activities are itemized here:

(1) *Activation By The Pineal's Sympathetic Innervation*

This has two parts: (1A) vasoconstrictor activity of sympathetic endings on pineal blood vessels (probably involving β-adrenergic receptors); and (1B) stimulatory and regulatory activity of sympathetic endings in the vicinity of pinealocyte perikarya and/or perivascular processes (involving α-adrenergic receptors). The activities occurring at 1B may be the most important ones in regulating pineal circadian metabolic rhythms and related secretory activities.

(2) *Intercellular Metabolite Exchanges and Controls*

Pinealocytes have three theoretically possible sites or mechanisms for uptake and exchange of materials and control of these activities (2A–2C in Fig. 66): (2A) The one supported by direct evidence is that involving the perivascular terminal of the pinealocyte (Figs. 9 and 66). This structure is not only characteristically perivascular and in some species free of a basement membrane, but also has an intense pinocytic activity observed in cultures. (2B) The possibility of a pinealocyte astrocyte metabolic exchange or interaction is based largely on the premise that this relationship may be functionally analogous, as well as evolutionarily homologous, to the central

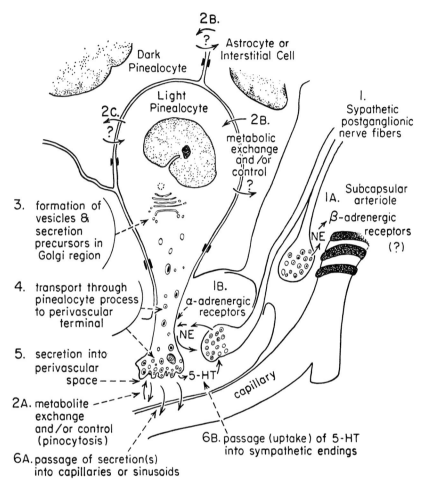

Figure 66. Postulated cellular basis of mammalian pineal endocrine secretory activity and its intercellular control mechanisms. Additional explanation is contained in the text; cell and tissue components are not drawn to the same scale.

nervous system's neuron-astrocyte relationship. Although close functional attachments typify these pineal cells, neither intercellular transport of materials nor metabolic interactions have been described for them. (2C) Interaction of light and dark pinealocytes seems possible on the basis of the close physical proximity and spatial organization of these cells and their ultrastructural definition stemming from multiple consistent differences in composition and structure. In fact, however, it is not known whether these cells represent different phases of activity of a single cell type or whether they are permanently differentiated in a mutually exclusive pattern.

(3–5) *Secretion Formation Transport and Release*

Two kinds of secretion precursor structures are seen in pinealocytes: small vesicles usually less than 1000 Å in diameter and probably containing indoleamines, and larger more irregular dense or granulated bodies or vesicles usually greater than 1000 Å in diameter and containing a tryptophan-rich, pineal-specific peptide or protein. The membrane systems of both apparently are elaborated and budded from the Golgi apparatus in the perikaryon, transported through the pinealocyte process and emptied, released or secreted into the perivascular space. The light pinealocytes resemble neurosecretory neurons in their intracellular spatial arrangement or subdivision of three processes, secretion formation, transport and release.[544] However, neuroendocrinologists adhering to a restrictive definition of neurosecretory cells usually do not consider pinealocytes members since there is no evidence that pinealocytes behave like neurons and since neuronal ancestry while possible is not proven for them.

(6) *Secretion Fates*

Pineal products secreted into the perivascular space have two possible fates within the organ (6A and 6B, Fig. 66). The indoleamines are taken up by sympathetic terminals in some species, as well as find passage into the bloodstream. The protein or peptide secretion presumably passes into the blood, but definitive evidence is lacking.

METABOLIC-FUNCTIONAL RELATIONS

The most distinctive general attribute of pineal metabolic activities is their high amplitude circadian rhythmicity with triggering mechanisms activated by lights-on and lights-off signals at particular times of the day. The premise of our further discussion here is that the pineal's various observed circadian rhythms can be temporally organized to portray the probable major events and phases in the gland's daily cellular and metabolic activities (Fig. 67). The picture that emerges is more instructive than merely the sum of its parts, the individual circadian rhythms. Plotting order of the circadian peaks was based on three principles: (1) association together of circadian cycles with the greatest rate increment ($\triangle\uparrow$ max) or decrement ($\triangle\downarrow$ max) at or following onset of light or onset of darkness; (2) association together of circadian cycles with gradual rate increments and decrements; (3) within these associations sequencing the cycles when possible according to either or both their order of cresting and known or suspected position in a metabolic or cytologic train.

The reconstructed pineal events and phases (Fig. 67) can be outlined as follows: During the time of darkness pineal content of norepinephrine (NE) in its sympathetic fibers and terminals increases to a peak, attained near or before the onset of light. At the onset of light a rapid and profound pineal vasoconstriction occurs, probably due to a sympathetic stimulation and release of NE at this time. Subsequent events observed *in vivo*, coupled with results *in vitro* with NE, suggest that activation of pineal uptake of tryptophan and other amino acids may occur following the light triggering of NE release. Thenceforward through the hours of light occur peaks of all remaining cycles with gradual and similarly slow circadian increases and decreases in parameter values. These cycles form two categories, one having to do with general anabolic activities and protein synthesis, and the other involving synthesis of 5-HT and 5-HIAA. The last segment of this daytime and *metabolic phase I* is primarily an inactive or storage subphase. With the exception of vasoconstriction, all cyclic pineal parameters that have sudden rate changes occur at or following the onset of darkness, which starts *metabolic phase II*.

This second phase, with its rapid changes in proximally cresting and troughing components, appears to involve at the outset triggered cellular release, uptake and synthetic

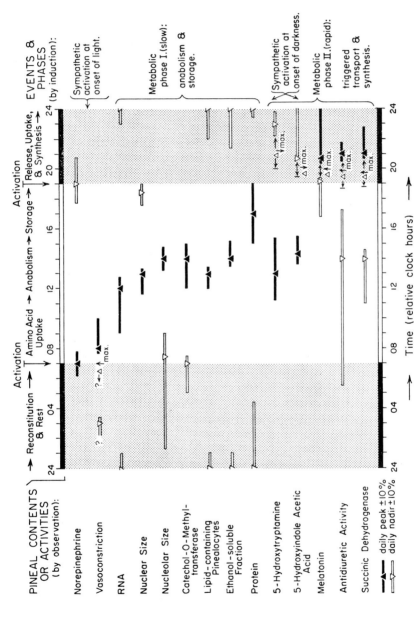

Figure 67. Integration and tentative sequencing of the cellular and metabolic circadian rhythms of the adult male rat's pineal gland. The component rhythms have been described or cited in earlier chapters. The integrated pattern serves as the basis for the induction of major events and phases in the gland's daily activity cycle. Rationale and implications are discussed in the text.

mechanisms. This is in contrast with the slower processes during phase I. A primary component of the trigger is probably the accumulated 5-HT within sympathetic terminals and pinealocytes. It is likely that pineal secretion of methoxyindoles and possibly of peptides or proteins occurs primarily after the onset of darkness. But, data are insufficient for an appraisal of the magnitude and duration of this secretory activity. The last segment or subdivision of phase II can provisionally be considered reconstitutive for the noradrenergic triggering mechanism and a resting subphase for the pinealocyte.

Finally, it should be emphasized that this circadian pineal rhythmicity is not peculiar to the laboratory rat and that the correlations of peaks and troughs with times of light or darkness may not relate to the nocturnality of this animal. Pineal indoleamine rhythms of great amplitude and with photodependent timing occur in a diurnal primate and diverse diurnal birds, with peaks and troughs occurring respectively during the same light and dark phases as in the rat. In all species studied so far, a major rate change occurs at or after the daily start of darkness.

PINEAL PHYSIOLOGY

The endocrine and physiological significance of the pineal gland has been investigated by studying the results of pineal extirpation and of administration of pineal substance or constituent compounds. The results of only the last of these approaches have been reviewed here. Recent reviews are available concerning other approaches and points of view.[293,466,619,636,840,841,1080] The intent here is to summarize by means of a diagrammatic model (Fig. 68) the chief postulated targets of pineal endocrine activity and the primary physiological control mechanisms that impinge upon them. Such a model facilitates visualization and study of the functionally interrelated series of systems. The inclusion of five major target systems does not imply that all are necessarily true or equally likely as targets of pineal secretory activity.

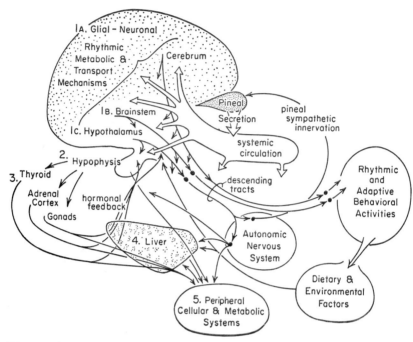

Figure 68. Diagrammatic model of postulated targets of pineal endocrine activity in mammals and the related physiological control mechanisms. (Modified from Quay.[807])

It means only that they have been overtly proposed by one or more groups of recent investigators and that they are still worthy of consideration in the design of experiments to be done, or in the interpretation of the results of completed experiments. It is only fair to admit, however, a partiality to the view that most if not all of the pineal's endocrine effects can be explained on the basis of the primary target being rhythmic metabolic and transport mechanisms within the central nervous system (1A in Fig. 68).[787,800,807,809] Various brain activities have been reported to be modified by pinealectomy or by administration of pineal extracts.[30,116,117,682,858,859] Diverse neuroendocrine and peripheral effects of pineal manipulations can be attributed to derivative or secondary effects as suggested by the diagram. Other investigators emphasize a possibly primary effect of the pineal on brainstem neurons, particularly those that are members of aminergic systems involved in arousal and sleep phasing (1B). While a yet larger group, including this reviewer, sees the hypothalamus as a pineal target, with secondary and tertiary effects downstream in the neuroendocrine axis, primarily on the hypophyseo-gonadal system (1C → 2 → 3).[4,150,214-217,458,639] Of a more fragmentary and less convincing nature is evidence for direct pineal effects on the hypophysis and individual, peripheral endocrine glands. The possibility of a pineal effect on liver metabolism and secondarily on blood chemistry is favored by active groups in eastern and southern Europe.[15,533,623,625,628,631,632,676,677,995,996] The numerous conceivable ramifications of general hepatic effects pose severe difficulties for the discriminating investigator. Also to be recognized are possibilities for pineal direct effects on yet other peripheral systems.[185,596,975] Evidence for these is firmer in lower animals, where, unlike the situation in mammals, certain pigment cells respond to very low concentrations of melatonin.[63,64,821]

The high amplitude circadian metabolic rhythms of the pineal gland have prompted the idea that this gland has a physiological role in the body's biological 24-hour "clock." Evidence for a direct pineal representation of this sort is stronger in birds than in mammals.[118,119,306,307,617,831] Although the hypothalamus appears to be the most necessary structure for mammalian circadian rhythms,[847,848] the pineal gland is a significant component in the mechanism governing rate of phase-shifts or changes in circadian behavioral rhythmicity.[486,805,809,811] An effect of pinealectomy on rate of circadian phase-shifting is life-long in the laboratory rat when the operation is done on the young animal.[816]

Antigonadotropic and circadian effects of the pineal gland coupled with the known physiological relations of these with environmental photoperiod suggest that the pineal mechanism may be significant in some seasonal breeders. Mostly indirect evidence supports this hypothesis.[163,807,809,840] It remains to be demonstrated in a natural population whether the presence of the organ is necessary for appropriate seasonal timing of reproductive activity.

PATHOLOGY

Published attempts to either implicate pineal malfunction in a disease process or to correlate pineal age changes or pathology with a disease or cause of death have been infrequent and generally not convincing. The kinds of pineal characteristics studied by early pathologists usually pertained not to pineal specific cells or activities but rather to vascular and glial features having a wide distribution and little if any association with pinealocyte activities. Such characteristics include incidence and relative amounts of corpora arenacea, glial formations, cysts and pigment granules. Possibly meriting greater attention is the observation by Walter (1923)[1023] that hypertrophy of human pinealocytes was associated with various disorders of intracranial circulation leading to brain pressure symptoms, as in cases of brain tumor and some cardiovascular diseases. The desirability of examing the pineal's less labile enzymatic activities in necropsy specimens remains. In Chapter Seven we noted that in one set of published data from human pineal specimens, relatively low pineal 5-HTP decarboxylase, acetylserotonin methyltransferase (HIOMT) and monoamine oxidase occurred in subjects with hypertensive and arteriosclerotic disease. This enzymatic correlation may be part of the same phenomenon observed cytopathologically by Walter fifty years ago.[1023]

The possible involvement of the pineal gland in abnormalities of rhythmic metabolic or behavioral activities has never been tested in human subjects. The suggestion has been made that experimental induction of circadian phase-shifting, as by modifying the patient's daily light, feeding and activity schedule, may possibly reveal a pineal deficit or hyperactivity where such occurs, as for example with tumors of the pineal region.[808]

REFERENCES

1. Abe, K., Robison, G.A., Liddle, G.W., Butcher, R.W., Nicholson, W.E., and Baird, C.E.: Role of cyclic AMP in mediating the effects of MSH, norepinephrine, and melatonin on frog skin color. *Endocrinology, 85:*674, 1969.
2. Abe, T., Yamada, Y., Hashimoto, P.H., and Shimizu, N.: Histochemical study of glucose-6-phosphate dehydrogenase in the brain of normal adult rat. *Med. J. Osaka Univ., 14:*67, 1963.
3. Abood, L.G., Gerard, R.W., and Tschirgi, R.D.: Spatial and chemical exchange of phosphate in the resting and active nervous system. In McElroy, W.D., and Glass, B. (Eds.): *Phosphorus Metabolism. A Symposium on the Role of Phosphorus in the Metabolism of Plants and Animals.* Baltimore, Johns Hopkins Press, 1952, vol. II, p. 798.
4. Abramof, I.R.K., Machado, A.B.M., and Machado, C.R.d.S.: Estudo citométrico do núcleo supraóptico em ratos pinealectomizados (I). *Ciéncia e Cultura 16:*177, 1964.
5. Adam, H.M.: Histamine in the central nervous system and hypophysis of the dog. In Kety, S.S., and Elkes, J. (Eds.): *Regional Neurochemistry. The Regional Chemistry, Physiology and Pharmacology of the Nervous System.* New York, Pergamon Press, 1961, p. 293.
6. Adams, C.W.M. (Ed.): *Neurohistochemistry.* Amsterdam, Elsevier Publ. Co., 1965.
7. Adams, C.W.M., Abdulla, Y.H., Bayliss, O.B., and Weller, R.O.: The reaction of Baker's chromate reagent with lipids. *J. Histochem. Cytochem., 13:*410, 1965.
8. Adams, W.C., Wan, L., and Sohler, A.: Effect of melatonin on anterior pituitary luteinizing hormone. *Endocrinology, 31:*295, 1965.
9. Addison, W.H.F., and Fraser, D.A.: Variability of pigmentation in the hypophysis and parathyroids of the gray rat (*Mus norvegicus*). *J. Comp. Neurol., 55:*513, 1932.
10. Adiga, P.R., Murthy, P.V.N., and McKenzie, J.M.: Stimulation by adenosine $3',5'$-cyclic monophosphate of protein synthess by adenohypophyseal polyribosomes. *Biochemistry, 10:*711, 1971.
11. Adolph, E.F.: Ontogeny of physiological regulations in the rat. *Q. Rev. Biol., 32:*89, 1957.
12. Agrawal, H.C., Davis, J.M., and Himwich, W.A.: Postnatal changes in free amino acid pool of rabbit brain, *Brain Res., 3:*374, 1967.
13. Agrawal, H.C., Davis, J.M., and Himwich, W.A.: Developmental changes in mouse brain: weight, water content and free amino acids. *J. Neurochem., 15:*917, 1968.
14. Albers, R.W.: The distribution of gamma-aminobutyrate and related enzyme systems. In Roberts, E., Baxter, C.F., van Harreveld,

A., Wiersma, C.A.G., Adey, W.R., and Killam, K.F. (Eds.): *Inhibition in the Nervous System and Gamma-Aminobutyric Acid.* New York, Pergamon Press, 1960, p. 196.

15. Alcozer, G., Giordano, G., and Masciocco, D.: Studi sull' epifisi; influenza dell'estratto acquoso di pineale su alcuni aspetti del metabolismo glicidico in soggetti sani ed eucrinici. *Archivio "E. Maragliano" di Patologia e Clinica (Genoa), 12:*1105, 1956.

16. Alexander, B., Dowd, A.J., and Wolfson, A.: Pineal hydroxyindole-O-methyltransferase (HIOMT) activity in female Japanese quail. *Neuroendocrinology, 6:*236, 1970.

17. Alexander, B., Dowd, A.J., and Wolfson, A.: Effects of prepuberal hypophysectomy and ovariectomy on hydroxyindole-*O*-methyltransferase activity in the female rat. *Endocrinology, 86:*1166, 1970.

18. Allison, J.H., and Stewart, M.A.: Carbohydrate changes in developing rat brain. *Transactions, American Society for Neurochemistry, 1:*24, 1970.

19. Altschule, M.D.: Some effects of aqueous extracts of acetone-dried beef-pineal substance in chronic schizophrenia. *N. Engl. J. Med., 257:*919, 1957.

20. Altschule, M.D., and Giancola, J.N.: Pineal-like effect of central nervous system tissue extracts. *Proc. Soc. Exp. Biol. Med., 104:*399, 1960.

21. Altschule, M.D., Siegel, E.P., Goncz, R.M., and Murnane, J.P.: Effect of pineal extracts on blood glutathione level in psychotic patients. *Arch. Neurol., 71:*615, 1954

22. Amprino, R.: Trasformazioni della ghiandola pineale dell'uomo e degli animali nell'accrescimento e nella senescenza. *Arch. Ital. Anat. Embriol., 34:*446, 1935.

23. Anderson, E.: Some cytological observations on the fine structure of a mammalian pineal organ. *Anat. Rec., 136:*328, 1960.

24. Anderson, E.: The anatomy of bovine and ovine pineals, light and electron microscopic studies. *Journal of Ultrastructure Research, suppl. 8:*1, 1965.

25. Angeletti, P.U.: Chemical sympathectomy in newborn animals. *Neuropharmacology, 10:*55, 1971.

26. Angeletti, P.U., and Levi-Montalcini, R.: Sympathetic nerve cell destruction in newborn mammals by 6-hydroxydropamine. *Proc. Natl. Acad. Sci. USA, 65:*114, 1970.

27. Angervall, L., Berger, S., and Röckert, H.: A microradiographic and x-ray crystallographic study of calcium in the pineal body and in intracranial tumours. *Acta. Pathol. Microbiol. Scand., 44:*113, 1958.

28. Anon.: Indexul bibliografic al lucrărilor stiintifice ale academicianului Stefan Milcu. *Stud. Cercet. Endocrinol., 14:*741, 1963.

29. Antón-Tay, F.: Pineal-brain relationships. In Wolstenholme, G.E.W., and Knight, J. (Eds.): *The Pineal Gland. A Ciba Foundation Symposium*. Edinburgh and London, Churchill Livingstone, 1971, p. 213.

30. Antón-Tay, F., Díaz, J.L., and Fernández-Guardiola, A.: On the effect of melatonin upon human brain. Its possible therapeutic implications. *Life Sci., 10:*841, 1971.

31. Antón-Tay, F., Sepulveda, J., and Gonzalez, S.: Increase of brain pyridoxal phosphokinase activity following melatonin administration. *Life Sci., 9:*1283, 1970.

32. Antón-Tay, F., and Wurtman, R.: Stimulation of hydroxyindole-O-methyltransferase activity in hamster pineal glands by blinding or continuous darkness. *Endocrinology, 82:*1245, 1968.

33. Antón-Tay, F., and Wurtman, R.J.: Regional uptake of ^{3}H-melatonin from blood or cerebrospinal fluid by rat brain. *Nature (Lond.), 221:*474, 1969.

34. Arieti, S.: The pineal gland in old age. *J. Neuropathol. Exp. Neurol. 13:*482, 1954.

35. Arnold, J.D., Berger, A., and Martin, D.C.: The role of the pineal in mediating photoperiodic control of growth and division synchrony and capillary sequestration of *Plasmodium berghei* in mice. *J. Parasitol., 55:*609, 1969.

36. Arnold, J.D., Berger, A.E., and Martin, D.C.: Chemical agents effective in mediating control of growth and division synchrony of *Plasmodium berghei* in pinealectomized mice. *J. Parasitol., 55:*617, 1969.

37. Arstila, A.U.: Electron microscopic studies on the structure and histochemistry of the pineal gland of the rat. *Neuroendocrinology, suppl. 2:*1, 1967.

38. Arstila, A.U., and Hopsu, V.K.: Studies on the rat pineal gland. I. Ultrastructure. *Ann. Acad. Sci. Fenn. (Med.), 113:*1, 1964.

39. Arstilia, A., and Rinne, U.: Electron microscopic studies on the perivascular secretory processes in the pineal gland of the rat. *Acta Neurol. Scand., 43 (suppl. 31):*211, 1967.

40. Arvy, L.: Contribution à la connaissance de la glande pinéale de *Bos taurus* L., d'*Ovis aries* L. et de *Sus scrofa* L.. *C.R. Acad. Sci. (Paris), 253:*1361, 1961.

41. Arvy, L.: *Histo-enzymologie des Glandes Endocrines*. Paris, Gauthier-Villars, 1963.

42. Arvy, L.: Activités enzymatiques histochimiquement décelables dans la glande pinéale, chez quelques artiodactyles. *Progr. Brain, Res., 10:*473, 1965.

43. Ashcroft, G.W., Eccleston, D., and Crawford, T.B.B.: 5-Hydroxyindole metabolism in rat brain. A study of intermediate metabolism using the technique of tryptophan loading—I. *J. Neurochem., 12:*483, 1965.

44. Axelrod, B.: Other pathways of carbohydrate metabolism. In Greenberg, D.M. (Ed.): *Metabolic Pathways*, New York, Academic Press, 1960, vol. 1, p. 205.

45. Axelrod, J.: Purification and properties of phenylethanolamine-N-methyl transferase. *J. Biol. Chem., 237:*1657, 1962.

46. Axelrod, J.: Noradrenaline: fate and control of its biosynthesis. *Science, 173:*598, 1971.

47. Axelrod, J., and Cohn, C.K.: Methyltransferase enzymes in red blood cells. *J. Pharmacol. Exp. Ther., 176:*650, 1971.

48. Axelrod, J., and Daly, J.: Pituitary gland: enzymic formation of methanol from S-adenosylmethionine. *Science, 150:*892, 1965.

49. Axelrod, J., and Lauber, J.K.: Hydroxyindole-O-methyltransferase in several avian species. *Biochem. Pharmacol., 17:*828, 1968.

50. Axelrod, J., MacLean, P.D., Albers, R.W., and Weissbach, H.: Regional distribution of methyl transferase enzymes in the nervous system and glandular tissues. In Kety, S.S., and Elkes, J., (Eds.): *Regional Neurochemistry.* Oxford, Pergamon Press, 1961, p. 307.

51. Axelrod, J., Mueller, R.A., Henry, J.P., and Stephens, P.M.: Changes in enzymes involved in the biosynthesis and metabolism of noradrenaline and adrenaline after psychosocial stimulation. *Nature (London.), 225:*1059, 1970.

52. Axelrod, J., Quay, W.B., and Baker, P.C.: Enzymatic synthesis of the skin-lightening agent, melatonin, in amphibians. *Nature (Lond.), 208:*386, 1965.

53. Axelrod, J., Shein, H.M., and Wurtman, R.J.: Stimulation of C^{14}-melatonin synthesis from C^{14}-tryptophan by noradrenaline in rat pineal in organ culture. *Proc. Natl. Acad. Sci. USA, 62:*544, 1969.

54. Axelrod, J., Snyder, S.H., Heller, A., and Moore, R.Y.: Light-induced changes in pineal hydroxyindole-O-methyltransferase: abolition by lateral hypothalamic lesions. *Science, 154:*898, 1966.

55. Axelrod, J., and Vesell, E.S.: Heterogeneity of N- and O-methyltransferases. *Mol. Pharmacol., 6:*78, 1970.

56. Axelrod, J., and Weissbach, H.: Enzymatic O-methylation of N-acetylserotonin to melatonin. *Science, 131:*1312, 1960.

57. Axelrod, J., and Weissbach, H.: Purification and properties of hydroxyindole-O-methyl transferase. *J. Biol. Chem., 236:*211, 1961.

58. Axelrod, J., Wurtman, R.J., and Snyder, S.: Control of hydroxyindole-O-methyltransferase activity in the rat pineal gland by environmental lighting. *J. Biol. Chem., 240:*949, 1965.

59. Axelrod, J., Wurtman, R.J., and Winget, C.M.: Melatonin synthesis

in the hen pineal gland and its control by light. *Nature (Lond.)*, *201:*1134, 1964.

60. Bäckström, M., and Wetterberg, L.: Catechol-O-methyltransferase, histamine-N-methyltransferase and methanol forming enzyme in the rat pineal gland. *Life Sci. [I]*, *11:*293, 1972.

61. Bagchi, S.P., and Zarycki, E.P.: The effect of p-chlorophenylalanine on the hydroxylation of phenylalanine in the pineal gland and brainstem. *Fed. Proc.*, *30:*381, 1971.

62. Bagnara, J.T.: Pineal regulation of the body lightening reaction in amphibian larvae. *Science, 132:*1481, 1960.

63. Bagnara, J.T.: The pineal and the body lightening reaction of larval amphibians. *Gen. Comp. Endocrinol.*, *3:*86, 1963.

64. Bagnara, J.T.: Pineal regulation of body blanching in amphibian larvae. *Progr. Brain Res.*, *10:*489, 1965.

65. Bailey, P.: Morphology of the roof plate of the forebrain and the lateral choroid plexuses in the human embryo. *J. Comp. Neurol.* *26:*79, 1916.

66. Bak, I.J., Hassler, R., and Kim, I.S.: Differential monoamine depletion by oxypertine in nerve terminals. Granulated synaptic vesicles in relation to depletion of norepinephrine, dopamine and serotonin. *Z. Zellforsch. Mikrosk. Anat.*, *101:*448, 1969.

67. Bak, I.J., Kim, J.H., and Hassler, R.: Electron microscopic autoradiography for demonstration of pineal serotonin in rat. *Z. Zellforsch. Mikrosk. Anat.*, *105:*167, 1970.

68. Bakay, L.: Dynamic aspects of the blood-brain barrier. In Richter, D. (Ed.): *Metabolism of the Nervous System*. London, Pergamon Press, 1957, p. 136.

69. Bakay, L.: Changes in barrier effect in pathological states. *Progr. Brain Research*, *29:*315, 1968.

70. Baker, J.R.: The histochemical recognition of lipine. *Quarterly Journal of Microscopical Science*, *87:*441, 1946.

71. Baker, P.C.: Melatonin levels in developing *Xenopus laevis. Comp. Biochem. Physiol.*, *28:*1387, 1969.

72. Baker, P.C., and Hoff, K.M.: The effect of light and dark background upon melatonin levels in larval *Xenopus. Comp. Gen. Pharmacol.* *2:*59, 1971.

73. Baker, P.C., and Quay, W.B.: 5-Hydroxytryptamine metabolism in early embryogenesis, and the development of brain and retinal tissues. A review. *Brain Res.*, *12:*273, 1969.

74. Baker, P.C., Quay, W.B., and Axelrod, J.: Development of hydroxyindole-O-methyl transferase activity in eye and brain of the amphibian, *Xenopus laevis. Life Sci.*, *4:*1981, 1965.

75. Baldessarini, R.J.: Factors influencing S-adenosylmethionine levels in mammalian tissues. In Himwich, H.E., Kety, S.S., and

Smythies, J.R. (Eds.): *Amines and Schizophrenia.* Oxford, Pergamon Press, 1967, p. 199.

76. Baldessarini, R.J., and Kopin, I.J.: Assay of tissue levels of S-adenosylmethionine. *Anal. Biochem., 6:*289, 1963.

77. Baldessarini, R.J., and Kopin, I.J.: S-Adenosylmethionine in brain and other tissues. *J. Neurochem., 13:*769, 1966.

78. Balemans, M.G.M., Ebels, I., and Vonk-Visser, D.M.A.: Separation of pineal extracts on Sephadex G-10. I. A spectrofluorimetric study of indoles in a cockerel pineal extract. *J. Neurovisc. Relat., 32:*65, 1970.

79. Bara, D., Skaliczki, J., and Ormos, J.: Comparative study of the histoenzymological properties of the supraoptic and paraventricular nuclei and of other nuclear regions of the hypothalamus, the epithalamus-epiphysis region and the subfornical organ. *Hormones, 2:*164, 1971.

80. Barchas, J., DaCosta, F., and Spector, S.: Acute pharmacology of melatonin. *Nature (Lond.), 214:*919, 1967.

81. Barchas, J.D., and Lerner, A.B.: Localization of melatonin in the nervous system. *J. Neurochem., 11:*489, 1964.

82. Barfuss, D.W., and Ellis, L.C.: Seasonal cycles in melatonin synthesis by the pineal gland as related to testicular function in the house sparrow *(Passer domesticus). Gen. Comp. Endocrinol., 17:*183, 1971.

83. Barfuss, D.W., Tait, G.R., and Ellis, L.C.: Melatonin synthesis in rat pineal glands inhibited by x-irradiation. *Proc. Soc. Exp. Biol. Med., 132:*35, 1969.

84. Bargmann, W.: Die Epiphysis cerebri. In von Möllendorff, W. (Ed.): *Handbuch der mikroskopischen. Anatomie des Menschen.* 6 (part 4):309, 1943.

85. Barman, T.E.: *Enzyme Handbook.* New York, Springer-Verlag, 1969, vols. 1 & 2.

86. Barry, J.: Etude histophysiologique des monoamines centrales chez le Lérot *(Eliomys quercinus)* en hibernation et en période d'activité sexuelle. *C. R. Acad. Sci. (Paris), 270:*2983, 1970.

87. Bartley, W., and Dean, B.: Extraction and estimation of glycogen and oligosaccharides from rat heart. *Anal. Biochem., 25:*99, 1968.

88. Bartoli, V., and Neri Serneri, G.G.: Contributo allo studio della funzione epifisaria II.—Modificazione dell'apparato genitale maschile e femminile dopo epifisectomia e dopo somministrazione di estratto epifisario acquoso. *Rass. Neurol. Veg., 12:*231, 1957.

89. Baschieri, L., de Luca, F., Camarossa, L., de Martino, C., Oliverio, A., and Negri, M.: Modifications of thyroid activity by melatonin. *Experientia, 19:*15, 1963.

90. Basinska, J., Sastry, P.S., and Stancer, H.C.: Lipid composition of human, bovine and sheep pineal glánds. *J. Neurochem.*, *16:*707, 1969.

91. Bayerová, G., and Bayer, A.: Beitrag zur cytochemischen Charakteristik einiger Zellarten in der menschlichen Epiphyse. *Acta Histochem. (Jena)*, *10:*276, 1960.

92. Bayerová, G., and Bayer, A.: Beitrag zur Fermenthistochemie der menschlichen Epiphyse. *Acta Histochem. (Jena)*, *28:*169, 1967.

93. Bayerová, G., Bayer, A., Malínský, J., and Zapletal, B.: On functional significance of epiphyseal pigment (electron-optic study). *Arkh. Anat., Gistol. Embriol.*, *45:*18, 1965.

94. Bayerová, G., Bayer, A., and Obručník, M.: Zur Frage der fluorescenz- und polarisationsmikroskopischen Untersuchungen an der menschlichen Epiphyse. *Acta Histochem. (Jena)*, *14:*276, 1962.

95. Bayerová, G., and Malínský, J.: Quantitative ultrastructural study of rat pinealocytes during postnatal development. *Folia Morphol. (Praha)*, *20:*56, 1972.

96. Beauvallet, M., Godefroy, F., and Fugazza, J.: Influence d'une surcharge du régime en chlorure de sodium sur la teneur en 5-hydroxytryptamine du cerveau et de l'épiphyse, chez le rat. *C. R. Soc. Biol. (Paris)*, *160:*1218, 1966.

97. Bedford, T.H.B.: The great vein of Galen and the syndrome of increased intracranial pressure. *Brain*, *57:*1, 1934.

98. Benda, C.: Die Zirbeldrüse (Epiphysis cerebri, Glandula pinealis). In Hirsch, M. (Ed.): *Handbuch der Inneren Sekretion. 1:*1098, 1932.

99. Bennett, D.S., and Giarman, N.J.: Schedule of appearance of 5-hydroxytryptamine (serotonin) and associated enzymes in the developing rat brain. *J. Neurochem.*, *12:*911, 1965.

100. Bensinger, R.E.: Control of activity of tryptophan hydroxylase. In Klein, D.C. (Ed.): *Pineal Gland: Proceedings of a Workshop.* New York, Raven Press, in press.

101. Benson, B., and Matthews, M.J.: Studies on a non-melatonin pineal antigonadotropin. *Endocrinology, 88(suppl.):*A-106, 1971.

102. Benson, B., Matthews, M.J., and Rodin, A.E.: A melatonin-free extract of bovine pineal with antigonadotropic activity. *Life Sci. (I)*, *10:*607, 1971.

103. Benson, B., Matthews, M.J., and Rodin, A.E.: Studies on a non-melatonin pineal anti-gonadotrophin. *Acta Endocrinol. (Kbh.)*, *69:*257, 1972.

104. Berblinger, W.: Die Glandula pinealis (Corpus pineale). *Handbuch der speziellen pathologischen Anatomie und Histologie. 8:*681, 1926.

105. Berg., G.R., and Klein, D.C.: Pineal gland melatonin production: site of action of norepinephrine and dibutyryl cyclic adenosine monophosphate. *Fed. Proc., 29:*615, 1970.

106. Berg, G.R., and Klein, D.C.: Pineal gland in organ culture. II. Role of adenosine 3',5'-monophosphate in the regulation of radiolabeled melatonin production. *Endocrinology, 89:*453, 1971.

107. Berg., G.R., and Klein, D.C., and Glinsmann, W.H.:'Pineal gland in organ culture: effect of norepinephrine and dibutyryl cyclic AMP on ^{32}P incorporation into phospholipids.*Fed. Proc.,30:*364, 1971.

108. Bergman, W.: Wirkung von Pinealisextracten auf das Gefässsystem des Frosches. *Archives Néerlandaises de Physiologie de l'Homme et des Animaux, 24:*391, 1940.

109. Bergmann, W., and Engel, P.: Ueber den Einfluss von Zirbelex-trakten auf Tumoren bei weissen Mäusen und bei Menschen. *Wien Klin. Wochenschr., 62:*79, 1950.

110. Bernád, I. and Csaba, G.: Localization of biogenic monoamines in tissue cultures of rat pineal.*Acta Biol. Acad. Sci. Hung., 21:*235, 1970.

111. Bertaccini, G., and Zamboni, P.: The relative potency of 5-hydroxytryptamine like substances. *Arch. Int. Pharmacodyn. Ther., 133:*138, 1961.

112. Bertler, Å., Falck, B., and Owman, C.: Cellular localization of 5-hydroxytryptamine in the rat pineal gland. *Kungl. Fysiografiska Sällskapets i Lund Förhandlingar, 33:*13, 1963.

113. Bertler, Å., Falck, B., and Owman, C.: Studies on 5-hydroxy-tryptamine stores in pineal gland of rat.*Acta Physiol. Scand., 63 (suppl. 239):*1, 1964.

114. Bianchini, P., and Osima, B.: Azione della pineale sulla ipertrofia gonadica compensatoria. *Boll. Soc. Ital., Biol. Sper., 38:*1547, 1962.

115. Bigelow, L., Vaughan, M.K., Vaughan, G.M., and Reiter, R.: Gonadal influence of aqueous pineal extracts: effects of pineal substances on compensatory ovarian hypertrophy in the mouse.*Fed. Proc., 31:*222, 1972.

116. Bindoni, M., and Rizzo, R.,: Effetti di lesioni elettrolitiche della ghiandola pineale sulla attivitá elettrica di alcune strutture encefaliche del coniglio. *Boll. Soc. Ital. Biol. Sper, 40:*2010, 1964.

117. Bindoni, M., and Rizzo, R.: Hippocampal evoked potentials and convulsive activity after electrolytic lesions of the pineal body, in chronic experiments on rabbits, *Arch. Sci. Biol. (Bologna), 49:*223, 1965.

118. Binkley, S., Kluth, E., and Menaker, M.: Pineal function in sparrows: circadian rhythms and body temperature. *Science, 174:*311, 1971.

119. Binkley, S., Kluth, E., and Menaker, M.: Pineal and locomotor activity: levels and arrhythmia in sparrows. *J. Comp. Physiol.,* 77:163, 1972.

120. Bloom, F.E., and Giarman, N.J.: The effects of *p*-Cl-phenylalanine on the content and cellular distribution of 5-HT in the rat pineal gland: combined biochemical and electron microscopic analyses. *Biochem. Pharmacol., 19:*1213, 1970.

121. Bloom, F.E., Iversen, L.L., and Schmitt, F.O.: Macromolecules in synaptic function. *Neurosciences Research Program Bulletin (MIT), 8:*325, 1970.

122. Bloom, W., and Fawcett, D.W.: *A Textbook of Histology.* Philadelphia, W.B. Saunders Co., 9th edition, 1968.

123. Bondareff, W.: Submicroscopic morphology of granular vesicles in sympathetic nerves of rat pineal body. *Z. Zellforsch. Mikrosk. Anat., 67:*211, 1965.

124. Bondareff, W.: Electron microscopic study of the pineal body in aged rats. *J. Gerontol., 20:*321, 1965.

125. Bondareff, W.: Submicroscopic localization of norepinephrine in sympathetic nerves of rat pineal. *Anat. Rec., 154:*498, 1966.

126. Bondareff, W.: Localization of α-methylnorepinephrine in sympathetic nerve fibers of the pineal body. *Exp. Neurol., 16:*131, 1966.

127. Bondareff, W., and Gordon, N.: Submicroscopic localization of norepinephrine in sympathetic nerves of rat pineal. *J. Pharmacol. Exp. Ther., 153:*42, 1966.

128. Borell, U., and Örström, A.: Metabolism in different parts of the brain, especially in the epiphysis, measured with radioactive phosphorus. *Acta Physiol Scand., 10:*231, 1945.

129. Borell, U., and Örström, A.: The turnover of phosphate in the pineal body compared with that in other parts of the brain. *Biochem. J., 41:*398, 1947.

130. Bostelmann, W.: Beitrag zur submikroskopischen Zytologie der Epiphysis cerebri und zur experimentellen Beeinflussung ihrer Zellelemente. *Zentralbl. Allg. Pathol., 107:*430, 1965.

131. Bostelmann, W.: Das ultrastrukturelle und enzymhistochemische Verhalten der Rattenzirbeldrüse nach Funktionsphasenwechsel durch Dauerbeleuchtung und ständige Dunkelheit. *Endokrinologie, 53:*365, 1968.

132. Bostelmann, W.: Der Einfluss der bilateralen Kastration auf die Feinstruktur der Zirbeldrüse. *Endokrinologie, 54:*56, 1969.

133. Bostelmann, W., and Bienengräber, A.: Enzymhistochemie der Epiphysis cerebri des Kaninchens. *Acta Neuropathol. (Berl.),* 2:461, 1963.

134. Bratiano, S., and Giugariu, D.: Les processus histophysiologiques d'involution de l'épiphyse humaine adulte.*Arch. Anat. Microsc. Morphol. Exp., 29:*261, 1933.
135. Brewer, G.F., and Quay, W.B.: Pineal and hypophyseal phosphate uptake after castration and administration of sex hormones.*Proc. Soc. Exp. Biol. Med., 98:*361, 1958.
136. Brooks, C.J.W., and Horning, E.C.: Gas chromatographic studies of catecholamines, tryptamines, and other biological amines. Part 1. Catecholamines and related compounds. *Anal. Chem., 36:*1540, 1964.
137. Brown, F.C., and Gordon, P.H.: A study of L-(^{14}C) cystathionine metabolism in the brain, kidney, and liver of pyridoxine-deficient rats. *Biochim. Biophys. Acta, 230:*434, 1971.
138. Brownstein, M.J., and Heller, A.: Hydroxyindole-O-methyl-transferase activity: effect of sympathetic nerve stimulation. *Science, 162:*367, 1968.
139. Budd, G.C., and Salpeter, M.M.: ^{3}H Norepinephrine-labeled axons in electron microscope radioautograms of pineal body and adrenal capsule.*J. Cell Biol., 39:*19a, 1968.
140. Bugnon, C., Lenys, D., and Lenys, R.: Organe sous-commissural et zone glomerulaire surrenalienne. *C.R. Assoc. Anat., Bull. Assoc. Anat., 131:*219, 1966.
141. Burgers, A.C.J., and van Oordt, G.J.: Regulation of pigment migration in the amphibian melanophore. *Gen. Comp Endocrinol., suppl. 1:*99, 1962.
142. Burstone, M.S.: *Enzyme Histochemistry and Its Application in the Study of Neoplasms.* New York, Academic Press, 1962.
143. Buss, H., and Gusek, W.: Zur Ultrastruktur der Epiphysis cerebri der Ratte unter dem Einfluss von Noradrenalin und Niamid. *Endokrinologie, 48:*76, 1965.
144. Cady, P., and Dillman, R.O.: Influence of catechol and indole amines upon pineal uptake of thyroxine. *Neuroendocrinology, 8:*228, 1971.
145. Calcinai, M.: L'acido ascorbico nei tessuti. Ricerche su materiale di autopsia e di esperimento esposizione critica. *Arch. Patol. Clin. Med., 19:*513, 1939.
146. Calvet, J.: Etude du chondriome dans les cellules épiphysaires de quelques mammifères.*C.R. Soc. Biol. (Paris), 113:*300, 1933.
147. Cardinali, D.P., and Rosner, J.M.: Retinal localization of the hydroxyindole-O-methyl transferase(HIOMT) in the rat. *Endocrinology, 89:*301, 1971.
148. Cardinali, D.P., and Rosner, J.M.: Ocular distribution of hydroxyindole-O-methyl transferase (HIOMT) in the duck*(Anas platyrhinchos). Gen. Comp. Endocrinol., 18:*407, 1972.

149. Cardinali, D.P., and Wurtman, R.J.: Hydroxyindole-O-methyl trans-ferases in rat pineal, retina and harderian gland. *Endocrinology, 91:*247, 1972.

150. Carnicelli, A., Saba, P., Cella, P.L., and Marescotti, V.: Effects of epiphysectomy on karyometry of hypothalamic nuclei in rats. *Folia Endocrinol. (Roma), 16:*229, 1963.

151. Carr, J.L.: Cystic hydrops of the pineal gland with a report of six cases. *J. Nerv. Ment. Dis., 99:*552, 1944.

152. Cassano, C., Torsoli, A., Peruzy, A.D. and De Martino, C.: Studi su l'epifisi. Indagini nell'animale da esperimento e nell'uomo. *Folia Endocrinol. (Roma), 14:*755, 1961.

153. Chamoles, N., Karcher, D., Zeman, W., and Lowenthal, A.: Studies on alpha albumin in nervous tissue. II. Topographical distri-bution in normal tissue. *Brain Res., 17:*315, 1970.

154. Chase, P.A., Seiden, L.S., and Moore, R.Y.: Behavioral and neuroen-docrine responses to light mediated by separate visual pathways in the rat. *Physiology and Behavior, 4:*949, 1969.

155. Cheesman, D.W.: Structural elucidation of a gonadotropin-inhibit-ing substance from the bovine pineal gland. *Biochim. Biophys. Acta, 207:*247, 1970.

156. Cheesman, D.W., and Fariss, B.L.: Isolation and characterization of a gonadotropin-inhibiting substance from the bovine pineal gland. *Proc. Soc. Exp. Biol. Med., 133:*1254, 1970.

157. Cheung, W.Y.: Cyclic nucleotide phosphodiesterase. In Greengard, P., and Costa, E. (Eds.): Role of Cyclic AMP in Cell Function. *Advances in Biochemical Psychopharmacology,* vol. *3:*51, 1970.

158. Chu, E.W., Wurtman, R.J., and Axelrod, J.: An inhibitory effect of melatonin on the estrous phase of the estrous cycle of the rodent. *Endocrinology,* 75, 238, 1964.

159. Ciaranello, R.D., Dankers, H.J., and Barchas, J.D.: The enzymatic formation of methanol from S-adenosylmethionine by various tissues of the rat. *Mol. Pharmacol., 8:*311, 1972.

160. Clabough, J.W.: Ultrastructural features of the pineal gland in nor-mal and light deprived golden hamsters. *Z. Zellforsch. Mikrosk. Anat., 114:*151, 1971.

161. Clabough, J., and Seibel, H.: Studies of the pineal glands of rats and hamsters during ontogenesis and under various experi-mental conditions. *Anat. Rec., 120:*463, 1968.

162. Clara, M.: Beiträge zue Histotopochemie des Vitamin C im Nerven-system des Menschen. *Z. Mikrosk. Anat. Forsch., 52:*359, 1942.

163. Clausen, H.J., and Poris, E.G.: The effect of light upon sexual activity in the lizard, *Anolis carolinesis,* with especial reference to the pineal body. *Anat. Rec., 69:*39, 1937.

164. Cleaver, J.E.: *Thymidine Metabolism and Cell Kinetics.* Amsterdam, North-Holland Publ. Co., 1967.

165. Clementi, F., Fraschini, F., Müller, E., and Zanoboni, A.: The pineal gland and the control of electrolyte balance and of gonadotropic secretion: functional and morphological observations. *Progr. Brain Res.*, *10:*585, 1965.

166. Clementi, F., Müller, E., and Zanoboni, A.: Pineal function and modifications of its ultrastructural aspects. *Excerpta Medica International Congress Series*, *83:*364, 1964.

167. Clive, D., and Snell, R.S.; Effect of melatonin on mammalian hair color. *J. Invest. Dermatol.*, *53:*159, 1969.

168. Cohen, R.A., Wurtman, R.J., Axelrod, J., and Snyder, S.H.: Some clinical, biochemical and physiological actions of the pineal gland. Combined clinical staff conference at the National Institutes of Health. *Ann. Intern. Med.*, *61:*1144, 1964.

169. Cole, E.R., and Crank, G.: Tryptamines I. The chromatography of melatonin. *J. Chromatogr.*, *61:*225, 1971.

170. Collier, R.: Über den Feinbau der Epiphysis cerebri von Nagetieren und die Frage seiner Funktionellen Veränderungen. *Z. Zellforsch. Mikrosk. Anat.*, *33:*51, 1943.

171. Collin, J.-P.: Differentiation and regression of the cells of the sensory line in the epiphysis cerebri. In Wolstenholme, G.E.W., and Knight, J. (Eds.): *The Pineal Gland.* Edinburgh and London, Churchill Livingstone, 1971, p. 79.

172. Collu, R., Fraschini, F., and Martini, L.: The effect of pineal methoxy-indoles on rat vaginal opening time. *J. Endocrinol.*, *50:*679, 1971.

173. Constantini, G.: Intoro ad alcune particolaritá di struttura della glandola pineale. *Pathologica*, *2:*439, 1910.

174. Conti, M., Serluca, F.P., and Mascia, C.: L'azione esercitata da un estratto acquoso di ghiandola pineale sulla distribuzione del radiofosforo a livello dell'apparato genitale femminile. *Radiobiologica Latina*, *6:*43, 1963.

175. Corrodi, H., and Jonsson, G.: Fluoreszenzmethoden zur histochemischen Sichtbarmachung von Monoaminen. 5. Identifizierung des fluoreszierenden Produktes aus Modellversuchen mit 5-Methoxytryptamin und Formaldehyd. *Acta Histochem. (Jena)*, *22:*247, 1965.

176. Corrodi, H., and Jonsson, G.: The formaldehyde fluorescence method for the histochemical demonstration of biogenic monoamines. A review on the methodology. *J. Histochem. Cytochem.*, *15:*65, 1967.

177. Cotzias, G.C., Tang, L.C., Miller, S.T., and Ginos, J.Z.: Melatonin and abnormal movements induced by L-dopa in mice. *Science*, *173:*450, 1971.

178. Coupland, R.E., and Weakley, B.A.: Developing chromaffin tissue in the rabbit: an electron microscopic study. *J. Anat.*, *102:*425, 1968.

179. Courville, C.B., Nusbaum, R.E., and Butt, E.M.: Changes in trace metals in brain in Huntington's chorea. *Arch. Neurol.*, 8:481, 1963.

180. Crane, F.L.: Distribution of ubiquinones. In Morton, R.A. (Ed.): *Biochemistry of Quinones*. New York, Academic Press, 1965, p. 183.

181. Crane, F.L., and Low, H.: Quinones in energy-coupling systems. *Physiol. Rev.*, 46:622, 1966.

182. Cronkite, E.P., Fliedner, T.M., Killmann, S.A., and Rubini, J.R.: Tritium-labelled thymidine (H^3TDR): its somatic toxicity and use in the study of growth rates and potentials in normal and malignant tissue of man and animals. *Tritium in the Physical and Biological Sciences*. International Atomic Energy Agency, Vienna, vol. 2:189, 1962.

183. Crozier, W.J., and Pincus, G.: The geotropic conduct of young rats. *J. Gen. Physiol.*, 10:257, 1926.

184. Crozier, W.J., and Pincus, G.: Photic stimulation of young rats. *J. Gen. Psychol.*, 17:105, 1937.

185. Csaba, G., Dunay, C., Fischer, J., and Bodoky, M.: Hormonal relationships of mastocytogenesis in lymphatic organs. III. Effect of the pineal body-thyroid-thymus system on mast cell production. *Acta Anat. (Basel)*, 71:565, 1968.

186. Cumings, J.N.: The copper and iron content of brain and liver in the normal and in hepato-lenticular degeneration. *Brain.* 71:410, 1948.

187. Cunningham, D.J.: Notes on hypertrophy of the sympathetic nervous system. *J. Anat.*, 12:294, 1878.

188. Cutore, G.: Il corpo pineale di alcuni mammiferi. *Arch. Ital. Anat. Embriol.*, 9:402, 1910.

189. Cutore, G.: Alcune notizie sul corpo pineale del *Macacus sinicus* L. e del *Cercopithecus griseus viridis* L. *Folia Neurobiol. (Haarlem)*, 6:267, 1912.

190. Czarnocki, J., Sastry, P.S., and Stancer, H.C.: The lipids of human pineal gland. In Richter, D. (Ed.): *Biochemical Factors Concerned in the Functional Activity of the Nervous System*. London, Pergamon Press, 1969, p. 47.

191. Das Gupta, T.K., and Terz, J.: Influence of pineal body on melanoma of hamsters. *Nature (Lond.)*, 213:1038, 1967.

192. Das Gupta, T.K., and Terz, J.: Influence of pineal gland on the growth and spread of melanoma in the hamster. *Cancer Res.*, 27:1306, 1967.

193. Debeljuk, L., Vilchez, J.A.: Schnitman, M.A., Paulucci, O.A., and Feder, V.M.: Further evidence for a peripheral action of melatonin. *Endocrinology*, 89:1117, 1971.

194. de Champlain, J., Krakoff, L.R., and Axelrod, J.: Catecholamine metabolism in experimental hypertension in the rat. *Circ. Res.*, *20:*136, 1967.

195. de Champlain, J., Mueller, R.A., and Axelrod, J.: Turnover and synthesis of norepinephrine in experimental hypertension in rats. *Circ. Res.*, 25:285, 1969.

196. DeFronzo, R.A., and Roth, W.D.: Evidence for the existence of a pineal-adrenal and a pineal-thyroid axis. *Acta Endocrinol. (Kbh.)*, 70:35, 1972.

197. Degen, P.H., DoAmaral, J.R., and Barchas, J.D.: A gas-liquid chromatographic assay of melatonin and indoleamines using heptafluorobutyryl derivatives. *Anal. Biochem.*, 45:634, 1972.

198. Deguchi, T., and Axelrod, J.: Induction and superinduction of serotonin N-acetyltransferase by adrenergic drugs and denervation in rat pineal organ. *Proc. Nat. Acad. Sci. USA*, 69:2208, 1972.

199. Deguchi, T., and Barchas, J.: Inhibition of transmethylations of biogenic amines by S-adenosylhomocysteine. *J. Biol. Chem.*, 246:3175, 1971.

200. Deguchi, T., and Barchas, J.: Effect of p-chlorophenylalanine on tryptophan hydroxylase in rat pineal. *Nature, New Biology*, 235:92, 1972.

201. del Rio Hortega, P.: Pineal gland. In Penfield, W. (Ed.): *Cytology and Cellular Pathology of the Nervous System.* New York, Hoeber, 1932, vol. 2:637.

202. Delvigs, P., McIsaac, W.M., and Taborsky, R.G.: The metabolism of 5-methoxytryptophol. *J. Biol. Chem.*, 240:348, 1965.

203. De Martino, C., Pavoni, P., and Peruzy, A.D.: Modificazioni istologiche e captazione del ^{32}P della ghiandola pineale nel ratto maschio di varie età. *Giornale di Gerontologia*, 9:275, 1961.

204. De Martino, C., Peruzy, A.D., Pavoni, P., Capone, M., and Lintas, P.L.: Captazione del ^{32}P ed aspetti istologici della ghiandola pineale nelle varie età. *Folia Endocrinol. (Roma)*, 15:363, 1962.

205. de Mennato, M.: Grassi e lipoidi nell'epifisi cerebrale. Modificazioni strutturali in rapporto a stati funzionali. *Nuova Rivista di Clinica ed Assistenza Psichiatrica e di Terapia Applicata (Napoli)*, 11:85, 1934.

206. Dempsey, E.W., and Wislocki, G.B.: An electron microscopic study of the blood-brain barrier in the rat, employing silver nitrate as a vital stain. *J. Biophys. Biochem. Cytol.*, 1:245, 1955.

207. Dengler, H.J., Wilson, C.W.M., Spiegel, H.E., and Titus, E.: Uptake of norepinephrine by isolated pineal bodies. *Biochem. Pharmacol.*, 11:795, 1962.

208. De Prospo, N.D., and Hurley, J.: A comparison of intracerebral and intraperitoneal injections of melatonin and its precursors on ^{131}I uptake by the thyroid glands of rats. *Agents and Actions*, 2:14, 1971.

209. De Prospo, N., and Hurley, J.: Effects of injecting melatonin and its precursors into the lateral cerebral ventricles on selected organs in rats. *J. Endocrinol.*, 49:545, 1971.

210. De Prospo, N.D., Safinski, R.J., De Martino, L.J., and McGuiness, E.T.: Melatonin and its precursor's effects on ^{131}I uptake by the thyroid gland under different photic conditions. *Life Sci.*, 8:837, 1969.

211. De Robertis, E., and Pellegrino de Iraldi, A.: A plurivesicular component in adrenergic nerve endings. *Anat. Rec.*, 139:299, 1961.

212. De Robertis, E., and Pellegrino de Iraldi, A.: Plurivesicular secretory processes and nerve endings in the pineal gland of the rat. *J. Biophys. Biochem. Cytol.*, 10:361, 1961.

213. Des Gouttes, M.N.L.: Évolution pondérale des glandes endocrines et des glandes génitales annexes chez le rat mâle de la naissance à la puberté. *Ann. Endocrinol. (Paris)*, 27:121, 1966.

214. de Vries, R.A.C.: *Some Aspects of the Functional Relationship of the Rat Pineal Gland to the Hypothalamic Magnocellular Neurosecretory Nuclei under Different Experimental Conditions.* Thesis, Purmerend, The Netherlands, Novy's Drukkerij, 1972.

215. de Vries, R.A.C.: Influence of pinealectomy on hypothalamic magnocellular neurosecretory activity in the female rat during normal light conditions, light-induced persistent oestrus, and after gonadectomy. *Neuroendocrinology*, 9:244, 1972.

216. de Vries, R.A.C.: Abolition of the effect of pinealectomy on hypothalamic magnocellular neurosecretory activity in male rats by hypothalamic pineal implants. *Neuroendocrinology*, 9:358, 1972.

217. de Vries, R.A.C., and Kappers, J.A.: Influence of the pineal gland on the neurosecretory activity of the supraoptic hypothalamic nucleus in the male rat. *Neuroendocrinology*, 8:359, 1971.

218. Diebel, N.D.: Yamamoto, M., and Bogdanove, E.M.: Lack of diurnal rhythms in pituitary and serum LH and FSH of male rats. *Fed. Proc.*, 29:440, 1970.

219. Dikstein, S., and Sulman, F.G.: Mechanism of melanophore dispersion. *Biochem. Pharmacol.*, 13:819, 1964.

220. Dill, R.E., and Walker, B.E.: Pineal cell proliferation in the mouse. *Proc. Soc. Exp. Biol. Med.*, 121:911, 1966.

221. Dreux, C.: Études sur la biochimie des methoxyindols dosage spectrofluorimetrique de la methoxy-5, N-acetyltryptamine (mélatonine). *Clin. Chim. Acta, 23:177, 1969.

222. Duffy, P.E., and Markesbery, W.R.: Granulated vesicle in sympathetic nerve endings in the pineal gland: observations on the effects of pharmacologic agents by electron microscopy. *Am. J. Anat.*, 128:97, 1970.

223. Duncan, D., and Micheletti, G.: Notes on the fine structure of the pineal organ of cats. *Tex. Rep. Biol. Med., 24*:576, 1966.

224. Earle, K.M.: X-ray diffraction and other studies of the calcareous deposits in human pineal glands. *J. Neuropathol. Exp. Neurol., 24*:108, 1964.

225. Ebadi, M.S., Weiss, B., and Costa, E.: A sensitive and specific method for assaying cyclic 3′, 5′-AMP in rat pineal gland. *Fed. Proc., 29*:263, 1970.

225a. Ebadi, M.S., Weiss, B., and Costa, E.: Diurnal periodicity of cyclic 3′,5′-adenosine monophosphate in rat pineal gland. *The Pharmacologist, 12*:489, 1970.

226. Ebadi, M.S., Weiss, B., and Costa, E.: Adenosine 3′, 5′-monophosphate in rat pineal gland: increase induced by light. *Science, 170*:188, 1970.

227. Ebadi, M.S., Weiss, B., and Costa, E.: Microassay of adenosine–3′, 5′-monophosphate (cyclic AMP) in brain and other tissues by the luciferin-luciferase system. *J. Neurochem.,18*:183, 1971.

228. Ebadi, M.S., Weiss, B., and Costa, E.: Distribution of cyclic adenosine monophosphate in rat brain. *Arch. Neurol., 24*:353, 1971.

229. Ebels, I.: Étude chemique des extraits épiphysaires fractionnés. *Biol. Med. (Paris), 56*:395, 1967.

230. Ebels, I., Balemans, M.G.M., and Verkley, A.J.: Separation of pineal extracts on Sephadex G-10. II. A spectrofluorimetric and thin layer chromatographic study of indoles in sheep pineal extract. *J. Neurovisc. Relat., 32*:270, 1972.

231. Ebels, I., Moszkowska, A., and Scémama, A.: Étude in vitro des extraits épiphysaires fractionnés. Resultats préliminaires. *C.R. Acad. Sci. (D) (Paris), 260*:5126, 1965.

232. Ebels, I., Moszkowska, A., and Scémama, A.: An attempt to separate a sheep pineal extract fraction showing antigonadotropic activity. *J. Neurovisc. Relat., 32*:1, 1970.

233. Ebels, I., and Prop, N.: A study of the effect of melatonin on the gonads, the oestrous cycle and the pineal organ of the rat. *Acta Endocrinol. (Kbh.), 49*:567, 1965.

234. Ebels, I., Versteeg, D.H.G., and Vliegenthart, J.F.G.: An attempt to isolate arginine vasotocin from sheep and bovine pineal body. *Koninkl. Nederl. Akad. Weten.-Amsterdam, Proc. Ser. B, 68*:1, 1965.

235. Edvinsson, L., Håkanson, R., Owman, C., and West, K.A.: Sympathetic influence on carbanhydrase activity in choroid plexus. *Exp. Cell Res., 67*:245, 1971.

236. Edvinsson, L., Owman, C., and West, K.A.: Changes in continuously recorded intracranial pressure of conscious rabbits at different time-periods after superior cervical sympathectomy. *Acta Physiol. Scand., 83*:42, 1971.

237. Eichberg, J., Schwartz, M., Shein, H., and Hauser, G.: Stimulation of ^{32}P incorporation into phosphatidylglycerol (PG) and phosphatidylinositol (PI) by catecholamines and propranolol in rat pineal organ cultures. *Fed. Proc., 31:*453, 1972.

238. Eigsti, O.J., and Dustin, P., Jr.: *Colchicine—in Agriculture, Medicine, Biology and Chemistry.* Ames, Iowa, Iowa State College Press, 1955.

239. Elden, C.A., Keyes, M.C., and Marshall, C.E.: Pineal body of the northern fur seal (*Callorhinus ursinus*): A model for studying the probable function of the mammalian pineal body. *Amer. J. Vet. Res., 32:*639, 1971.

240. Eldred, S.H., Bell, H.W., and Sherman, L.J.: A pilot study comparing the effects of pineal extract and a placebo in patients with chronic schizophrenia. *N. Engl. J. Med., 263:*1330, 1960.

241. Ellis, L.C.: Some interrelationships between experimental lighting, melatonin synthesis, and x-irradiation induced changes in the germinal epithelium of rat testes. *Fed. Proc.,* 29:452, 1970.

242. Ellis, L.C.: Inhibition of rat testicular androgen synthesis in vitro by melatonin and serotonin. *Endocrinology, 90:*17, 1972.

243. Ellis, L.C., Barfuss, D.W., and van Kampen, K.R.: Modification of rat testicular response to x-irradiation by various lighting regimes: 1. The pineal gland and melatonin synthesis as a possible mediator of the response. *Life Sci., 9:*1011, 1970.

244. Ellis, R.A., and Montagna, W.: Histology and cytochemistry of human skin. XV. Sites of phosphorylase and amylo-1, 6-glucosidase activity. *J. Histochem. Cytochem., 6:*201, 1958.

245. Ellison, N., Weller, J.L., and Klein, D.C.: Development of a circadian rhythm in the activity of pineal serotonin N-acetyltransferase. *J. Neurochem., 19:*1335, 1972.

246. Engel, P.: Untersuchungen über die Wirkung der Zirbeldrüse. *Z. Gesamte Exp. Med., 93:*69, 1934.

247. Engel, P.: Ueber den Einfluss von Hypophysenvorderlappen-hormonen und Epiphysen-hormon auf das Wachstum von Impftumoren. *Z. Krebsforsch., 41:*281, 1934.

248. Engel, P.: Ensayos sobre la glandula pineal. *Anales de la Sociedad de Biologia de Bogota, 1:*60, 1943.

249. Eränkö, O.: The practical histochemical demonstration of catecholamines by formaldehyde-induced fluorescence. *J. Microsc., 87:*259, 1967.

250. Eränkö, O., and Eränkö, L.: Loss of histochemically demonstrable catecholamines and acetylcholinesterase from sympathetic nerve fibers of the pineal body of the rat after chemical sympathectomy with 6-hydroxydopamine. *Histochemical Journal, 3:*357, 1971.

251. Eränkö, O., Rechardt, L., Eränkö, L., and Cunningham, A.: Acetylcholinesterase (AChE) activity in the sympathetic nerve

fibres of the pineal body (PB) of the rat. *Scand. J. Clin. Lab. Invest., 25(suppl. 113):*82, 1970.

252. Eränkö, O., Rechardt, L., Eränkö, L., and Cunningham, A.: Light and electron microscopic histochemical observations on cholinesterase-containing sympathetic nerve fibres in the pineal body of the rat. *Histochemical Journal, 2:*479, 1970.

253. Fabre, L.F., Jr., Banks, R.C., McIsaac, W.M., and Farrell, G.: Effects of ubiquinone and related substances on secretion of aldosterone and cortisol. *Am. J. Physiol., 208:*1275, 1965.

254. Fahn, S., and Côté, L.J.: Regional distribution of choline acetylase in the brain of the rhesus monkey. *Brain Res., 7:*323, 1968.

255. Fajer, A., Hoxter, G., and Fraga, E.: Electrophorectic pattern of the soluble proteins of a pineal body extract. *Nature (Lond.), 196:*274, 1962.

256. Falck, B., Hillarp, N.-Å, Thieme, G., and Torp, A.: Fluorescence of catechol amines and related compounds condensed with formaldehyde. *J. Histochem. Cytochem., 10:*348, 1962.

257. Falck, B., and Owman, C.: A detailed methodological description of the fluorescence method for the cellular demonstration of biogenic monoamines. *Acta Universitatis Lundensis, Sect. II, No. 7:*1, 1965.

258. Falck, B., Owman, C., and Rosengren, E.: Changes in rat pineal stores of 5-hydroxytryptamine after inhibition of its synthesis or break-down. *Acta Physiol. Scand., 67:*300, 1966.

259. Fales, H.M., and Pisano, J.J.: Gas chromatography of biologically important amines. *Anal. Biochem., 3:*337, 1962.

260. Farrell, G.: Epiphysis cerebri in the control of steroid secretion. *Fed. Proc., 19:*601, 1960.

261. Farrell, G.: Adrenoglomerulotropin. *Circulation, 21:*1009, 1960.

262. Farrell, G.: In discussion. *Recent Progr. Horm. Res., 19:*367, 1963.

263. Farrell, G., and McIsaac, W.M.: Adrenoglomerulotropin. *Arch. Biochem. Biophys., 94:*543, 1961.

264. Farrell, G., McIsaac, W.M., and Taylor, A.N.: Neurohumoral factors from the brain stem and epiphysis. *International Congress on Hormonal Steroids, Excerpta Medica. Int. Congr. Series, 51:*17, 1962.

265. Farrell, G., McIsaac, W.M., and Taylor, A.N.: Neurohumoral factors from the brainstem and epiphysis. In Martini, L., and Pecile, A. (Eds.): *Hormonal Steroids, Biochemistry, Pharmacology, and Therapeutics.* New York, Academic Press, 1964, vol. 1:141.

266. Fasano, A.V., Kasprow, B.A., Kovarik, F.A., and Velardo, J.T.: Enzyme study of the pineal gland of the albino rat during the estrous cycle. *The Physiologist, 14:*141, 1971.

267. Feldberg, W., and Fleischhauer, K.: Penetration of bromophenol blue from the perfused cerebral ventricles into the brain tissue. *J. Physiol (Lond.), 150:*451, 1960.

268. Feldstein, A., Chang, F.H., and Kucharski, J.M.: Tryptophol, 5-hydroxytryptophol and 5-methoxytryptophol induced sleep in mice. *Life Sci.*, *9:*323, 1970.
269. Feldstein, A., Williamson, O.: Serotonin metabolism in pineal homogenates. *Advances in Pharmacology*, *6A:*91, 1968.
270. Fenger, F.: The composition and physiologic activity of the pineal gland. *JAMA*, *67:*1836, 1916.
271. Fenwick, J.C.: Demonstration and effect of melatonin in fish. *Gen. Comp. Endocrinol.*, *14:*86, 1970.
272. Fernstrom, J.D., and Wurtman, R.J.: Brain serotonin content: Physiological dependence on plasma tryptophan levels. *Science*, *173:*149, 1971.
273. Fillion, G.M.B., Lluch, S., and Uvnäs, B.: Release of noradrenaline from the dog heart *in situ* after intravenous and intracoronary administration of 5-hydroxytryptamine. *Acta Physiol. Scand.*, *83:*115, 1971.
274. Fisher, E.: Preparation of an active fraction of the pineal gland. *Endocrinology*, *33:*116, 1943.
275. Fiske, V.M.: Serotonin rhythm in the pineal organ: control by the sympathetic nervous system. *Science*, *146:*253, 1964.
276. Fiske, V.M., Bryant, G.K., and Putnam, J.: Effect of light on the weight of the pineal in the rat. *Endocrinology*, *66:*489, 1960.
277. Fiske, V.M., and Huppert, L.C.: Melatonin action on pineal varies with photoperiod. *Science*, *162:*279, 1968.
278. Florkin, M., and Stotz, E.H. (Eds.): *Comprehensive Biochemistry. Report of the Commission on Enzymes of the International Union of Biochemistry.* Amsterdam, Elsevier Publ. Co., 1964, vol. 13.
279. Folbergrová, J., Passonneau, J.V., Lowry, O.H., and Schulz, D.W.: Glycogen, ammonia and related metabolites in the brain during seizures evoked by methionine sulphoximine. *J. Neurochem.*, *16:*191, 1969.
280. Folch, J., Ascoli, I., Lees, M., Meath, J.A., and LeBaron, F.N.: Preparation of lipide extracts from brain tissue. *J. Biol. Chem.*, *191:*833, 1951.
281. Folch, J., and LeBaron, F.N.: Chemical composition of the mammalian nervous system. In Richter, D. (Ed.): *Metabolism of the Nervous System.* London, Pergamon Press, 1957, p. 67.
282. Fontana, J.A., and Lovenberg, W.: A cyclic AMP-dependent protein kinase of the bovine pineal gland. *Proc. Nat. Acad. Sci. USA*, *68:*2787, 1971.
283. Fontana, J.A., and Lovenberg, W.: Pineal protein kinase and the regulation of hydroxyindole metabolism. *Fed. Proc.*, *31:*440, 1972.
284. Ford, D.H.: Uptake of ^{131}I-labeled triiodothyronine in the pineal

body as compared with the cerebral grey and other tissues of the rat. *Progr. Brain Res.*, *10*:530, 1965.

285. Ford, D.H., and Gross, J.: The metabolism of I^{131}-labeled thyroid hormones in the hypophysis and brain of the rabbit. *Endocrinology*, *62*:416, 1958.

286. Fore, H., and Morton, R.A.; Microdetermination of manganese in biological material by a modified catalytic method. *Biochem. J.*, *51*:594, 1952.

287. Fore, H., and Morton, R.A.: Manganese in rabbit tissues. *Biochem. J.*, *51*:600, 1952.

288. Fore, H., and Morton, R.A.: Manganese in eye tissues. *Biochem. J.*, *51*:603, 1952.

289. Fradá, G., and Micale, O.: Studio clinics—radiologico sulla calcificationi pineali in gravidanza. *Radiol. Med. (Torino)*, *28*:209, 1941.

290. Franchimont, P.: Action de la mélatonine et de la glomérulotrophine sur les fonctions génitale et surrénalienne du rat. *Arch. Int. Physiol Biochim.*, *72*:735, 1964.

291. Fraschini, F.: Role of indoleamines in the control of the secretion of pituitary gonadotropins. In Martini, L., and Meites, J. (Eds.): *Neurochemical Aspects of Hypothalamic Function*. New York, Academic Press, 1970, p. 141.

292. Fraschini, F., Collu, R., and Martini, L.: Mechanisms of inhibitory action of pineal principles on gonadotropin secretion. In Wolstenholme, G.E.W., and Knight, J. (Eds.): *The Pineal Gland*. Edinburgh and London, Churchill Livingstone, 1971, p. 259.

293. Fraschini, F., and Martini, L.: Rhythmic phenomena and pineal principles. In Martini, L., Motta, M., and Fraschini, F. (Eds.): *The Hypothalamus*. New York, Academic Press, 1970, p. 529.

294. Fraschini, F., Mess, B., and Martini, L.: Pineal gland, melatonin and the control of luteinizing hormone secretion. *Endocrinology*, *82*:919, 1968.

295. Fraschini, F., Mess, B., Piva, F., and Martini, L.: Brain receptors sensitive to indole compounds: function in control of luteinizing hormone secretion. *Science*, *159*:1104, 1968.

296. Frauchiger, E., and Sellei, K.: Dunnschichtschromatographie der Lipoide in der Glandula pinealis. *Schweiz. Arch. Neurol. Neurochir. Psychiatr.*, *98*:240, 1966.

297. Freysz, L., Bieth, R., and Mandel, P.: Kinetics of the biosynthesis of phospholipids in neurons and glial cells isolated from rat brain cortex. *J. Neurochem.*, *16*:1417, 1969.

298. Friede, R.L.: The relation of the formation of lipofuscin to the distribution of oxidative enzymes in the human brain. *Acta Neuropathol. (Berl.)*, *2*:113, 1962.

299. Friede, R.L.: *Topographic Brain Chemistry*. New York, Academic Press, 1966.

300. Friedman, J.J.: Muscle blood flow and ^{86}Rb as a capillary flow indicator. *Am. J. Physiol.*, *214:*488, 1968.
301. Frigerio, A.: Contributo alla conoscenza della ghiandola pineale. *Riv. Patol. Nerv. Ment.*, *19:*499, 1914.
302. Fuentes, J.A., and Longo, V.G.: An investigation on the central effects of harmine, harmaline and related β-carbolines. *Neuropharmacology*, *10:*15, 1971.
303. Fujita, T., Tanayama, S., Shirakawa, Y., and Suzuoki, Z.: Metabolic fate of ubiquinone-7. I. Absorption, excretion and tissue distribution in rats. *J. Biochem. (Tokyo)*, *69:*53, 1971.
304. Galasescu, P., and Urechia, C.-J.: Les cellules acidophiles de la glande pineale. *C. R. Soc. Biol. (Paris)*, *68:*623, 1910.
305. Gardner, J.H.: Development of the pineal body in the hooded rat. *Anat. Rec.*, *103:*538, 1949.
306. Gaston, S.: The influence of the pineal organ on the circadian activity rhythm in birds. In Menaker, M. (Ed.): *Biochronometry.* Washington, D.C., National Academy of Sciences, 1971, p. 541.
307. Gaston, S., and Menaker, M.: Pineal function: the biological clock in the sparrow. *Science, 160:*1125, 1968.
308. Gerebtzoff, M.A.: *Cholinesterases, a Histochemical Contribution to the Solution of some Functional Problems.* London, Pergamon Press, 1959, p. 159.
309. Gershon, M.D., and Ross, L.L.: Location of sites of 5-hydroxytryptamine storage and metabolism by radioautography. *J. Physiol. (Lond.)*, *186:*477, 1966.
310. Gessner, P.K., McIsaac, W.M., and Page, I.H.: Pharmacological actions of some methoxyindole alkylamines. *Nature (Lond.)*, *190:*179, 1961.
311. Gfeller, E., Green, A., and Snyder, S.H.: Regional differences in [3H]noradrenaline accumulation in monkey brain (*Macaca irus*). *Brain Res.*, *11:*263, 1968.
312. Ghosal, S., Bhattacharya, S.K., and Mehta, R.: Naturally occurring and synthetic β-carbolines as cholinesterase inhibitors. *J. Pharm. Sci.*, *61:*808, 1972.
313. Gianferrari, L.: Influenza dell'alimentazione con capsule surrenali, ipofisi ed epifisi su la pigmentazione cutanea ed il ritmo respiratorio di *Salmo fario. Arch. Sci. Biol. (Bologna)*, *3:*39, 1922.
314. Giarman, N.J., and Day, M.: Presence of biogenic amines in the bovine pineal body. *Biochem. Pharmacol, 1:*235, 1959.
315. Giarman, N.J., Day, S.M., and Pepeu, G.: Presence of neuro-humors in bovine pineal glands. *Fed. Proc.*, *18:*394, 1959.
316. Giarman, N.J., Freedman, D.X., and Picard-Ami, L.: Serotonin content of the pineal glands of man and monkey. *Nature (Lond.)*, *186:*480, 1960.

317. Gilbert, M.S.: The early development of the human diencephalon. *J. Comp. Neurol.*, *62*:81, 1935.

318. Giles, R.E., and Miller, J.W.: The catechol-O-methyl transferase activity and endogenous catecholamine content of various tissues in the rat and the effect of administration of U-0521 (3',4'-dihydroxy-2-methyl propiophenone). *J. Pharmacol. Exp. Ther.*, *158*:189, 1967.

319. Giordano, G., Balestreri, R., Jacopino, G.E., Foppiani, E., and Bertolini, S.: L'action *in vitro* de la mélatonine sur l'hormono-synthèse coritco-surrénale du rat. *Ann Endocrinol. (Paris)*, *31*: 1071, 1970.

320. Giroud, A., Ratsimamanga, A.R., Lebloud, C.P., Rabinowicz, M., and Drieux, H.: Répartition générale de l'acide ascorbique dans l'organisme et déductions. *Bull. Soc. Chim. Biol. (Paris)*, *19*:1105, 1937.

321. Gladstone, R.J., and Wakeley, C.P.G.: Development and histogenesis of the human pineal organ. *J. Anat.*, *69*:427, 1935.

322. Glick, D., and Biskind, G.R.: Studies in histochemistry. VII. Relationship between concentration of vitamin C and development of pineal gland. *Proc. Soc. Exp. Biol. Med.*, *34*:866, 1936.

323. Globus, J.H., and Silbert, S.: Pinealomas. *Arch. Neurol.*, *25*:937, 1931.

324. Glücksmann, A.: Cell deaths in normal vertebrate ontogeny. *Biol. Rev.*, *26*:59, 1951.

325. Godina, G.: La struttura dell'epiphysis cerebri in rapporto alla castrazione ed alla gravidanza. *Riv. Patol. Nerv. Ment.*, *54*:74, 1939.

326. Goldman, H.: The nervous control of blood flow to the pineal body. *Life Sci.*, *6*:2071, 1967.

327. Goldman, H., and Nikitovitch-Winer, M.B.: Rapid flow of blood through pituitary autographts in the rat. *Am J. Physiol.*, *217*:567, 1969.

328. Goldman, H., and Wurtman, R.J.: Flow of blood to the pineal body of the rat. *Nature (Lond.)*, *203*:87, 1964.

329. Goldstein, M., Lauber, E., and McKereghan, M.R.: The inhibition of dopamine-β-hydroxylase by tropolone and other chelating agents. *Biochem. Pharmacol.*, *13*:1103, 1964.

330. Gomori, G.: Histochemical localization of true lipase. *Proc. Soc. Exp. Biol. Med.*, *72*:697, 1949.

331. Goodyer, C.G.: H-Estradiol uptake studies in the neonatal female rat. *Anat. Rec.*, *172*:318, 1972.

332. Goridis, C., and Neff, N.H.: Evidence for a specific monoamine oxidase associated with sympathetic nerves. *Neuropharmacology*, *10*:557, 1971.

333. Goridis, C., and Neff, N.H.: Evidence for specific monoamine oxidases in human sympathetic nerve and pineal gland. *Proc. Soc. Exp. Biol. Med.*, *140*:573, 1972.

334. Grahame-Smith, D.G.: Tryptophan hydroxylation in brain. *Biochem. Biophys. Res. Commun.*, *16*:586, 1964.

335. Green, J.P.: Histamine. In Lajtha, A. (Ed.): *Handbook of Neurochemistry.* New York, Plenum Press, 1970, vol. 4, p. 221.

336. Green, J.P., Day, M., and Robinson, J.D., Jr.: Some acidic substances in neo-plastic mast cells and in the pineal body. *Biochem. Pharmacol.*, *11*:957, 1962.

337. Greenberg, D.M.: The acid-soluble phosphates in animal metabolism. In McElroy, W.D., and Glass, B. (Eds.): *Phosphorus Metabolism. A Symposium on the Role of Phosphorus in the Metabolism of Plants and Animals.* Baltimore, Johns Hopkins Press, 1952, vol. 2:3.

338. Greengard, P.: On the role and mechanism of action of cyclic AMP in neural function. *Fifth Internat. Congress on Pharmacology, Invited Presentations*, 236, 1972.

339. Greer, M., and Williams, C.M.: Gas-chromatographic determination of melatonin and 6-hydroxymelatonin. *Clin. Chim. Acta, 15*:165, 1967.

340. Grieder, A., Odartchenko, N., Cottier, H., Cronkite, E.P., and Schindler, R.: Specificity of tritiated thymidine as a precursor of DNA under conditions of prolonged administration. *Proc. Soc. Exp. Biol. Med.*, *134*:1026, 1970.

341. Griffith, G.C., Butt, E.M., and Walker, J.: The inorganic element content of certain human tissues. *Annals of Internal Medicine, 41*:501, 1954.

342. Gromova, E., Kraus, M., and Křeček, J.: Effect of melatonin and 5-hydroxytryptamine on aldosterone and corticosterone production by adrenal glands of normal and hypophysectomized rats. *J. Endocrinol.*, *39*:345, 1967.

343. Guidotti, A., Badiani, G., and Pepeu, G.: Taurine distribution in cat brain. *J. Neurochem.*, *19*:431, 1972.

344. Gusek, W.: Neue Befunde zur Morphologie und Frunktion der Epiphysis cerebri. *Ergebnisse der Allgemeinen Pathologie und Pathologischen Anatomie. 50*:103, 1968.

345. Gusek, W., Buss, H., and Wartenberg, H.: Weitere Untersuchungen zur Feinstruktur der Epiphysis cerebri normaler und vorbehandelter Ratten. *Progr. Brain Res.*, *10*:317, 1965.

346. Gusek, W., and Santoro, A.: Elektronenoptische Beobachtungen zur Ultramorphologie der Pinealzellen bei der Ratte. *Biologica Latina, 8*:451, 1960.

347. Gusek, W., and Santoro, A.: Zur Ultrastruktur der Epiphysis cerebri der Ratte. *Endokrinologie, 41*:105, 1961.

348. Gustavson, K.H.: *The Chemistry and Reactivity of Collagen.* New York, Academic Press, 1956.

349. Hackman, R.H., and Goldberg, M.: Microchemical detection of melanins. *Anal. Biochem., 41:*279, 1971.

350. Haddy, F.J., and Scott, J.B.: Metabolically linked vasoactive chemicals in local regulation of blood flow. *Physiol. Rev., 48:*688, 1968.

351. Hadfield, G.: Siderosis of the globus pallidus: its relation to bilateral necrosis. *J. Pathol., 32:*135, 1929.

352. Hadley, M.E., and Bagnara, J.T.: Integrated nature of chromatophore responses in the *in vitro* frog skin bioassay. *Endocrinology, 84:*69, 1969.

353. Hafeez, M.A., and Quay, W.B.: Pineal acetylserotonin methyltransferase activity in the teleost fishes, *Hesperoleucus symmetricus* and *Salmo gairdneri,* with evidence for lack of effect of constant light and darkness. *Comp. Gen. Pharmacol., 1:*257, 1970.

354. Håkanson, R., and Hoffman, G.J.: A sensitive radiometric assay for tryptophan-5-hydroxylase. *Biochem. Pharmacol., 16:*1677, 1967.

355. Håkanson, R., des Gouttes, M.-N.L., and Owman, C.: Activities of tryptophan hydroxylase, DOPA decarboxylase, and monoamine oxidase as correlated with the appearance of monamines in developing rat pineal gland. *Life Sci., 6:*2577, 1967.

356. Håkanson, R., and Owman, C.: Effect of denervation and enzyme inhibition on DOPA decarboxylase and monoamine oxidase activities of rat pineal gland. *J. Neurochem., 12:*417, 1965.

357. Håkanson, R., and Owman, C.: Pineal DOPA decarboxylase and monoamine oxidase activities as related to the monoamine stores. *J. Neurochem., 13:*597, 1966.

358. Halaris, A.: Effect of continuous illumination on mitochondria of the rat pineal body. *Acta Endocrinol. [suppl.] (Kbh.), 138:*239, 1969.

359. Halaris, A., and Matussek, N.: Effect of continuous illumination on mitochondria of the rat pineal body. *Experientia, 25:*486, 1969.

360. Halaris, A., Rüther, E., and Matussek, N.: Effect of a benzoquinolizine (RO-4-1284) on granulated vesicles of the rat brain. *Z. Zellforsch. Microsk. Anat., 76:*100, 1967.

361. Halberg, F.: Physiologic 24-hour periodicity; general and procedural considerations with reference to the adrenal cycle. *Zeitschrift für Vitamin-, Hormon-, und Fermentforschung, 10:*225, 1959.

362. Hallgren, B., and Sourander, P.: The effect of age on the non-haemin iron in the human brain. *J. Neurochem., 3:*41, 1958.

363. Halpern, C.C., and Martin, C.R.: Effect of melatonin and thymectomy on food and fluid intake and renal excretion rhythms of adrenalectomized rats. *Fed. Proc., 31:*27, 1972.

364. Halpert, B., Erickson, E.E., and Fields, W.S.: Intracranial involvement from carcinoma of the lung. *Arch. Pathol., 69:*93, 1960.

365. Hamberger, B., Malmfors, T., and Sachs, C.: Standardization of paraformaldehyde and of certain procedures for the histochemical demonstration of catecholamines. *J. Histochem. Cytochem.,* 13:147, 1965.

366. Hamburger, V., and Levi-Montalcini, R.: Proliferation, differentiation and degeneration in the spinal ganglia of the chick embryo under normal and experimental conditions. *J. Exp. Zool.,* 111:457, 1949.

367. Handa, S., and Burton, R.M.: Lipids of retina: I. Analysis of gangliosides in beef retina by thin layer chromatography. *Lipids,* 4:205, 1969.

368. Harper, A.E., Benevenga, N.J., and Wohlhueter, R.M.: Effects of ingestion of disproportionate amounts of amino acids. *Physiol. Rev.,* 50:428, 1970.

369. Hartmann, F.: Über die Innervation der Epiphysis cerebri einiger Säugetiere. *Z. Zellforsch. Microsk. Anat.,* 46:416, 1957.

370. Hassler, R., and Bak, I.J.: Effects of amine-depleting and amine-storing substances on the axonterminals of the pineal gland. In Uyeda, R. (Ed.): *Electron Microscopy,* Tokyo, Maruzen Co., Ltd., 1966, vol. 2, p. 521.

371. Haug, F.-M. Š.: Electron microscopical localization of the zinc in hippocampal mossy fibre synapses by a modified sulfide silver procedure. *Histochemie,* 8:355, 1967.

372. Hayhow, W.R., Webb, C., and Jervie, A.: The accessory optic fiber system in the rat. *J. Comp. Neurol.,* 115:187, 1960.

373. Hedlund, L., Ralph, C.L., Chepko, J., and Lynch, H.J.: A diurnal serotonin cycle in the pineal body of Japanese quail: photoperiod phasing and the effect of superior cervical ganglionectomy. *Gen. Comp. Endocrinol.,* 16:52, 1971.

374. Heidel, G.: Die Häufigkeit des Vorkommens von Kalkkonkrementen im Corpus pineale des Kindes. *Anat. Anz., 116:*139, 1965.

375. Heinecke, H.: Kernkugeln in den Parenchymzellen der Schweineepiphyse. *Z. Mikrosk. Anat. Forsch.,* 65:282, 1959.

376. Heiniger, H.J.: Histochemische Untersuchungen über den Ribonucleinsäuregehalt der Pineocyten der Glandula pinealis bei Schwein und Mensch. *Acta Neuropathol. (Berl.),* 4:340, 1965.

377. Heinzelman, R.V., and Szmuszkovicz, J.: Recent studies in the field of indole compounds. *Prog. Drug Res.,* 6:75, 1963.

378. Heller, A.: Neuronal control of brain serotonin. *Fed. Proc.,* 31:81, 1972.

379. Heller, H.: Neurohypophysial hormones. In von Euler, U.S., and Heller, H. (Eds.): *Comparative Endocrinology.* New York, Academic Press, 1963, vol. 1, p. 26.

380. Hellman, B., and Larsson, S.: Utilization of uniformly labelled ^{14}C-glucose in the pineal body of goats. *Acta Endocrinol. (Kbh),* 38:353, 1961.

381. Henneberg, B.: Normentafel zur Entwicklungsgeschichte der Wan-
     derratte *(Rattus norvegicus* Erxleben). In Keibel, F. (Ed.): *Nor-
     mentafel zur Entwicklungsgeschichte der Wirbeltiere.* Jena,
     Fischer, 1937, No. 15.
382. Hernández, F., Iglesias, J.F., and de Morentin, J.M.: Histochemical
     study of ubiquinones in the central nervous system of mice.
     *J. Anat., 110:*73, 1971.
383. Hernández, J., and Illnerová, H.: 5-Hydroxytryptophan decarboxy-
     lase activity in the rat pineal gland during the first 20 days of
     postnatal life: effect of light, *Neuroendocrinology, 6:*343, 1970.
384. Herring, P.T.: The pineal region of the mammalian brain: its
     morphology and histology in relation to function. *Q. J. Exp.
     Physiol., 17:*125, 1927.
385. Hertting, G., and Axelrod, J.: The fate of H³–norepinephrine at
     the sympathetic nerve endings. *Nature (Lond.), 192:*172, 1961.
386. Hertz-Eschel, M., and Rahamimoff, R.: Effect of melatonin on
     uterine contractility. *Life Sci., 4:*1367, 1965.
387. Hevesy, G.: *Radioactive Indicators, Their Application in
     Biochemistry, Animal Physiology, and Pathology.* New York,
     Interscience Publ. Inc., 1948.
388. Hidaka, H., Nagatsu, T., and Yagi, K.: Micro-determination of
     monoamine oxidase using serotonin as substrate. *J. Biochem.
     (Tokyo), 62:*621, 1967.
389. Hines, M.: Studies in the growth and differentiation of the telen-
     cephalon in man. The fissura hippocampi. *J. Comp. Neurol.,
     34:*73, 1922.
390. Hipkin, L.J.: Effect of 5-methoxytryptophol and melatonin on
     uterine weight responses to human chorionic gonadotrophin.
     *J. Endocrinol. (Lond.), 48:*287, 1970.
391. Hirsch, H.E.: Enzyme levels of individual neurons in relation to
     lipofuscin content. *J. Histochem. Cytochem., 18:*268, 1970.
392. Ho, B.T.: Inhibitors of hydroxyindole-O-methyltransferase. In
     Klein, D.C. (Ed.): *Pineal Gland: Proceedings of a Workshop.*
     New York, Raven Press, in press.
393. Ho, B.T., Fritchie, G.E., Noel, M.B., and McIsaac, W.M.:
     Hydroxyindole-O-methyltransferase V. Effects of substituents
     on hydrolysis of N-acyltryptamines in rats. *J. Pharm. Sci., 60:*634,
     1971.
394. Ho, B.T., McIsaac, W.M., and Tansey, L.W.: Hydroxyindole-
     O-methyltransferase I: substrate binding. *J. Pharm. Sci., 58:*130,
     1969.
395. Ho, B.T., McIsaac, W.M., and Tansey, L.W.: Hydroxyindole-
     O-methyltransferase. III: Influence of the phenyl moiety on the
     inhibitory activities of some N-acyltryptamines. *J. Pharm. Sci.,
     58:*563, 1969.

396. Ho, B.T., McIsaac, W.M., Tansey, L.W., and Kralik, P.M.: Hydroxyindole-O-methyltransferase II. Inhibitory activities of some N-acyltryptamines. *J. Pharm. Sci.*, *57:*1998, 1968.

397. Ho, B.T., McIsaac, W.M., Walker, K.E., and Estevez, V.: Inhibitors of monoamine oxidase. Influence of methyl substitution on the inhibitory activity of β-carbolines. *J. Pharm. Sci.*, *57:*269, 1968.

398. Ho, B.T., Noel, M.B., McIsaac, W.M.: Hydroxyindole-O-methyltransferase IV: Inhibitory activities of some N-acrylyltryptamines and N-crotonyltryptamines. *J. Pharm. Sci.*, *59:*573, 1970.

399. Ho, B.T., Noel, M.B., and Tansey, L.W.: Hydroxyindole-O-methyltransferase VI: Inhibitory activities of substituted benzoyltryptamines and benzenesulfonyltryptamines. *J. Pharm. Sci.*, *60:*636, 1971.

400. Ho, B.T., Taylor, D., Askew, W.E., and McIsaac, W.M.: Effect of 6-methoxy-1, 2, 3, 4-tetrahydro-β-carboline on the regional and subcellular distribution of serotonin in mouse and rat brains. *Life Sci.*, *11:*493, 1972.

401. Ho, B.T., Taylor, D., and McIsaac, W.M.: Studies on the mechanism of action of 6-methoxytetrahydro-β-carboline in elevating brain serotonin. In Ho, B.T., and McIsaac, W.M. (Eds.): *Brain Chemistry and Mental Disease.* New York, Plenum Press, 1971, Adv. Behav. Biol., vol. *1*, p. 97.

402. Hochstetter, F.: *Beiträge zur Entwicklungsgeschichte des menschlichen Gehirns.* Vienna and Leipzig, Franz Deuticke, 1919.

403. Hochstetter, F.: Über eine Varietät der Vena cerebralis basialis des Menschen nebst Bemerkungen über die Entwicklung bestimmter Hirnvenen. *Z. Anat. Entwicklungsgesch.*, *108:*311, 1938.

404. Hoffmann, K.: Melatonin inhibits photoperiodically induced testis development in a dwarf hamster. *Naturwissenschaften, 59:*218, 1972.

405. Hokin, L.E.: Effects of acetylcholine on the incorporation of ^{32}P into various phospholipids in slices of normal and denervated superior cervical ganglia of the cat. *J. Neurochem., 13:*179, 1966.

406. Hokin, L.E.: Phospholipid metabolism and functional activity of nerve cells. In Bourne, G.H. (Ed.): *The Structure and Function of Nervous Tissue.* New York and London, Academic Press, 1969, vol. *3*, p. 161.

407. Hopsu, V.K., and Arstila, A.U.: An apparent somato-somatic synaptic structure in the pineal gland of the rat. *Exp. Cell Res., 37:*484, 1965.

408. Horányi, B.: Das Corpus pineale im Senium. *Wien Z. Nervenheilkd.*, *17:*129, 1960.

409. Hosaka, T., Nakai, A., and Kushima, S.: Innervation of the pineal

body and the supracommissural and subcommissural organs of the japanese monkey. *Ika Shika Daigaku (Tokyo)*, 4:365, 1957.

410. Houssay, A.B., Pazo, J.H., and Epper, C.E.: Effects of the pineal gland upon the hair cycles in mice. *J. Invest. Dermatol., 47:*230, 1966.

411. Hu, F.: The influence of certain hormones and chemicals on mammalian pigment cells. *J. Invest. Dermatol., 46:*117, 1966.

412. Hu, K.H., and Friede, R.L.: Topographic determination of zinc in human brain by atomic absorption spectrophotometry. *J. Neurochem., 15:*677, 1968.

413. Hülsemann, M.: Development of the innervation in the human pineal organ. Light and electron microscopic investigations. *Z. Zellforsch. Mikrosk. Anat., 115:*396, 1971.

414. Hungerford, G.F., and Panagiotis, N.M.: Response of pineal lipid to hormone imbalances. *Endocrinology, 71:*936, 1962.

415. Hungerford, G.F., and Pomerat, C.M.: Observations on the growth of rat pineal gland in tissue culture. *Anat. Rec., 142:*347, 1962.

416. Hungerford, G.F., and Pomerat, C.M.: Rat pineal parenchymal cells as observed in tissue culture. *Z. Zellforsch. Mikrosk. Anat., 57,* 809, 1962.

417. Hungerford, G.F., and Pomerat, C.M.: Observations on the rat pineal in tissue culture. *Progr. Brain Res., 10:*465, 1965.

418. Hutchins, D.A., and Rogers, K.J.: Physiological and drug-induced changes in the glycogen content of mouse brain. *Br. J. Pharmacol., 39:*9, 1970.

419. Huxley, J.S., and Hogben, L.T.: Experiments on amphibian metamorphosis and pigment responses in relation to internal secretions. *Proc. R. Soc. Lond. [Biol.],* 93:36, 1922.

420. Huxley, M., and Tapp, E.: Effects of biogenic amines on the growth of rat tumours. *Life Sci. [II],* 11:19, 1972.

421. Huxley, M., and Tapp, E.: The histochemical measurements of the lipid content of the pineal gland in rats suffering from malignancy. *Brain Res., 37:*23, 1972.

422. Hyyppä, M.: Hypothalamic monoamines and pineal dopamine during the sexual differentiation of the rat brain. *Experientia,* 27:336, 1971.

423. Hyyppä, M., Lehtinen, P., and Rinne, U.K.: Effect of L-DOPA on the hypothalamic, pineal and striatal monoamines and on the sexual behaviour of the rat. *Brain Res., 30:*265, 1971.

424. Ichiyama, A., Nakamura, S., Nishizuka, Y., and Hayaishi, O.: Tryptophan-5-hydroxylase in mammalian brain. *Advances in Pharmacology, 6A:*5, 1968.

425. Illnerová, H.: 5-Hydroxytryptophan decarboxylase activity in the rat pineal body during ontogenesis. *Physiologia Bohemoslovaca, 18:*119, 1969.

426. Illnerová, H.: Effect of environmental lighting on serotonin rhythm in rat pineal gland during postnatal development. *Life Sci.* [*I*], *10:*583, 1971.

427. Illnerová, H.: Effect of light on the serotonin content of the pineal gland. *Life Sci.* [*I*], *10:*955, 1971.

428. Ito, T., and Matsushima, S.: A quantitative morphological study of the postnatal development of the pineal body of the mouse. *Anat. Rec., 159:*447, 1967.

429. Ito, T., and Matsushima, S.: Electron microscopic observations on the mouse pineal, with particular emphasis on its secretory nature. *Arch. Histol. Jap., 30:*1, 1968.

430. Ito, T., and Matsushima, S.: Effects of gonadectomy and hypophysectomy on the pineal body in the mouse: a quantitative morphological study. *Anat. Rec., 162:*479, 1968.

431. Iverson, L.L.: *The Uptake and Storage of Noradrenaline in Sympathetic Nerves.* Cambridge, Cambridge Univ. Press, 1967.

432. Izawa, Y.: Studies on the pineal body I. On the postnatal growth of the pineal body of the albino rat with observations on its histology. *J. Comp. Neurol., 39:*1, 1925.

433. Jackson, R.L., and Lovenberg, W.: Isolation and characterization of multiple forms of hydroxyindole-O-methyltransferase. *J. Biol. Chem., 246:*4280, 1971.

434. Jacobson, J.G., and Smith, L.H., Jr.: Biochemistry and physiology of taurine and taurine derivatives. *Physiol. Rev., 48:*424, 1968.

435. Jaim-Etcheverry, G., and Zieher, L.M.: Ultrastructural cytochemistry and pharmacology of 5-hydroxytryptamine in adrenergic nerve endings. III. Selective increase of norepinephrine in the rat pineal gland consecutive to depletion of neuronal 5-hydroxytryptamine. *J. Pharmacol. Exp. Ther., 178:*42, 1971.

436. Jarvik, M.E.: Drugs used in the treatment of psychiatric disorders. In Goodman, L.S., and Gilman, A. (Eds.): *The Pharmacological Basis of Therapeutics.* New York, Macmillan Co., 1965, 3rd. edition.

437. Jensen, E.V., and Jacobson, H.I.: Basic guides to the mechanism of estrogen action. *Recent Progr. Horm. Res., 18:*387, 1962.

438. Jequier, E., Robinson, D.S., Lovenberg, W., and Sjoerdsma, A.: Further studies on tryptophan hydroxylase in rat brainstem and beef pineal. *Biochem. Pharmacol., 18:*1071, 1969.

439. Jöchle, W.: Über die Wirkung eines Epiphysenextraktes (Glanepin) auf Sexualentwicklung and Sexualcyklus junger weiblicher Ratten unter normalen Hallungsbedingungen und bei Dauerbeleuchtung. *Endokrinologie, 33:*287, 1956.

440. Johanson, C.: The central veins and deep dural sinuses of the brain. *Acta Radiol. (Stockh.), suppl. 107:*1, 1954.

441. Johnson, J.L., and Aprison, M.H.: The distribution of glutamic acid,

a transmitter candidate, and other amino acids in the dorsal sensory neuron of the cat. *Brain Res., 24:*285, 1970.

442. Jones, R.L., McGeer, P.L., and Greiner, A.C.: Metabolism of exogenous melatonin in schizophrenic and non-schizophrenic volunteers. *Clin. Chim. Acta, 26:*281, 1969.

443. Jonsson, G.: *The formaldehyde fluorescence method for the histochemical demonstration of biogenic amines. A methodological study.* Stockholm, Haeggströms Tryckeri AB, 1967, p. 1.

444. Joó, F., and Csillik, B.: Topographic correlation between the hematoencephalic barrier and the cholinesterase activity of brain capillaries. *Exper. Brain Res., 1:*147, 1966.

445. Jordan, H.E.: The histogenesis of the pineal body of the sheep. *Am. J. Anat., 12:*249, 1911.

446. Jordan, H.E.: A note on the cytology of the pineal body of the sheep. *Anat. Rec., 22:*275, 1921.

447. Jouan, P., Boisseau, J., and More, E.: Isolement des acides amines et des peptides de la glande pinéale de mouton. *Rev. Roum. Endocrinol., 5:*117, 1968.

448. Jouan, P., Dai, T.V., and Cormier, M.: Sur la nature des phospholipides de la glande pineale (épiphyse) du porc. *Bull. Soc. Chim. Biol. (Paris), 46:*1121, 1964.

449. Jouan, P., Garreau, A., and Samperez, S.: Extraction et séparation des peptides de la glande pinéale du mouton. *Ann. Endocrinol. (Paris), 26:*535, 1965.

450. Jouan, P., and Rocaboy, J.-C.: Étude de quelques activités enzymatiques de l'épiphyse du porc. *C. R. Soc. Biol. (Paris), 159:*591, 1965.

451. Jouan, R., and Rocaboy, J.-C.: Étude de l'activité peptidasique de la glande pineale du porc. *C. R. Soc. Biol. (Paris), 160:*859, 1966.

452. Jouan, P., and Samperez, S.: Recherches sur l'action de la N-acétyl, 5-methoxytryptamine (mélatonine) vis-à-vis de la sécretion adrenocorticotrope hypophysaire chez le rat. *C. R. Soc. Biol. (Paris), 159:*1270, 1965.

453. Jouan, P., Samperez, S., Boisseau, J., and Dupuis, A.: Méthode d'isolement de la 5-hydroxytryptamine et des dérivés indoliques par chromatographie sur gel de Séphadex G. 25. *Rev. Roum. Endocrinol., 5:*161, 1968.

454. Jouan, P., Samperez, S., and Garreau, A.: Isolement de la 5-hydroxytryptamine (serotonine) des épiphyses de rats par filtration sur gel de Sephadex G. 25. *Ann. Endocrinol. (Paris), 27:*561, 1966.

455. Kaasik, A.E., Nilsson, L., Siesjö, B.K.: The effect of asphyxia upon the lactate, pyruvate and bicarbonate concentrations of brain tissue and cisternal CSF, and upon the tissue concentrations of phosphocreatine and adenine nucleotides in anesthetized rats. *Acta Physiol. Scand., 78:*433, 1970.

456. Kachi, T., Matsushima, S., and Ito, T.: Diurnal changes in glycogen content in the pineal cells of the male mouse. *Z. Zellforsch. Mikrosk. Anat., 118:*310, 1971.

457. Kallenbach, H., and Malz, W.: Über den Einfluss der Epiphyse auf das Wachstum transplantabler Impftumoren. *Endokrinologie, 34:*293, 1957.

458. Kamberi, I.A., Mical, R.S., and Porter, J.C.: Effect of anterior pituitary perfusion and intraventricular injection of catecholamines and indoleamines on LH release. *Endocrinology, 87:*1, 1970.

459. Kaplan, H.A., and Ford, D.H.: *The Brain Vascular System.* Amsterdam, Elsevier Publ. Co., 1966.

460. Kappers, J.A.: The development, topographical relations and innervation of the epiphysis cerebri in the albino rat. *Z. Zellforsch. Mikrosk. Anat., 52:*163, 1960.

461. Kappers, J.A.: Melatonin, a pineal compound. Preliminary investigations on its function in the rat. *Gen. Comp. Endocrinol., 2:*610, 1962.

462. Kappers, J.A.: Epiphysis. In Crosby, E.C., Humphrey, T., and Lauer, E.W. (Eds.) *Correlative Anatomy of the Nervous System.* New York, Macmillan Co., 1962.

463. Kappers, J.A.: Survey of the innervation of the pineal organ in vertebrates. *Amer. Zool., 4:*47, 1964.

464. Kappers, J.A.: Survey of the innervation of the epiphysis cerebri and the accessory pineal organs of vertebrates. *Progr. Brain Res., 10:*87, 1965.

465. Kappers, J.A.: On the innervation of the pineal organs and on their function in relation to their innervation. In Bargmann, W. (Ed.): *Aus der Werkstatt der Anatomen.* Stuttgart, Georg Thieme Verlag, 1965, p. 93.

466. Kappers, J.A.: The mammalian pineal organ. *J. Neurovisc. Relat., suppl. 9:*140, 1969.

467. Kappers, J.A., Prop, N., and Zweens, J.: Qualitative evaluation of pineal fats in the albino rat by histochemical methods and paper chromatography and the changes in pineal fat contents under physiological and experimental conditions. *Progr. Brain Res., 5:*191, 1964.

468. Karahasanoğlu, A.M., and Özand, P.T.: The purification and properties of bovine pineal S-adenosylmethionine: N-acetylserotonin O-methyl transferase. *J. Neurochem., 19:*411, 1972.

469. Karasek, M.: Electron microscopic cytologic studies of the pineal in albino rats treated with serpasil and niamid. *Polish Endocrinology, 16:*187, 1965.

470. Karasek, M.: Morphologic and histochemical studies on the pineal gland in white rats during regeneration of the adrenals. *Polish Endocrinology, 19:*236, 1968.

471. Karasek, M.: Ultrastructure of the epiphysis in white rats under

normal conditions and after hypophysectomy. *Polish Endo-crinology, 22:*13, 1971.

472. Karler, A.: Report summarizing work on the Bergmann pineal prep-arations. *Zeitschrift für Vitamin-, Hormon- und Ferment-forschung, 12:*350, 1963.

473. Kashiwamata, S.: Brain cystathionine synthase: vitamin-B_6 require-ment for its enzymic reaction and changes in enzymic activity during early development of rats. *Brain Res., 30:*185, 1971.

474. Kastin, A.J., Redding, T.W., and Schally, A.V.: MSH activity in rat pituitaries after pinealectomy. *Proc. Soc. Exp. Biol. Med., 124:*1275, 1967.

475. Kastin, A.J., and Schally, A.V.: *In vivo* assay for melanocyte lighten-ing substances. *Experientia, 22:*389, 1966.

476. Kastin, A.J., and Schally, A.V.: Autoregulation of release of melanocyte stimulating hormone from the rat pituitary. *Nature (Lond.), 213:*1238, 1967.

477. Kastin, A.J., Schally, A.V., Viosca, S., Barrett, L., and Redding, T.W.: MSH activity in the pituitaries of rats exposed to constant illumination. *Neuroendocrinology, 2:*257, 1967.

478. Kawamura, R., and Hosono, H.: Fettbefunde der innersek-retorischen Organe. *Transactions of the Japanese Path. Soc., 23:*232, 1933.

479. Kawashima, T., Takeuchi, K., Nakamura, M., and Ogata, T.: The relationship between histochemical enzyme activities of brain tumors and clinical features of the patients.*Acta Med. Okayama., 19:*293, 1965.

480. Kenny, G.C.: The "nervus conarii" of the monkey. (An experimental study). *J. Neuropathol. Exp. Neurol., 20:*563, 1961.

481. Kety, S.S.: Theory of blood-tissue exchange and its application to measurement of blood flow. *Methods in Medical Research, 8:*223, 1960.

482. Kevorkian, J., and Wessel, W.: So-called "nuclear pellets" ("kernkugeln") of pineocytes. *Arch. Pathol., 68:*513, 1959.

483. Key, B.J., and White, R.P.: Neuropharmacological comparison of cystathionine, cysteine, homoserine and alpha-ketobutyric acid in cats. *Neuropharmacology, 9:*349, 1970.

484. Khelimsky, A.M.: On the origin of cerebral sand from the colloid of epiphysis. *Probelmy Endokrinologii i Gormonoterapii, 4:*86, 1958.

485. Khelimsky, A.M.: *Epiphysis (Pineal Gland).* Moscow, "Medicine," 1969, p. 1.

486. Kincl, F.A., Chang, C.C., and Zbuzkova, V.: Observation on the influence of changing photoperiod on spontaneous wheel-running activity of neonatally pinealectomized rats. *Endo-crinology, 87:*38, 1970.

487. Kinson, G.A., and Peat, F.: The influences of illumination, melatonin and pinealectomy on testicular function in the rat. *Life Sci., 10:*259, 1971.

488. Kinson, G.A., and Robinson, S.: Gonadal function of immature male rats subjected to light restriction, melatonin administration and removal of the pineal gland. *J. Endocrinol., 47:*391, 1970.

489. Kirk, J.E.: Variations with age in the tissue contents of vitamins and hormones. *Vitamins and Hormones, 20:*67, 1962.

490. Kitay, J.I., and Altschule, M.D.: *The Pineal Gland. A Review of the Physiologic Literature.* Cambridge, Mass., Harvard University Press, 1954.

491. Kitay, J.I., and Altschule, M.D.: Effects of pineal extract administration on ovary weight in rats. *Endocrinology, 55:*782, 1954.

492. Klatzo, I., Miquel, J., Ferris, P.J., Prokop, J.D., and Smith, D.E.: Observations on the passage of the fluorescein labeled serum proteins (FLSP) from the cerebrospinal fluid. *J. Neuropathol, Exp. Neurol., 23:*18, 1964.

493. Klaus, S.N., and Snell, R.S.: The response of mammalian epidermal melanocytes in culture to hormones. *J. Invest. Dermatol., 48:*352, 1967.

494. Klein, D.C.: Biochemistry of the pineal gland. II. In Klein, D.C. (Ed.): *Pineal Gland: Proceedings of a Workshop.* New York, Raven Press, 1972.

495. Klein, D.C., and Berg, G.R.: Pineal gland: stimulation of melatonin production by norepinephrine involves cyclic AMP-mediated stimulation of N-acetyltransferase. In Greengard, P., and Costa, E. (Eds.): *Role of Cyclic AMP in Cell Function.* New York, Raven Press, 1970.

496. Klein, D.C., Berg, G.R., and Weller, J.: Melatonin synthesis: adenosine 3′,5′-monophosphate and norepinephrine stimulate N-acetyltransferase. *Science, 168:*979, 1970.

497. Klein, D.C., Berg, G.R., Weller, J., and Glinsmann, W.: Pineal gland: dibutyryl cyclic adenosine monophosphate stimulation of labeled melatonin production. *Science, 167:*1738, 1970.

498. Klein, D.C., and Lines, S.V.: Pineal hydroxyindole-O-methyl transferase activity in the growing rat. *Endocrinology, 84:*1523, 1969.

499. Klein, D.C., and Notides, A.: Thin-layer chromatographic separation of pineal gland derivatives of serotonin–^{14}C, *Anal. Biochem., 31:*480, 1969.

500. Klein, D.C., Reiter, R.J., and Weller, J.L.: Pineal N-acetyltransferase activity in blinded and anosmic male rats. *Endocrinology, 89:*1020, 1971.

501. Klein, D.C., and Rowe, J.: Pineal gland in organ culture. I. Inhibition by harmine of serotonin–^{14}C oxidation, accompanied by stimulation of melatonin–^{14}C production. *Mol. Pharmacol., 6:*164, 1970.

502. Klein, D.C., and Weller, J.L.: Indole metabolism in the pineal gland: a circadian rhythm in N-acetyltransferase. *Science, 169:*1093, 1970.

503. Klein, D.C., and Weller, J.: Pineal gland in culture: serotonin N-acetyltransferase activity is stimulated by norepinephrine and dibutyryl cyclic adenosine monophosphate. *Fed. Proc., 29:*615, 1970.

504. Klein, D.C., and Weller, J.: Input and output signals in a model neural system: the regulation of melatonin production in the pineal gland. *In Vitro, 6:*197, 1970.

505. Klein, D.C., and Weller, J.L.: Pineal N-acetylserotonin. *Fed. Proc., 31:*222, 1972.

506. Klein, D.C., and Weller, J.L., and Moore, R.Y.: Melatonin metabolism: neural regulation of pineal serotonin: acetyl coenzyme A N-acetyltransferase activity. *Proc. Nat. Acad. Sci. USA, 68:*3107, 1971.

507. Klüver, H.: Porphyrins in relation to the development of the nervous system. In Waelsch, H. (Ed.): *Biochemistry of the Developing Nervous System.* New York, Academic Press, 1955, p. 137.

508. Kobayashi, F., Hara, K., and Miyake, T.: Further studies on the causal relationship between the secretion of estrogen and the release of luteinizing hormone in the rat. *Endocrinol. Jap., 16:*501, 1969.

509. Kolmer, W.: Ganglienzellen als konstanter Bestandteil der Zirbel von Affen. *Zeitschrift für Gesamte Neurologie und Psychiatrie, 121:*423, 1929.

510. König, A., and Engelhardt, D.C.: Die Tagesperiodik des neurohypophysären Adiuretins männlicher Ratten unter Dauerlicht. *Journal of Interdisciplinary Cycle Research, 1:*349, 1970.

511. König, A., and Meyer, A.: Tagesperiodische Schwankungen einer antidiuretischen Aktivität aus der Epiphysis cerebri ausgewachsener männlicher Ratten. *Naturwissenschaften, 54:*93, 1967.

512. König, A., and Meyer, A.: The effect of continuous illumination on the circadian rhythm of the antidiuretic activity of the rat pineal. *Journal of Interdisciplinary Cycle Research, 2:*255, 1971.

513. Kopin, I.J., and Gordon, E.K.: Metabolism of H^3-norepinephrine released by tyramine and reserpine. *J. Pharmacol. Exp. Ther., 138:*351, 1962.

514. Kopin, I.J., Pare, C.M.B., Axelrod, J., and Weissbach, H.: 6-Hydroxylation, the major metabolic pathway for melatonin. *Biochim. Biophys. Acta., 40:*377, 1960.

515. Kopin, I.J., Pare, C.M.B., Axelrod, J., and Weissbach, H.: The fate of melatonin in animals. *J. Bilo. Chem., 236:*3072, 1961.

516. Kovács, K., David, M.A., and Weisz, P.: Aldosteronotrophic and

corticosteronotrophic substances in normal human brain. *Med. Exp. (Basel)*, 3:113, 1960.

517. Krabbe, K.H.: Histologische und embryologische Untersuchungen über die Zirbeldrüse des Menschen. *Anatomische Hefte, 54:* 187, 1916.

518. Krabbe, K.H.: Bidrag til kundskaben om corpus pineal hos pattedyrene. *Biologiske Meddelelser udgivnae af Det Kgl. Danske Videnskabernes Selskab.*, 2:1, 1920.

519. Krakoff, L.R., de Champlain, J., and Axelrod, J.: Abnormal storage of norepinephrine in experimental hypertension in the rat. *Circ. Res.*, 21:583, 1967.

520. Krass, M.E., and LaBella, F.S.: Biochemical evidence for a secretory role of the pineal body. Oxidation of $(1-^{14}C)$—and $(6-^{14}C)$ glucose *in vitro* by pineal body, pituitary, and brain from young and adult animals. *J. Neurochem.*, 13:1157, 1966.

521. Krass, M.E., and LaBella, F.S.: Hexosemonophosphate shunt in endocrine tissues. Quantitative estimation of the pathway in bovine pineal body, anterior pituitary, posterior pituitary, and brain. *Biochim. Biophys. Acta, 148:* 384, 1967.

522. Krisman, C.R.: A method for the colorimetric estimation of glycogen with iodine. *Anal. Biochem.*, 4:17, 1962.

523. Kroon, D.B.: Certain cells in the hypothalamic neurosecretory nuclei which are stainable by the acid-haematein test for phospholipids according to Baker. *Z. Zellforsch. Mikrosk. Anat., 61:* 317, 1963.

524. Krstić, R.: Intramitochondriellen lamellarkörper in Pinealzellen. *Biochimica e Biologia Sperimentale*, 6:19, 1967.

525. Krstić, R.: Die Einwirking von Kälte auf mit zinkjodid-osmium tetroxyd reagierende synaptische Bläschen in den Nervenendigungen im Corpus pineale der Ratte. *Z. Anat. Entwicklungsgesch., 135:* 301, 1972.

526. Kugler, J.H., and Wilkinson, W.J.C.: Glycogen fractions and their role in the histochemical detection of glycogen. *J. Histochem. Cytochem.*, 8:195, 1960.

527. Kunkel, A.: The influence of melatonin on the male gonad in Sprague-Dawley rats. *Polish Endocrinology, 20:* 32, 1969.

528. Kveder, S., and McIsaac, W.M.: The metabolism of melatonin (N-acetyl-5-methoxytryptamine) and 5-methoxytryptamine. *J. Biol. Chem.*, 236:3214, 1961.

529. Kveder, S., McIsaac, W.M., and Page, I.H.: The metabolism of N-Acetyl-5-[β-^{14}C] methoxytryptamine. *Biochem. J.,* 76:28P, 1960.

530. LaBella, F.S., and Krass, M.E.: Oxidation of ^{14}C-1- and ^{14}C-6-glucose in vitro by bovine pineal body (PB) anterior pituitary (AP), posterior pituitary (PP), and brain (B.). *Fed. Proc.*, 25:254, 1966.

531. LaBella, F.S., and Shin, S.: Estimation of cholinesterase and choline

acetyltransferase in bovine anterior pituitary, posterior pituitary, and pineal body. *J. Neurochem., 15:*335, 1968.

532. LaBella, F.S., Vivian, S., and Queen, G.: Abundance of cystathionine in the pineal body. Free amino acids and related compounds of bovine pineal, anterior and posterior pituitary and brain. *Biochim. Biophys. Acta, 158:*286, 1968.

533. Lacassagne, A., Chamorro, A., Hurst, L., and Giao, N.B.: Effet de l'epiphysectomie sur l'hépatocancérogenèse chimique chez le rat. *C. R. Acad. Sci. [D] (Paris), 269:*1043, 1969.

534. Laduron, P., and Belpaire, F.: Transport of noradrenaline and dopamine-β-hydroxylase in sympathetic nerves. *Life Sci., 7:*1, 1968.

535. Laduron, P., and Belpaire, F.: Tissue fractionation and catecholamines—II. Intracellular distribution patterns of tyrosine hydroxylase, DOPA decarboxylase, dopamine-β-hydroxylase, phenylethanolamine N-methyltransferase and monoamine oxidase in adrenal medulla. *Biochem. Pharmacol., 17:*1127, 1968.

536. Langman, J.: Histogenesis of the central nervous system. In Bourne, G.H. (Ed.): *The Structure and Function of Nervous Tissue.* New York, Academic, 1968, vol. *1,* p. 33.

537. Larrabee, M.G., Klingman, J.D., and Leicht, W.S.: Effects of temperature, calcium and activity on phospholipid metabolism in a sympathetic ganglion. *J. Neurochem., 10:*549, 1963.

538. Larrabee, M.G., and Leicht, W.S.: Metabolism of phosphatidyl inositol and other lipids in active neurones of sympathetic ganglia and other peripheral nervous tissues. The site of the inositide effect. *J. Neurochem., 12:*1, 1965.

539. Lauber, J.K., Boyd, J.E., and Axelrod, J.: Enzymatic synthesis of melatonin in avian pineal body: extraretinal response to light. *Science, 161:*489, 1968.

540. Lazo-Wasem, E.A., and Graham, C.E.: Quantitative *in vivo* assay of pineal melanophore contracting principle (melatonin). *Fed. Proc., 19:*150, 1960.

541. Leduc, E.H., and Wislocki, G.B.: The histochemical localization of acid and alkaline phosphatases, non-specific esterase and succinic dehydrogenase in the structures comprising the hematoencephalic barrier of the rat. *J. Comp. Neurol., 97:*241, 1952.

542. Le Gros Clark, W.E.: The nervous and vascular relations of the pineal gland. *J. Anat., 74:*471, 1940.

543. Lenti, G., Molinatti, G.M., and Pizzini, A.: Sull'azione svolta da un estratto liofilizzato di ghiandola pineale sull'apparato genitale del topo e del ratto (ricerche sui rapporti epifisi-ipofisi). *Folia Endocrinol. (Roma), 10:*11, 1957.

544. Leonhardt, H.: Über axonähnliche Fortsätze, Sekretbildung und

Estrusion der hellen Pinealozyten des Kaninchens. Z. *Zellforsch. Mikrosk. Anat., 82:*307, 1967.

545. Leopold, P.G.: Über den histotopochemischen Nachweis von Vitamin C in Zentralnervensystem (mit Berucksichtigung der Epiphysis Cerebri.) Zugleich ein Beitrag zur Frage der Spezifität der Vitamin C-Reaktion. Z. *Zellforsch. Mikrosk. Anat., 31:*502, 1941.

546. Lerner, A.B., and Case, J.D.: Pigment cell regulatory factors. *J. Invest. Dermatol., 32:*211, 1959.

547. Lerner, A.B., Case, J.D., Biemann, K., Heinzelman, R.V., Szmuszkovicz, J., Anthony, W.C., and Krivis, A.: Isolation of 5-methoxyindole-3-acetic acid from bovine pineal glands. *J. Am. Chem. Soc., 81:*5264, 1959.

548. Lerner, A.B., Case, J.D., and Heinzelman, R.V.: Structure of melatonin. *J. Am. Chem. Soc., 81:*6084, 1959.

549. Lerner, A.B., Case, J.D., Mori, W., and Wright, M.R.: Melatonin in peripheral nerve. *Nature (Lond.), 183:*1821, 1959.

550. Lerner, A.B., Case J.D., and Takahashi, Y.: Isolation of melatonin and 5–methoxyindole–3–acetic acid from bovine pineal glands. *J. Biol. Chem., 235:*1992, 1960.

551. Lerner, A.B., Case, J.D., Takahashi, Y., Lee, T.H., and Mori, W.: Isolation of melatonin, the pineal gland factor that lightens melanocytes. *J. Am. Chem. Soc., 80:*2587, 1958.

552. Lerner, A.B., and Wright, M.R.: *In vitro* frog skin assay for agents that darken and lighten melanocytes. *Methods of Biochem. Analysis, 8:*294, 1960.

553. Leske, R., and Mayersbach, H.v.: The role of histochemical and biochemical preparation methods for the detection of glycogen. *J. Histochem. Cytochem., 17:*527, 1969.

554. Levi–Montalcini, R.: The origin and development of the visceral system in the spinal cord of the chick embryo. *J. Morphol., 86:*253, 1950.

555. Levi–Montalcini, R.: Control mechanisms in the sympathetic nervous system. In Paoletti, R., and Davison, A.N. (Eds.): *Chemistry and Brain Development.* New York, Plenum Press, 1971, p. 185.

556. Levi–Montalcini, R., and Angeletti, P.U.: Biological properties of a nerve-growth promoting protein and its antiserum. In: Kety, S.S., and Elkes, J. (Eds.): *Regional Neurochemistry.* New York, Pergamon Press, 1961, p. 362.

557. Levi–Montalcini, R., and Angeletti, P.U.: Immunosympathectomy. *Pharmacol. Rev., 18:*619, 1966.

558. Levin, P.M.: A nervous structure in the pineal body of the monkey. *J. Comp. Neurol., 68:*405, 1938.

559. Levitt, M., Spector, S., Sjoerdsma, A., and Udenfriend, S.: Elucida-

tion of the rate–limiting step in norepinephrine biosynthesis in the perfused guinea–pig heart. *J. Pharmacol. Exp. Ther., 148:*1, 1965.

560. Lignac, G.O.E.: Über die Entstehung von Sandkörnern und Pigment in der Zirbeldrüse. *Beitr. Pathol. Anat., 72:*366, 1925.

561. Lilja, B.: Displacement of the calcified pineal body in roentgen pictures as an aid in diagnosing intracranial tumors. *Acta Radiol. (Stockh.), suppl. 37:*1, 1939.

562. Lin, H.–S.: Microcylinders within mitchondrial cristae in the rat pinealocyte. *J. Cell Biol., 25:*435, 1965.

563. Linden I., and Smith, B.H.: Neuronal uptake of ^{3}H–thymidine. *Curr. Mod. Biol., 2:*274, 1968.

564. Lingjaerde, P., Malm, O.J., Natvig, R.A., and Skaug, O.E.: The effect of adrenalectomy on the uptake of radioactive phosphorus in the rat. *Acta Endocrinol. (Kbh.), 28:*558, 1958.

565. Lingjaerde, P., Malm, O.J., and Skaug, O.E.: Some biochemical aspects of the effect of chlorpromazine in the rat. *Confin. Neurol., 18:*124, 1958.

566. Lingjaerde, P., Malm, O.J., and Skaug, O.E.: P^{32} uptake in pinealectomized-adrenalectomized rats. *Acta Endocrinol. (Kbh.), 31:*305, 1959.

567. Lingjaerde, P., and Skaug, O.E.: Effect of 5–hydroxytryptamine on the uptake of P^{32} in the rat. *J. Biol. Chem., 226:*33, 1957.

568. Lloyd, K.G., and Hornykiewicz; ,O.: Occurrence and distribution of aromatic L–amino acid (L–dopa) decarboxylase in the human brain. *J. Neurochem., 19:*1549, 1972.

569. Löfgren, F.O.: Vertebral angiography in the diagnosis of tumors in the pineal region. *Acta Radiol. (Stockh.), 50:*108, 1958.

570. Lott, I.T., Quarles, R.H., and Klein, D.C.: Glycoproteins are synthesized and secreted by pineal glands in culture. *Fed. Proc., 30:*364, 1971.

571. Louis, C.J., Kenny, G.C., and Anderson, R.M.: Autoradiographic localization of 5–hydroxytryptamine in monkey pineal gland. *Experientia, 26:*756, 1970.

572. Lovenberg, W., Jequier, E., and Sjoerdsma, A.: Tryptophan hydroxylation: measurement in pineal gland, brainstem, and carcinoid tumor. *Science, 155:*217, 1967.

573. Lovenberg, W., Jequier, E., and Sjoerdsma, A.: Trytophan hydroxylation in mammalian systems. *Advances in Pharmacology, 6A:*21, 1968.

574. Lovenberg, W., Weissbach, H., and Udenfriend, S.: Aromatic L–amino acid decarboxylase. *J. Biol. Chem., 237:*89, 1962.

575. Lues, G.: Die Feinstruktur des Zirbeldrüse normaler, trächtiger und experimentell beeinflusster Meerschweinchen. *Z. Zellforsch. Mikrosk. Anat., 114:*38, 1971.

576. Lynch, H.J.: Diurnal oscillations in pineal melatonin content. *Life Sci.,* [*I*], *10:*791, 1971.

577. Lynch, H.J., and Ralph, C.L.: Diurnal variation in pineal melatonin and its non–relationship to HIOMT activity. *Am. Zool., 10:*300, 1970.

578. Lynch, H.J., and Wurtman, R.J., and Greenhouse, G.: Relative merits of *Rana pipiens* and *Xenopus laevis* larvae in the quantitative assay of melatonin. *Am. Zool., 11:*650, 1971.

579. Macdonald, R.A.: Human and experimental hemochromatosis and hemosiderosis. In Wolman, M. (Ed.): *Pigments in Pathology.* New York, Academic Press, 1969, p. 115.

580. Machado, A.B.M.: Ultrastructure of the pineal body of the newborn rat. *Anat. Rec., 154:*381, 1966.

581. Machado, A.B.M.: Electron microscopy of developing sympathetic fibres in the rat pineal body. The formation of granular vesicles. *Progr. Brain Res., 34:*171, 1971.

582. Machado, A.B.M., Faleiro, L.C.M., and Da Silva, W.D.: Study of mast cell and histamine contents of the pineal body. Z. *Zellforsch. Mikrosk. Anat., 65:*521, 1965.

583. Machado, A.B.M., and Lemos, V.P.J.: Histochemical evidence for a cholinergic sympathetic innervation of the rat pineal body. *J. Neurovisc. Relat., 32:*104, 1971.

584. Machado, A.B.M., and Machado, C.R.d.S.: Occurrence and distribution of alcaline phosphatase in the human subcommissural organ. *Anat. Rec., 151:*463, 1965.

585. Machado, A.B.M., Machado, C.R.S., and Wragg, L.E.: Catecholamines and granular vesicles in adrenergic axons of the developing pineal body of the rat. *Experientia, 24:*464, 1968.

586. Machado, C.R.S.: Histochemical study of catecholamines and 5–HT in the developing pineal body. *Anat. Res., 157:*282, 1967.

587. Machado, C.R.S.. Machado, A.B.M., and Wragg, L.E.: Circadian serotonin rhythm control: sympathetic and nonsympathetic pathways in rat pineals of different ages. *Endocrinology, 85:*846, 1969.

588. Machado, C.R.S., Wragg, L.E., and Machado, A.B.M.: A histochemical study of sympathetic innervation and 5–hydroxytryptamine in the developing pineal body of the rat. *Brain Res., 8:*310, 1968.

589. Machado, C.R.S., Wragg, L.E., and Machado, A.B.M.: Circadian rhythm of serotonin in the pineal body of immunosympathectomized immature rats. *Science, 164:*442, 1969.

590. MacKinnon, P.C.B., and Simpson, R.A.: Preliminary observations on the uptake and incorporation of C^{14} uridine into RNA in brains of female rats from birth to senility. In Mitchell, R.P. (Ed.): *Endocrinology and Human Behavior.* London, Oxford Univ. Press, 1968, p. 330.

591. Mahoney, K., Vogel, W.H., Salvenmoser, F., and Boehme, D.H.: Activity of choline acetyltransferase in various human adult and fetal tissues. *J. Neurochem., 18:*1357, 1971.

592. Maickel, R., and Miller, F.: The fluorometric determination of indolealkylamines in brain and pineal gland. *Advances in Pharmacology, 6A:*71, 1968.

593. Manocha, S.L.: Histochemical distribution of alkaline and acid phosphatase and adenosine triphosphatase in the brain of squirrel monkey *(Saimiri sciureus). Histochemie, 21:*221, 1970.

594. Manocha, S.L.: Histochemical distribution of acetylcholinesterase and simple esterases in the brain of squirrel monkey (*Saimiri sciureus). Histochemie, 21:*236, 1970.

595. Manocha, S.L., and Bourne, G.H.: Histochemical mapping of monoamine oxidase and lactic dehydrogenase in the pons and mesencephalon of squirrel monkey (*Saimiri sciureus). J. Neurochem., 13:*1047, 1967.

596. Marcean, R., Nanu, L., Ionescu, V., and Milcu, I.: Actiunea pinealectomiei asupra permeabilității tesutului conjunctiv subcutanat la sobolan. *Stud. Cercet. Endocrinol., 19:*289, 1968.

597. Marczynski, T.J., Yamaguchi, N., Ling, G.M., and Grodzinska, L.: Sleep induced by the administration of melatonin (5-methoxy-N-acetyltryptamine) to the hypothalamus in unrestrained cats. *Experientia, 20:*435, 1964.

598. Maren, T.H.: Carbonic anhydrase: chemistry, physiology and inhibition. *Physiol. Rev., 47:*595, 1967.

599. Markina, V.V.: Determination of lipids and the lipase activity level in the epiphysis of adrenalectomized rats kept on a diet containing different amounts of sodium. *Biull. Eksp. Biol. Med., 69:*34, 1970.

600. Marston, H.R.: Cobalt, copper and molybdenum in the nutrition of animals and plants. *Physiol. Rev., 32:*66, 1952.

601. Matthews, M.J., Benson, B., and Rodin, A.E.: Antigonadotropic activity in a melatonin-free extract of human pineal glands. *Life Sci.* [*I*], *10:*1375, 1971.

602. McCord, C.P., and Allen, F.P.: Evidences associating pineal gland function with alterations in pigmentation. *J. Exp. Zool., 23:*207, 1917.

603. McGeer, E.G., Gibson, S., Wada, J.A., and McGeer, P.L.: Distribution of tyrosine hydroxylase activity in adult and developing brain. *Can. J. Biochem., 45:*1943, 1967.

604. McGeer, E.G., and McGeer, P.L.: Circadian rhythm in pineal tyrosine hydroxylase. *Science, 153:*73, 1966.

605. McGuire, J., and Möller, H.: Response of melanocytes of dermis and epidermis to lightening agents. *Nature (Lond.)., 208:*493, 1965.

606. McGuire, J., and Möller, H.: Differential responsiveness of dermal and epidermal melanocytes of *Rana pipiens* to hormones. *Endocrinology*, 78:367, 1966.

607. McIlwain, H.: *Biochemistry and the Central Nervous System*. Boston, Little Brown, 1959, 2nd edition.

608. McIsaac, W.M.: A biochemical concept of mental disease. *Postgrad. Med., 30:*111, 1961.

609. McIsaac, W.M.: Formation of 1-methyl-6-methoxy-1,2,3,4-tetra-hydro-2-carboline under physiological conditions. *Biochim. Biophys. Acta*, 52:607, 1961.

610. McIsaac, W.M., and Estevez, V.: Structure-action relationship of β-carbolines as monoamine oxidase inhibitors. *Biochem. Pharmacol.*, 15:1625, 1966.

611. McIsaac, W.M., Farrell, G., Taborsky, R.G., and Taylor, A.N.: Indole compounds: isolation from pineal tissue. *Science*, 148:102, 1965.

612. McIsaac, W.M., Khairallah, P.A., and Page, I.H.: 10-Methoxyharmalan, a potent serotonin antagonist which affects conditioned behavior. *Science*, 134:674, 1961.

613. McIsaac, W.M., Taborsky, R.G., and Farrell, G.: 5-Methoxytryptophol: effect on estrus and ovarian weight. *Science*, 145:63, 1964.

614. McIsaac, W.M., Taylor, D., Walker, K.E., and Ho, B.T.: 6-Methoxy-1,2,3,4-tetrahydro-β-carboline—a serotonin elevator.*J. Neurochem.*, 19:1203, 1972.

615. McKennee, C.T., Timiras, P.S., and Quay, W.B.: Concentrations of 5-hydroxytryptamine in rat brain and pineal after adrenalectomy and cortisol administration. *Neuroendocrinology, 1:* 251, 1966.

616. Meister, A.: *Biochemistry of the Amino Acids*. New York, Academic Press, 1965, 2nd edition, 2 vols.

617. Menaker, M.: The pineal organ and circadian rhythmicity. *Gen. Comp. Endocrinol.*, 18:608, 1972.

618. Merritt, J.H., and Sulkowski, T.S.: Alterations of pineal gland biorhythms by N-methyl-3-piperidyl benzilate. *J. Pharmacol. Exp. Ther.*, 166:119, 1969.

619. Mess, B.: Endocrine and neurochemical aspects of pineal function. *Int. Rev. Neurobiol.*, 11:171, 1968.

620. Meyburg, P.: Zur Frage nach der Herkunft der Parenchymzellen des Pinealorganes. *Schweiz. Arch. Neurol. Neurochir. Psychiatr.*, 95:245, 1965.

621. Meyer, C.J., Wurtman, R.J., Altschule, M.D., and Lazo-Wasem, E.A.: The arrest of prolonged estrus in "middle-aged" rats by pineal gland extract. *Endocrinology*, 68:795, 1961.

622. Mikami, S.: Cytological and histochemical studies of the pineal bodies of domestic animals. *Tohoku Journal of Agricultural Research*, 2:41, 1951.

623. Milcou, I., Nanu, L., and Marcean, R.: De l'existence d'une hormone hypoglycémiante épiphysaire synergique de l'insuline. *Ann. Endocrinol. (Paris)*, *18:*612, 1957.

624. Milcou, I., Nanu, L., Marcean, R., and Sitaru, S.: L'action de l'extrait pinéal et de la pinéalectomie, sur le glycogène hepatique et musculaire après infusion prolongée de glucose. *Stud. Cercet. Endocrinol.*, *14:*651, 1963.

625. Milcou, S., Milcou, I., and Nanu, L.: Le rôle de la glande pinéale dans le métabolisme des glucides. *Ann. Endocrinol. (Paris)*, *24:*233, 1963.

626. Milcou, S.M., and Petrea, I.: Caractère secrétoire des cellules de la glande pinéale vue au microscope électronique. *Ann. Endocrinol. (Paris)*, *22:*902, 1961.

627. Milcou, S.M., and Petrea, I.: Some aspects of the endocrinosecretory cytodynamic in the pineal gland at the electron microscope. In: *Electron Microscopy 1964*, Prague, Publ. House Czech Acad. Sci., 1965, vol.B, p. 481.

628. Milcou, S.M., Vrejoin, G., Marcean, R., and Nanu, L.: L'action de l'hormone hypoglycémiante épiphysaire sur le pancréas endocrinien chez les animaux alloxanisés. *Ann. Endocrinol. (Paris)*, *18:*621, 1957.

629. Milcu, I., Damian, E., Ionescu, M., and Popescu, I.: Cercetări privind actiunea antisexuală a melatoninei. *Stud. Cercet. Endocrinol.*, *17:*229, 1966.

630. Milcu, I., Marcean, R., and Ionescu, V.: Controlul actiunii melatoninei asupra glicemiei. *Stud. Cercet. Endocrinol.*, *18:*405, 1967.

631. Milcu, I., Nanu, L., and Marcean, R.: Cercetări *in vitro* privind efectul metabolic al epifizhormonului. *Stud. Cercet. Endocrinol.*, *11:*467, 1960.

632. Milcu, I., Nanu-Ionescu, L., Marcean, R., and Ionescu, V.: The influence of the pineal gland on nitrogen metabolism. *J. Endocrinol.*, *45:*175, 1969.

633. Milcu, S.M., Pavel, S., and Neacsu, C.: Biological and chromatographic characterization of a polypeptide with pressor and oxytocic activities isolated from bovine pineal gland. *Endocrinology*, *72:*563, 1963.

634. Milcu, S.M., Petrescu, R.R., and Tască, C.: The effect of thyroxine and cortisol on some dehydrogenases and lysosomal enzymes activities in rat pineal cultures. *Histochemie*, *15:*312, 1968.

635. Milcu, S.M., and Vrejoiu, G.: Structure of the pineal gland in aged subjects. *Rom. Med. Rev.*, *3:*13, 1959.

636. Milin, R., Devercerski, V., and Krstić, R.: Corpus pineale-glande de nature sensoneuroendocrine. *Akad. Nauka I Umjetnosti Bosne I Hercegovine, Odjeljenje Medicinskih Nauka,37:*69, 1969.

637. Milin, R., Stern, P., and Hukovic, S.: Sur la présence de la serotonine dans la glande pineale. *Akad. Savet. Fnrj., Bull. Sci., Ljusl. Yougoslavie, 4:*75, 1959.

638. Miline, R., Krstić, R., and Devečerski, V.: Sur le comportement de la glande pineale dans des conditions de stress. *Acta Anat. (Basel), 71:*352, 1968.

639. Miline, R., Werner, R., Scepovic, M., Devečerski, V., and Miline, J.: Influence du froid sur le comportement du noyau supraoptique chez les rats épiphysectomisés. *C.R. Assoc. Anat., Bull. Assoc. Anat., 145:*289, 1970.

640. Miller, A.L., and Pitts, F.N., Jr.: Brain succinate semialdehyde dehydrogenase-III. Activities in twenty-four regions of human brain. *J. Neurochem., 14:*579, 1967.

641. Miller, F.P., and Maickel, R.P.: Fluorometric determination of indole derivatives. *Life Sci., 9:*747, 1970.

642. Millhouse, O.E.: A golgi study of the descending medial forebrain bundle. *Brain Res., 15:*341, 1969.

643. Milofsky, A.: The fine structure of the pineal in the rat, with special reference to parenchyma. *Anat. Rec., 127:*435, 1957.

644. Misugi, K., Liss, L., and Bradel, E.J.: Electron microscopic study of an ectopic pinealoma. *Acta Neuropathol. (Berl.), 9:*346, 1967.

645. Mitchell, G.A.G.: The cranial extremities of the sympathetic trunks. *Acta Anat. (Basel), 18:*195, 1953.

646. Mizuno, H., and Sensui, N.: Lack of effects of melatonin administration and pinealectomy on the milk ejection response in the rat. *Endocrinol. Jap., 17:*417, 1970.

647. Mokrasch, L.C.: Free amino acid content of normal and neoplastic rodent astroglia. *Brain Res., 25:*672, 1971.

648. Molinoff, P., and Axelrod, J.: Octopamine: normal occurrence in sympathetic nerves of rats. *Science, 164:*428, 1969.

649. Molinoff, P., and Axelrod, J.: Biochemistry of catecholamines. *Ann. Rev. Biochem., 40:*465, 1971.

650. Molinoff, P.B., and Axelrod, J.: Distribution and turnover of octopamine in tissues. *J. Neurochem., 19:*157, 1972.

651. Moore, R.Y.: Pineal response to light: mediation by the accessory optic system in the monkey. *Nature (Lond.), 222:*781, 1969.

652. Moore, R.Y., Heller, A., Bhatnager, R.K., Wurtman, R.J., and Axelrod, J.: Central control of the pineal gland: visual pathways. *Arch. Neurol., 18:*208, 1968.

653. Moore, R.Y., Heller, A., Wurtman, R.J., and Axelrod, J;: Visual pathway mediating pineal response to environmental light. *Science, 155:*220, 1967.

654. Moore, R.Y., and Smith, R.A.: Postnatal development of a norepinephrine response to light in the rat pineal and salivary glands. *Neuropharmacology, 10:*315, 1971.

655. Moreau, M.H.: Radiological localization of the pineal gland. *Acta Radiol. [Diagn.] (Stockh.)*, 5:65, 1966.

656. Moreau, N.: *Contribution a l'Etude de Certaines Correlations Endocriniennes de l'Epiphyse (Avec: La Glande Diencephalique, La Prehypophyse, La Corticosurrenale, La Thyroide)*. These, Faculte de Med., Univ. Nancy, 1964, p. 1.

657. Morgane, P.J.: The function of the limbic and rhinic forebrain-limbic midbrain systems, and reticular formation in the regulation of food and water intake. *Ann. N.Y. Acad. Sci.*, 157:806, 1969.

658. Mori, M., Sugimura, M., and Matsuura, H.: Histochemical observations of monoamine oxidase activity in human tumors. *Ann. Histochim.*, 15:97, 1970.

659. Mori, W., and Lerner, A.: A microscopic bioassay for melatonin. *Endocrinology*, 67:443, 1960.

660. Moszkowska, A.: Contribution a l'étude de l'antagonisme epiphyso-hypophysaire. *J. Physiol. (Paris)*, 43:827, 1951.

661. Moszkowska, A.: Contribution à l'étude du mécanisme de l' antagonisme épiphyso-hypophysaire. *Progr. Brain Res.*, 10:564, 1965.

662. Moszkowska, A.: Étude des extraits épiphysaires fraction-nés—Physiologie. *Biol. Med. (Paris)*, 56:403, 1967.

663. Moszkowska, A., and des Gouttes, M.N.: L'action des extraits épiphysaires sur la réponse du tractus génital de la Ratte exposée à la lumière continue. *C.R. Soc. Biol. (Paris)*, 156:1750, 1962.

664. Moszkowska, A., and Ebels, I.: A study of the antigonadotropic action of synthetic arginine vasotocin. *Experientia*, 24:610, 1968.

665. Moszkowska, A., Ebels, I., and Scémama, A.: Étude *in vitro* des extraits fractionnes d'épiphyses d'agneau. *C.R. Soc. Biol. (Paris)*, 159:2298, 1965.

666. Moszkowska, A., Kordon, C., and Ebels, I.: Biochemical fractions and mechanisms involved in the pineal modulation of pituitary gonadotropin release. In Wolstenholme, G.E.W., and Knight, J. (Eds.): *The Pineal Gland*. Edinburgh and London, Churchill Livingstone, 1971.

667. Motta, M., Fraschini, F., and Martini, L.: Endocrine effects of pineal gland and of melatonin. *Proc. Soc. Exp. Biol. Med.*, 126:431, 1967.

668. Mukherji, M., Ray, A.K., and Sen, P.B.: Histochemical identification of noradrenaline in fluorescence microscopy by borohy-dride–periodic acid sequence. *J. Histochem. Cytochem.*, 14:479, 1966.

669. Munns, T.W.: Effect of different photoperiods on melatonin synth-esis in the pineal gland of the canary *(Serinus canarius)* and testicular activity. *Anat. Rec.*, 166:352, 1970.

670. Musacchio, J., Kopin, I.J., and Snyder, S.: Effects of disulfiram on tissue norepinephrine content and subcellular distribution of dopamine, tyramine and their β-hydroxylated metabolites. *Life Sci., 3:*769, 1964.

671. Musacchio, J.M., and Wurzburger, R.: Aggregation of beef adrenal tyrosine hydroxylase. *Fed. Proc., 28:*287, 1969.

672. Mussini, E., and Marcucci, F.: Free amino acids in brain after treatment with psychotropic drugs. In Holden, J.T. (Ed.):, *Amino Acid Pools. Distribution, Formation and Function of Free Amino Acids.* Amsterdam, Elsevier, 1962, p. 486.

672a. Nagle, C.A., Cardinali, D.P., and Rosner, J.M.: Light regulation of rat retinal hydroxyindole–O–methyl transferase (HIOMT) activity. *Endocrinology, 91:*423, 1972.

673. Nair, R.M.G., Kastin, A.J., and Schally, A.V.: Isolation and structure of another hypothalamic peptide possessing MSH–release–inhibiting activity. *Biochem. Biophys. Res. Commun., 47:*1420, 1972.

674. Nakatani, M., Ohara, Y., Katagiri, E., and Nakano, K.: Studien über die zirbellosen weiblichen weissen Ratten. *Trans. Soc. Pathol. Jap., 30:*232, 1940.

675. Namin, P.: *L'Angiographic Vertébrale.* Paris, G. Doin et Cie, 1955, p. 1.

676. Nanu–Ionescu, L., and Ionescu, V.: The pineal gland and the insulin metabolism. I. The plasmatic level of total insulinic activity and of free and bound insulin during experimental apinealism. *Stud. Cercet. Endocrinol., 20:*237, 1969.

677. Nanu–Ionesco, L., Marcean, R., and Ionesco, V.: Modèle expérimental pour l'étude du métabolisme azoté chez la souris. Application du contrôle de l'activité d'un extrait pinéal. *Rev. Roum. Endocrinol., 6:*293, 1969.

678. Narang, G.D., Singh, D.V., and Turner, C.W.: Effect of melatonin on thyroid hormone secretion rate and feed consumption of female rats. *Proc. Soc. Exp. Biol. Med., 125:*184, 1967.

679. Nasr, H., Hamed, M.Y., and Soliman, F.A.: Studies on pineal body functions. I. The relation between the pineal body and some anterior pituitary hormones in male rabbits. *Zentralbl. Veterinärmedizin., 8:*192, 1961.

680. Neff, N.H., and Barret, R.E., and Costa, E.: Kinetic and fluorescent histochemical analysis of the serotonin compartments in rat pineal gland. *Eur. J. Pharmacol., 5:*348, 1969.

681. Niemi, M., and Ikonen, M.: Histochemical evidence of aminopeptidase activity in rat pineal gland. *Nature (Lond.), 185:*9280, 1960.

682. Nir, I., Behroozi, K., Assael, M., Ivriani, I., and Sulman, F.G.: Changes in the electrical activity of the brain following pinealectomy. *Neuroendocrinology, 4:*122, 1969.

683. Nir, I., Hirschmann, N., Mishkinsky, J., and Sulman, F.G.: The effect of light and darkness on nucleic acids and protein metabolism of the pineal gland. *Life Sci.*, 8:279, 1969.
684. Nir, I., Hirschmann, N., and Sulman, F.G.: The effect of light and darkness on lactic acid content of the pineal gland. *Proc. Soc. Exp. Biol. Med.*, 133:452, 1970.
685. Nir, I., Hirschmann, N., and Sulman, F.G.: Diurnal rhythms of pineal nucleic acids and protein. *Neuroendocrinology*, 7:271, 1971.
686. Nir, I., Hirschmann, N., and Sulman, F.G.: Influence of the oestrous cycle on the nucleic acid and protein content of the rat pineal gland. *Experientia*, 28:88, 1972.
687. Nir, I., Hirschmann, N., and Sulman, F.G.: Pineal gland changes of rats exposed to heat. *Experientia*, 28:701, 1972.
688. Nir, I., Kaiser, N., Hirschmann, N., and Sulman, F.G.: The effect of 17β—estradiol on pineal metabolism. *Life Sci.*, 9:851, 1970.
689. Nishimura, T., Tanimukai, H., and Nishinuma, K.: Distribution of carbonic anhydrase in human brain. *J.Neurochem.*, 10:257, 1963.
690. Norton, W.T., and Poduslo, S.E.: Neuronal perikarya and astroglia of rat brain: chemical composition during myelination. *J. Lipid Res.*, 12:84, 1971.
691. Nováková, V., Sandritter, W., Křeček, J., and Zelenková: Veranderungen des Nucleinsäuregehaltes von Zellen der Epiphyse während der postnatalen Entwicklung bei Ratten. *Virchows Arch.* [*Zellpathol.*], 2:292, 1969.
692. Nováková, V., Sterc, J., Sandritter, W., and Křeček, J.: The day–night difference in total RNA content of parenchymal cells of rat pineal gland. *Beitr. Pathol. Anat.*, 144:211, 1971.
693. Novales, R.R., and Novales, B.J.: Analysis of antagonisms between pineal melatonin and other agents which act on the amphibian melanophore. *Progr. Brain Res.*, 10:507, 1965.
694. Obrunčník, M., and Bayerová, G.: The scope of fluorescent and polarized–light–microscopical investigation in the human pineal body. *Cesk. Morfol.*, 10:329, 1962.
695. Oksche, A., Ueck, M., and Rüdeberg: Comparative ultrastructural studies of sensory and secretory elements in pineal organs. *Memoirs Soc. Endocrinol.*, 19:7, 1971.
696. Olson, R.E., Gursey, D., and Vester, J.W.: Evidence for a defect in tryptophan metabolism in chronic alcoholism. *N. Engl. J. Med.*, 263:1169, 1960.
697. Olsson, R.: Subcommissural ependyma and pineal organ development in human fetuses. *Gen. Comp. Endocrinol.*, 1:117, 1961.
698. O'Rahilly, R.: The development of the epiphysis cerebri and the subcommissural complex in staged human embryos. *Anat. Rec.*, 160:488, 1968.

699. Orfino, G.: Ultrastructure of the pineal gland as observed under electronmicroscope. *Policlinico [Med.], 70:*179, 1963.
700. Orlandi, N., and Guardini, G.: Sulla struttura della pineale umana. *Rivista Sud-americana de Endocrinologia, Inmunologia y Quimioterapia, 12:*465, 1929.
701. Ortega, P., Malamud, N., and Shimkin, M.G.: Metastasis to the pineal body. *Arch. Pathol., 52:*518, 1951.
702. O'Steen, W.K., and Dill, R.E.: Intracellular monoamine oxidase and lipids in diffusion chamber cultures of the pineal organ. *J. Histochem. Cytochem., 12:*615, 1964.
703. Ota, M., Hsieh, K.S., Sato, N., and Obara, K.: Gonado-tropin–inhibiting substance in urine. IV. The absence of the inhibitor in urine of pinealectomized rat. *Proc. 42nd. Ann. Meeting, Japan Endocrinol. Soc.,* 137, 1969.
704. Otani, T., Creaven, P.J., Farrell, G., and McIsaac, W.M.: Studies on the biosynthesis of 5–methoxytryptophol in the pineal. *Biochim. Biophys. Acta, 184:*184, 1969.
705. Otani, T., Györkey, F., and Farrell, G.: Enzymes of the human pineal body. *J. Clin. Endocrinol. Metab., 28:*349, 1968.
706. Ouyang, R., and Rozdilsky, B.: Metastasis of carcinoma to pineal body. Report of two cases. *Arch. Neurol., 15:*399, 1966.
707. Owman, C.: Sympathetic nerves probably storing two types of monoamines in the rat pineal gland. *Int. J. Neuropharmacology, 3:*105, 1964.
708. Owman, C.: New aspects of the mammalian pineal gland. *Acta Physiol. Scand., 63 (suppl. 240):*1, 1964.
709. Owman, C.: Localization of neuronal and parenchymal monoamines under normal and experimental conditions in the mammalian pineal gland. *Progr. Brain Res., 10:*423, 1965.
710. Owman, C.: On the significance of the 5–hydroxytryptamine stores in the pineal gland. *Adv. Pharmacol., 6A:*167, 1968.
711. Owman, C., and West, K.A.: Effect of superior cervical sympathec-tomy on experimentally induced intracranial hypertension. *Brain Res., 18:*469, 1970.
712. Palkovits, M.: Morphology and function of the subcommissural organ. *Studia Biologica Academiae Scientiarum Hungaricae. 4:*1, 1965.
713. Panagiotis, N.M., and Hungerford, G.F.: Response of the pineal and adrenal glands to sodium restriction. *Anat. Rec., 139:*262, 1961.
714. Panagiotis, N.M., and Hungerford, G.F.: Response of the pineal and adrenal glands to sodium restriction. *Endocrinology, 69:*217, 1961.
715. Panagiotis, N.M., and Hungerford, G.F.: Response of the pineal

gland to hypophysectomy, hormone administration and dietary sodium restriction. *Anat. Rec., 142*:264, 1962.

716. Panagiotis, N.M., and Hungerford, G.F.: Responses of pineal sympathetic nerve processes and endings to angiotensin. *Nature (Lond.), 211*:374, 1966.

717. Panda, J.N., and Turner, C.W.: The role of melatonin in the regulation of thyrotrophin secretion. *Acta Endocrinol. (Kbh.), 57*:363, 1968.

718. Pavel, S.: Evidence for the presence of lysine vasotocin in the pig pineal gland. *Endocrinology, 77*:812, 1965.

719. Pavel, S.: Endocrine functions of arginine vasotocin from mammalian pineal gland. *Gen. Comp. Endocrinol., 9*:481, 1967.

720. Pavel, S.: Tentative identification of arginine vasotocin in human cerebrospinal fluid. *J. Clin. Endocrinol. Metab., 31*:369, 1970.

721. Pavel, S., and Petrescu, S.: Inhibition of gonadotrophin by a highly purified pineal peptide and by synthetic arginine vasotocin. *Nature (Lond.), 212*:1054, 1966.

722. Pavel, T.: Investigations on a new pineal hormone with a peptidic structure. *Stud. Cercet, Endocrinol., 14*:665, 1963.

723. Pearse, A.G.E.: *Histochemistry Theoretical and Applied.* Boston, Little, Brown, first edition, 1953.

724. Pearse, A.G.E.: *Histochemistry Theoretical and Applied.* Boston, Little, Brown, 1960, second edition.

725. Pearse, A.G.E.: *Histochemistry Theoretical and Applied.* Boston, Little, Brown, 1968, third edition, vol. 1.

726. Pelc, S.R.: Labelling of DNA and cell division in so–called non–dividing tissues. *J. Cell Biol, 22*:21, 1964.

727. Pelc, S.R.: Metabolic DNA and the problem of ageing. *Exp. Gerontol., 5*:217, 1970.

728. Pelham, R.W., Mull, D.R., and Ralph, C.L.: A melatonin–like principle in chicken serum. *Am. Zool., 11*:650, 1971.

729. Pelham, R.W., Ralph, C.L., and Campbell, I.M.: Mass spectral identification of melatonin in blood. *Biochem. Biophys. Res. Commum., 46*:1236, 1972.

730. Pellegrino de Iraldi, A.: Granular vesicles in pinealocytes of the hamster. *Ant. Rec., 154*:481,1966.

730a. Pellegrino de Iraldi, A., and Arnaiz, G.R.d.L.: 5-Hydroxytryptophan-decarboxylase activity in normal and denervated pineal gland of rats. *Life Sci., 3*:589, 1964.

731. Pellegrino de Iraldi, A., and DeRobertis, E.: Ultrastructure and function of catecholamine containing systems. *Proc. 2nd Internat. Congr. Endocrinol. [1], Excerpta Medica Found.,* p. 355, 1965.

732. Pellegrino de Iraldi, A., and DeRobertis, E.: The neurotubular system of the axon and the origin of granulated and non-granulated

vesicles in regenerating nerves. Z. *Zellforsch. Mikrosk. Anat.*, 87:330, 1968.

733. Pellegrino de Iraldi, A., and Gueudet, R.: Action of reserpine on the osmium tetroxide zinc iodide reactive site of synaptic vesicles in pineal nerves of the rat. Z. *Zellforsch. Mikrosk. Anat.*, 91:178, 1968.

734. Pellegrino de Iraldi, A., and Gueudet, R.: Catecholamine and serotonin in granulated vesicles of nerve endings in the pineal gland of the rat. *Int. J. Neuropharmacology*, 8:9, 1969.

735. Pellegrino de Iraldi, A., and Suburo, A.M.: Action of p–chlorophenylalanine on the synaptic vesicles from rat pineal nerves. *Experientia*, 27:289, 1971.

736. Pellegrino de Iraldi, A., and Suburo, A.M.: Functional structure of the adrenergic nerve ending. *Acta Cientifica Venezolana*, 22(*Suppl. 2*):172, 1971.

737. Pellegrino de Iraldi, A., and Suburo, A.M.: Two compartments in the granulated vesicles of the pineal nerves. In Wolstenhome, G.E.W., and Knight, J. (Eds.):*The Pineal Gland*. Edinburgh and London, Churchill Livingstone, 1971, p. 177.

738. Pellegrino de Iraldi, A., and Zieher, L.M.: Noradrenaline and dopamine content of normal, decentralized and denervated pineal gland of the rat. *Life Sci.*, 5:149, 1966.

739. Pellegrino de Iraldi, A., and Zieher, L.M., and DeRobertis, E.: The 5-hydroxytryptamine content and synthesis of normal and denervated pineal gland. *Life Sci.*, 4:691, 1963.

740. Pende, V.: La calcifcazione della glandola pineale: correlazioni con le endocrinopatie. Studio clinico radiologico su 1121 casi.*Folia Endocrinol. (Roma)*, 6:191, 1953.

741. Penney, D.P., and Reiter, R.J.: Fine structural localization of a possible acyl transferase in the pineal gland of male golden hamster. *J. Histochem. Cytochem.*, 15:793, 1967.

742. Pennington, S.N.: A note on the chromatography of melatonin. *J. Chromatogr.*, 32:406, 1968.

743. Pepeu, G., and Giarman, N.J.: Serotonin in the developing mammal. *J. Gen. Physiol.*, 45:575, 1962.

744. Pérez–Cruet, J., Tagliamonte, A., Tagliamonte, P., and Gessa, G.L.: Changes in brain serotonin metabolism associated with fasting and satiation in rats. *Life Sci.*, 11:31, 1972.

745. Perrelet, A., Orci, L., and Rouiller, C.: Clarification of the osmiophilic granules of the rat pinealocytes by p–chlorophenylalanine. *Experientia*, 24:1047, 1968.

746. Piezzi, R.S., and Wurtman, R.J.: Pituitary serotonin content: effects of melatonin or deprivation of water. *Science*, 169:285, 1970.

747. Pletscher, A., Gey, K.F., and Burkard, W.P.: Inhibitors of monoamine

oxidase and decarboxylase of aromatic amino acids. *Handbuch der experimentellen Pharmakologie, 29:*593, 1966.

748. Polvani, F.: Studio anatomico della glandola pineale umana. *Folia Neurobiologica, 7:*655, 1963.

749. Porta, E.A., and Hartroft, W.S.: Lipid pigments in relation to aging and dietary factors (lipofuscins). In Wolman, M. (Ed.): *Pigments in Pathology.* New York and London, Academic Press, 1969, p. 191.

750. Potter, L.T., and Axelrod, J.: Subcellular localization of catecholamine in tissues of the rat. *J. Pharmacol. Exp. Ther., 142:*291, 1963.

751. Prieto Díaz, H., and Musacchio, I.T.L.: Observaciones citológicas de los pinealocitos (lipidos). *Actas y Trabajos del Primer Congreso Sudamericano de Zoologia. Univ. Nac. de la Plata, (Argentina), 5:*251, 1959.

752. Prop, N.: Fats in the pineal gland of the rat. *Acta Morphol. Neerl. Scand., 5:*285, 1963.

753. Prop, N.: Lipids in the pineal body of the rat. *Progr. Brain Res., 10:*454, 1965.

754. Prop, N., and Ebels, I.: Effects of sheep and young calf pineal extracts and continuous light on the pineal gland, the gonads and the oestrous cycle of the rat. *Acta Endocrinol. (Kbh.), 57:*585, 1968.

755. Prop, N., and Kappers, J.A.: Demonstration of some compounds present in the pineal organ of the albino rat by histochemical methods and paper chromatography. *Acta Anat. (Basel), 45:*90, 1961.

756. Pun, J.Y., and Lombrozo, L.: Microelectrophoresis of brain and pineal proteins in polyacrylamide gel. *Anal. Biochem., 9:*9, 1964.

757. Pysh, J.J., and Khan, T.: Variations in mitochondrial structure and content of neurons and neuroglia in rat brain: an electron microscopic study. *Brain Res., 36:*1, 1972.

758. Quarles, R.H.: Metabolism of glycoproteins by pineal glands in organ culture. In Klein, D.C. (Ed.): *Pineal Gland: Proceedings of a Workshop.* New York, Raven, 1972.

759. Quarles, R.H., and Brady, R.O.: Metabolism of glycoproteins and gangliosides in developing rat brain. *Transactions of the American Society for Neurochemistry, 1:*62, 1970.

760. Quarles, W.G.: *X–ray Structure Investigation of Some Substituted Indoles, and the X–ray Crystal of 1, 1'–Bishomocubane.* Ph.D. thesis, Lawrence Radiation Laboratory, University of California, Berkeley, 1970.

761. Quast, P.: Zur Histologie der Zirbeldrüse des Menschen. Untersuchungen über den Pigment–, Eisen–, Glykogen, und Lipoidstoffwechsel. *Verh. Anat. Ges., 66:*65, 1928.

762. Quast, P.: Beiträge zur Histologie und Cytologie der normalen Zirbeldrüse des Menschen. II. Zellen und Pigment des interdrüse. Zugleich ein Beitrag zur Morphologie und Mikrochemie der Abnutzungspigmente. Z. Mikrosk. Anat. Forsch., 23:335, 1930.

763. Quast, P.: Beitrage zur Histologie und Cytologie der normalen Zirbeldrüse des Menschen. II. Zellen und Pigment des interstitiellen Gewebes der Zirbeldrüse. Z. Mikrosk. Anat. Forsch., 24:38, 1931.

764. Quastel, J.H.: Effects of anaesthetics, depressants and tranquilizers on cerebral metabolism. In Hochster, R.M., and Quastel, J.H. (Eds.): Metabolic Inhibitors, A Comprehensive Treastise, New York, Academic Press, 1963, vol. 2, p. 517.

765. Quastel, M.R., and Rahamimoff, R.: Effect of melatonin on spontaneous contractions and response to 5-hydroxytryptamine of rat isolated duodenum. Br. J. Pharmacol., 24:455, 1965.

766. Quay, W.B.: The demonstration of a secretory material and cycle in the parenchymal cells of the mammalian pineal organ. Exp. Cell Res.,10:541, 1956.

767. Quay, W.B.: Volumetric and cytologic variation in the pineal body of Peromyscus leucopus (Rodentia) with respect to sex, captivity and day-length. J. Morphol., 98:471, 1956.

768. Quay, W.B.: Cytochemistry of pineal lipids in rat and man and their changes with age. Anat. Rec., 127:351, 1957.

769. Quay, W.B.: Cytochemistry of pineal lipids in rat and man. J. Histochem. Cytochem., 5:145, 1957.

770. Quay, W.B.: Localization, changes with age and experimental augmentation of pineal succinoxidase activity. Anat. Rec., 130:360, 1958.

771. Quay, W.B.: Effect of neural and vasomotor stimulants and depressants on the acid hematein-positive cells of the rodent pineal organ. Anat. Rec., 127:438, 1958.

772. Quay, W.B.: Pineal blood content and its experimental modification. Am. J. Physiol., 195:391, 1958.

773. Quay, W.B.: Experimental modifications and changes with age in pineal succinic dehydrogenase activity. Am. J. Physiol., 196:951, 1958.

774. Quay, W.B.: Experimental and comparative studies of succinic dehydrogenase activity in mammalian choroid plexuses, ependyma and pineal organ. Physiological Zoology, 33:206, 1960.

775. Quay, W.B.: Photic modification of mammalian pineal weight and composition and its anatomical basis. Anat. Rec., 139:265, 1961.

776. Quay, W.B.: Reduction of mammalian pineal weight and lipid during continuous light. Gen. Comp. Endocrinol., 1:211, 1961.

777. Quay, W.B.: The respiration of ependyma and pineal cells *in vitro* with diverse substrates and concentrations of inorganic ions. *Amer. Zool.*, 2:439, 1962.

778. Quay, W.B.: Experimental and cytological studies of pineal cells staining with acid hematein in the rat (*Rattus norvegicus*). *Acta Morphol. Neerl. Scand.*, 5:87, 1962.

779. Quay, W.B.: Differential extractions for the spectrophotofluorometric measurement of diverse 5-hydroxy- and 5-methoxyindoles. *Anal. Biochem.*, 5:51, 1963.

780. Quay, W.B.: Pineal and ependymal respriation with diverse substrates and inorganic ions. *Am. J. Physiol.*, 204:245, 1963.

781. Quay, W.B.: Cytologic and metabolic parameters of pineal inhibition by continuous light in the rat (*Rattus norvegicus*). Z. Zellforsch. Mikrosk. Anat., 60:479, 1963.

782. Quay, W.B.: Circadian rhythm in rat pineal serotonin and its modifications by estrous cycle and photoperiod. *Gen. Comp. Endocrinol.*, 3:473, 1963.

783. Quay, W.B.: Effect of dietary phenylalanine and tryptophan on pineal and hypothalamic serotonin levels. *Proc. Soc. Exp. Biol. Med.*, 114:718, 1963.

784. Quay, W.B.: Circadian and estrous rhythms in pineal melatonin and 5-hydroxyindole-3-acetic acid. *Proc. Soc. Exp. Biol. Med.*, 115:710, 1964.

785. Quay, W.B.: Circadian and estrous rhythms in pineal and brain serotonin. *Progr. Brain Res.*, 8:61, 1964.

786. Quay, W.B.: Histological structure and cytology of the pineal organ in birds and mammals. *Progr. Brain Res.*, 10:49, 1965.

787. Quay, W.B.: Experimental evidence for pineal participation in homeostasis of brain composition. *Progr. Brain Res.*, 10:646, 1965.

788. Quay, W.B.: Retinal and pineal hydroxyindole-O-methyl transferase activity in vertebrates. *Life Sci.*, 4:983, 1965.

789. Quay, W.B.: Daily rhythms and photic responses of pineal hydroxyindole derivatives in the pigeon (*Columba livia*). *Am. Zool.*, 5:218, 1965.

790. Quay, W.B.: Photic relations and experimental dissociation of circadian rhythms in pineal composition and running activity in rats. *Photochem. Photobiol.*, 4:425, 1965.

791. Quay, W.B.: Indole derivatives of pineal and related neural and retinal tissues. *Pharmacol. Rev.*, 17:321, 1965.

792. Quay, W.B.: 24-hour rhythms in pineal 5-hydroxytryptamine and hydroxyindole-O-methyl transferase activity in the macaque. *Proc. Soc. Exp. Biol. Med.*, 121:946, 1966.

793. Quay, W.B.: Rhythmic and light-induced changes in levels of pineal

5-hydroxyindoles in the pigeon (*Columba livia*). *Gen. Comp. Endocrinol.*, 6:371, 1966.

794. Quay, W.B.: The significance of darkness and monoamine oxidase in the nocturnal changes in 5-hydroxytryptamine and hydroxyindole-O-methyltransferase activity of the macaque's epiphysis cerebri. *Brain Res.*, 3:277, 1967.

795. Quay, W.B.: Lack of day-night rhythm and effect of darkness in rat pineal content of N-acetylserotonin O-methyltransferase. *The Physiologist*, 10:286, 1967.

795a. Quay, W.B.: Individuation and lack of pineal effect in the rat's circadian locomotor rhythm. *Physiology and Behavior*, 3:109, 1968.

796. Quay, W.B.: Comparative physiology of serotonin and melatonin. *Adv. Pharmacol.*, 6A:283, 1968.

797. Quay, W.B.: Specificity and structure-activity relationships in the *Xenopus* larval melanophore assay for melatonin. *Gen. Comp. Endocrinol.*, 11:253, 1968.

798. Quay, W.B.: Specificity of fluorometry of 5-hydroxytryptamine by means of products with ninhydrin. *J. Pharm. Sci.*, 57:1568, 1968.

799. Quay, W.B.: Relation of pineal acetylserotonin methyltransferase activity to daily photoperiod and light intensity. *Arch. Anat. Histol. Embryol. (Strasb.)*, 51:565, 1968.

800. Quay, W.B.: The role of the pineal gland in environmental adaptation. In Bajusz, E. (Ed.): *Physiology and Pathology of Adaptation Mechanisms: Neural- Neuroendocrine- Humoral.* Oxford, Pergamon Press, 1969.

801. Quay, W.B.: Evidence for a pineal contribution in the regulation of vertebrate reproductive systems. *Gen. Comp. Endocrinol.*, suppl. 2:101, 1969.

802. Quay, W.B.: Fluorometry of tissue contents of 5-hydroxytryptamine. *Fluorescence News (American Instrument Co.)*, 4:5, 1969.

803. Quay, W.B.: Catecholamines and tryptamines. *J. Neurovisc. Relat.*, suppl. 9:212, 1969.

804. Quay, W.B.: Comparative histology and histochemistry of the primate pineal region with particular reference to the orangutan (*Pongo pygmaeus*). *Anat. Rec.*, 166:364, 1970.

805. Quay, W.B.: Physiological significance of the pineal during adaptation to shifts in photoperiod. *Physiology and Behavior*, 5:353, 1970.

806. Quay, W.B.: Epiphyseal responses to light and darkness in birds and mammals. In Benoit, J., and Assenmacher, I. (Eds.): *La Photoregulation de la Reproduction chez les Oiseaux et les Mammiferes.* Paris, Colloques Internationaux du Centre National de la Recherche Scientifique, 1970, p. 549.

807. Quay, W.B.: Endocrine effects of the mammalian pineal. *Am. Zool.*, *10:*237, 1970.
808. Quay, W.B.: Diagnosis of destructive lesions of the pineal. *Lancet*, *7662:*42, 1970.
809. Quay, W.B.: The significance of the pineal. *Memoirs of the Society for Endocrinology*, *18:*423, 1970.
810. Quay, W.B.: Pineal structure and composition in the orangutan (*Pongo pygmaeus*). *Anat. Rec.*, *168:*93, 1970.
811. Quay, W.B.: Precocious entrainment and associated characteristics of activity patterns following pinealectomy and reversal of photoperiod. *Physiology and Behavior*, *5:*1281, 1970.
812. Quay, W.B.: Pineal organ. In Wimsatt, W.A. (Ed.): *Biology of Bats.* New York, Academic Press, 1970, vol. 2, p. 311.
813. Quay, W.B.: Structure and histochemistry of corpora amylacea in the brain of an orangutan (*Pongo pygmaeus*). *J. Comp. Pathol.*, *81:*89, 1971.
814. Quay, W.B.: Effects of cutting nervi conarii and tentorium cerebelli on pineal composition and activity shifting following reversal of photoperiod. *Physiology and Behavior*, *6:*681, 1971.
815. Quay, W.B.: Factors in the measurement of pineal acetylserotonin methyltransferase activity in the lizard *Sceloporus occidentalis*. *Gen. Comp. Endocrinol.*, *17:*220, 1971.
816. Quay, W.B.: Pineal homeostatic regulation of shifts in the circadian activity rhythm during maturation and aging. *Trans. N. Y. Acad. Sci.*, *34:*239, 1972.
817. Quay, W.B.: Studies on circadian differences and controls in carbonic anhydrase activities of brain regions, choroid plexuses and pineal organ. *Fifth Intern. Congr. Pharmacol., Abstracts of Volunteer Papers*, p. 187, 1972.
818. Quay, W.B.: Pineal vasoconstriction at daily onset of light: its physiological correlates and control. *The Physiologist*, *15:*241, 1972.
819. Quay, W.B.: Twenty-four-hour rhythmicity in carbonic anhydrase activities of choroid plexuses and pineal gland. *Anat. Rec.*, *174:*279, 1972.
820. Quay, W.B.: not published, original observations.
821. Quay, W.B., and Bagnara, J.T.: Relative potencies of indolic and related compounds in the body-lightening reaction of larval *Xenopus. Arch. Int. Pharmacodyn. Ther.*, *150:*137, 1964.
822. Quay, W.B., and Baker, P.C.: Form, weight and indole content of pineal organs of red and grey kangaroos. *Australian Journal of Zoology*, *13:*727, 1965.
823. Quay, W.B., and Halevy, A.: Experimental modification of the rat pineal's content of serotonin and related indole amines. *Physiological Zoology*, *35:*1, 1962.

824. Quay, W.B., and Kahn, R.H.: Pineal histology and cytochemistry in organ culture. *La Cellule.*, 63:247, 1963.

825. Quay, W.B., and Levine, B.E.: Pineal growth and mitotic activity in the rat and the effects of colchicine and sex hormones. *Anat. Rec.*, 129:65, 1957.

826. Quay, W.B., and Renzoni, A.: Twenty-four-hour rhythms in pineal mitotic activity and nuclear and nucleolar dimensions. *Growth*, 30:315, 1966.

827. Quay, W.B., and Smart, L.I.: Substrate specificity and post-mortem effects in mammalian pineal acetylserotonin methyltrasferase activity. *Arch. Int. Physiol. Biochim.*, 75:197, 1967.

828. Quay, W.B., Stebbins, R.C., Kelley, T.D., and Cohen, N.W.: Effects of environmental and physiological factors on pineal acetylserotonin methyltransferase activity in the lizard *Sceloporus occidentalis*. *Physiological Zoology*, 44:241, 1971.

829. Quercy, R., Rigaldies, R., Carles, J., and Quercy, D.: Sur la région épiphysaire.—I. Le sac dorsal. II. Les calculs de l'épiphyse et du sac dorsal. *Rev. Neurol. (Paris)*, 79:401, 1947.

830. Rahamimoff, R., Bruderman, I., and Golshani, G.: Effect of melatonin on 5-hydroxytryptamine induced contraction of isolated cat trachea. *Life Sci.*, 4:2281, 1965.

831. Ralph, C.L.: Structure and alleged functions of avian pineals. *Am. Zool.*, 10:217, 1970.

832. Ralph, C.L., Hedlund, L., and Murphy, W.A.: Diurnal cycles of melatonin in bird pineal bodies. *Comp. Biochem. Physiol.*, 22:591, 1967.

833. Ralph, C.L., and Lynch, H.J.: A quantitative melatonin bioassay. *Gen. Comp. Endocrinol.*, 15:334, 1970.

834. Ralph, C.L., Mull, D., and Lynch, H.J.: Locomotor activity rhythms of rats under constant conditions as predictors of melatonin content of their pineals. *Am. Zool.*, 10:302, 1970.

835. Ralph, C.L., Mull, D., Lynch, H.J., and Hedlund, L.: A melatonin rhythm persists in rat pineals in darkness. *Endocrinology*, 89:1361, 1971.

836. Rasmussen, H.: Cell communication, calcium ion, and cyclic adenosine monophosphate. *Science*, 170:404, 1970.

837. Reams, W.L., Jr., Shervette, R.E., and Dorman, W.H.: Refractoriness of mouse dermal melanocytes to hormones. *J. Invest. Dermatol.*, 50:338, 1968.

838. Reiss, M., Badrick, F.E., and Halkerston, J.M.: The influence of the pituitary on phosphorus metabolism of brain. *Biochem. J.*, 44:257, 1949.

839. Reiss, M., Davis, R.H., Sideman, M.B., Mauer, I., and Plichta, E.S.: Action of pineal extracts on the gonads and their function. *J. Endocrinol.*, 27:107, 1963.

840. Reiter, R.J.: The role of the pineal in reproduction. In Balin, H., and Glasser, S. (Eds.): *Reproductive Biology.* Amsterdam, Excerpta Medica, 1972, p. 71.

841. Reiter, R.J., and Fraschini, F.: Endocrine aspects of the mammalian pineal gland: A review. *Neuroendocrinology,* 5:219, 1969.

842. Reiter, R.J., Hoffman, R.A., and Hester, R.J.: Inhibition of I^{131} uptake by thyroid glands of male rats treated with melatonin and pineal extract. *Am. Zool.,* 5:727, 1965.

843. Reiter, R.J., Morgan, W.W., and Talbot, J.A.: Pineal interaction with the brain: evidence from thyroparathyroidectomized rats. *Fed. Proc.,* 31:221, 1972.

844. Reiter, R.J., Sorrentino, S., Jr., and Jarrow, E.L.: Central and peripheral neural pathways necessary for pineal function in the adult female rat. *Neuroendocrinology,* 8:321, 1971.

845. Richards, D.A.: The therapeutic effect of melatonin on canine melanosis. *J. Invest. Dermatol.,* 44:13, 1965.

846. Richards, J.G., and Tranzer, J.P.: Electron microscopic localization of 5-hydroxydopamine, a "false" adrenergic neurotransmitter, in the autonomic nerve endings of the rat pineal gland. *Experientia,* 25:53, 1969.

847. Richter, C.P.: Biological clocks and the endocrine glands. Proc. 2nd. Intern. Congr. Endocrinol. Part I. *Excerpta Medica Found.,* p. 119, 1965.

848. Richter, C.P.: *Biological Clocks in Medicine and Psychiatry.* Springfield, Illinois, Charles C. Thomas Publ., 1965.

849. Roberts, E., and Simonsen, D.G.: Free amino acids in animal tissue. In Holden, J.T. (Ed.): *Amino Acid Pools. Distribution, Formation and Function of Free Amino Acids.* Amsterdam, Elsevier Publ. Co., 1962, p. 284.

850. Roberts, S.: Regulation of cerebral metabolism of amino acids—II. Influence of phenylalanine deficiency on free and protein-bound amino acids in rat cerebral cortex: relationship to plasma levels. *J. Neurochem.,* 10:931, 1963.

851. Robison, G.A., Butcher, R.W., and Sutherland, E.W.: *Cyclic AMP.* New York and London, Academic Press, 1971.

852. Robison, G.A., Schmidt, M.J., and Sutherland, E.W.: On the development and properties of the brain adenyl cyclase system. In Greengard, P., and Costa, E. (Eds.): *Role of Cyclic AMP in Cell Function.* New York, Raven Press, 1970, p. 11.

853. Rodin, A.E., and Overall, J.: Statistical relationships of weight of the human pineal to age and malignancy. *Cancer, 20:*1203, 1967.

854. Rodin, A.E., and Turner, R.A.: The perivascular space of the pineal gland. *Tex. Rep. Biol. Med., 24:*153, 1966.

855. Rodriguez de Lores Arnaiz, G., and Pellegrino de Iraldi, A.: Cholinesterase in cholinergic and adrenergic nerves: A study

of the superior cervical ganglia and the pineal gland of the rat. *Brain Res., 42:*230, 1972.

856. Rodriguez-Perez, A.P.: Contribucion al conocimiento de la inervation de las glandulas endocrinas. IV. Primeros resultados experimentales en torno a la inervación de la epífisis. *Trab. Inst. Cajal Invest. Biol., 54:*225, 1962.

857. Roe, J.H.: Chemical determination of ascorbic, dehydroascorbic, and diketogulonic acids. *Methods of Biochemical Analysis, 1:*115, 1954.

858. Roldán, E., and Antón-Tay, F.: EEG and convulsive threshold changes produced by pineal extract administration. *Brain Res., 11:*238, 1968.

859. Roldán, E., Antón-Tay, F., and Escobar, A.: Studies on the pineal gland. IV. The effect of pineal extract on the electroencephalogram. *Bol. Estud. Med. Biol., 22:*145, 1964.

860. Romieu, M., and Jullien, G.: Observations sur l'anatomie microscopique de la glande pinéale du nouveau-né humain. *C. R. Soc. Biol. (Paris), 136:*691, 1942.

861. Roozemond, R.C.: The effect of fixation with formaldehyde and glutaraldehyde on the composition of phospholipids extractable from rat hypothalamus. *J. Histochem. Cytochem., 17:*482, 1969.

862. Roozemond, R.C.: Phospholipid composition of some parts of rat hypothalamus, and its relation with some histochemical observations. *J. Neurochem., 17:*179, 1970.

863. Roozemond, R.C.: The staining and chromium binding of rat brain tissue and of lipids in model systems subjected to Baker's acid hematein technique. *J. Histochem. Cytochem., 19:*244, 1971.

864. Rossiter, R.J.: Chemical constituents of brain and nerve. In Elliott, K.A.C., Page, I.H., and Quastel, J.H. (Eds.): *Neurochemistry.* Springfield, Illinois, Charles C Thomas Publ., 1955, p. 11.

865. Roth, W.D.: Comments on J. Ariens Kappers' review and observations on pineal activity. *Am. Zool., 4:*53, 1964.

866. Roth, W.D.: Metabolic and morphologic studies on the rat pineal organ during puberty. *Progr. Brain Res., 10:*552, 1965.

867. Roth, W.D., Wurtman, R.J., and Altschule, M.D.: Morphologic changes in the pineal parenchymal cells of rats exposed to continuous light or darkness. *Endocrinology, 71:*888, 1962.

868. Roux, P.: *La Glande Pinéale ou Épiphyse.* Rennes, Oberthur, 1937.

869. Rubin, B.D., and Traum, R.E.: The effect of melatonin on ovarian compensatory hypertrophy in the rat. *J. Endocrinol., 50:*179, 1971.

870. Rudman, D., Del Rio, A.E., Garcia, L.A., Barnett, J., Bixler, T., and Hollins, B.: Lipolytic substances in bovine thyroid, parotid and pineal glands. *Endocrinology, 87:*27, 1970.

871. Rudman, D., Del Rio, A.E., Hollins, B., and Houser, D.H.: Observa-

tions on the lipolytic and melanotropic activities of the pineal gland. *J. Biol. Chem., 246:*324, 1971.

872. Rudman, D., Del Rio, A.E., Hollins, B., Houser, D.H., Sutin, J., and Mosteller, R.C.: Comparison of lipolytic and melanotropic factors in bovine choroid plexus and in bovine pineal gland. *Endocrinology, 90:*1139, 1972.

873. Ruggeri, E.: Modificazioni del contenuto lipo-mitocondriale delle cellule della pineale dopo ablazione completa degli organi genitali. *Riv. Patol. Nerv. Ment., 19:*649, 1914.

874. Rust, C.C., and Meyer, R.K.: Hair color, molt, and testis size in male, short-tailed weasels treated with melatonin. *Science, 165:*921, 1961.

875. Salama, A.I., Insalaco, J.R., and Maxwell, R.A.: Concerning the molecular requirements for the inhibition of the uptake of racemic ^{3}H-norepinephrine into rat cerebral cortex slices by tricyclic antidepressants and related compounds. *J. Pharmacol. Exp. Ther., 178:*474, 1971.

876. Saliichuk, L.I.: On the formation of epiphyseal sand at different age periods in the development of man. *Probl. Endokrinol. (Mosk), 10:*44, 1964.

877. Sandborn, E.B.: *Cells and Tissues by Light and Electron Microscopy.* New York and London, Academic Press, vol. 2, 1970.

878. Sano, I., Gamo, T., Kakimoto, Y., Taniguchi, K., Takesada, M., and Nishinuma, N.: Distribution of catechol compounds in human brain. *Biochim. Biophys. Acta, 32:*586, 1959.

879. Sano, Y., and Mashimo, T.: Elektronemikroskopische Untersuchungen an der Epiphysis cerebri beim Hund. *Z. Zellforsch. Mikrosk. Anat., 69:*129, 1966.

880. Sano, I., Taniguchi, K., and Gamo, T.: Die Katechinamine im Zentralnervensystem. *Klin. Wochenschr., 38:*57, 1960.

881. Santamarina, E.: Melanin pigmentation in bovine pineal gland and its possible correlation with gonadal function. *Can. J. Biochem. Physiol., 36:*227, 1958.

882. Santamarina, E., and Meyer-Arendt, J.: Identification of melanin in the bovine pineal gland. *Acta Histochem. (Jena), 3:*1, 1956.

883. Santamarina, E., and Venzke, W.G.: Physiological changes in the mammalian pineal gland correlated with the reproductive system. *Am. J. Vet. Res., 14:*555, 1953.

884. Santari, G., and Salvati, A.: Ulteriori ricerche sull'azione degli estratti epifisari nei confronti della fecondità del ratto. *Rass. Int. Clin. Ter., 39:*362, 1959.

885. Sapirstein, L.A.: Regional blood blow by fractional distribution of indicators. *Am. J. Physiol., 193:*161, 1958.

886. Satodate, R., Sasaki, K., and Ota, M.: The pineal gland of intact, hypophysectomized, or ovariectomized rats. Light and electron microscopic studies. *Arch. Neurol., 23:*278, 1970.

887. Saunders, J.W., Jr.: Death in embryonic systems. *Science, 154:*604, 1966.

888. Sawyer, W.H.: Evolution of antidiuretic hormones and their functions. *Am. J. Med., 42:*678, 1967.

889. Sawyer, W.H., Munsick, R.A., and van Dyke, H.B.: Antidiuretic hormones. *Circulation, suppl. 21, Part 2:*1027, 1959.

890. Schmidt, M.J., and Sanders-Bush, E.: Tryptophan hydroxylase activity in developing rat brain. *J. Neurochem., 18:*2549, 1971.

891. Schoenfeld, R.I.: Melatonin: effect on punished and nonpunished operant behavior of the pigeon. *Science, 171:*1258, 1971.

892. Schott, H.F., Masuoka, D.T., and Vivonia, C.: In utero sensitivity of rat pineal to nerve growth factor antiserum. *Life Sci., 9:*713, 1970.

893. Schubert, M., and Hamerman, D.: *A Primer on Connective Tissue Biochemistry.* Philadelphia, Lea and Febiger, 1968.

894. Shani (Mishkinsky), J., Knaggs, G.S., and Tindal, J.S.: The effect of noradrenaline, dopamine, 5-hydroxytryptamine and melatonin on milk yield and composition in the rabbit. *J. Endocrinol., 50:*543, 1971.

895. Shein, H.M., Larin, F., and Wurtman, J.R.: Lack of a direct effect of morphine on the synthesis of pineal ^{14}C-indoles in organ culture. *Life Sci., 9:*29, 1970.

896. Shein, H.M., Wilson, S., Larin, F., and Wurtman, R.J.: Stimulation of [^{14}C] serotonin synthesis from [^{14}C] tryptophan by mescaline in rat pineal organ cultures. *Life Sci. [II], 10:*273, 1971.

897. Shein, H.M., and Wurtman, R.J.: Cyclic adenosine monophosphate: stimulation of melatonin and serotonin synthesis in cultured rat pineals. *Science, 166:*519, 1969.

898. Shein, H.M., and Wurtman, R.J.: Stimulation of [^{14}C] tryptophan 5-hydroxylation by norepinephrine and dibutyryl adenosine 3',5' monophosphate in rat pineal organ cultures. *Life Sci. [I], 10:*935, 1971.

899. Shein, H.M.: Wurtman, R.J., and Axelrod, J.: Synthesis of serotonin by pineal glands of the rat in organ culture. *Nature (Lond.), 213:*730, 1967.

900. Sheridan, J.J., Sims, K.L., and Pitts, F.N., Jr.: Brain γ-aminobutyrate-α-oxoglutarate transaminase—II. Activities in twenty-four regions of human brain. *J. Neurochem., 14:*571, 1967.

901. Sheridan, M.N.: Further observations of the fine structure of the hamster pineal gland. *Anat. Rec., 163:*262, 1969.

902. Sheridan, M.N., and Keppel, J.F.: The effect of p-chlorophenylalaine (PCPA) and 6-hydroxydopamine (6-HD) on ultrastructural features of hamster pineal parenchyma. *Anat. Rec., 169:*427, 1971.

903. Sheridan, M.N., and Reiter, R.J.: The fine structure of the hamster pineal gland. *Am. J. Anat., 122:*357, 1968.

904. Shimizu, N., and Morikawa, N.: Histochemical studies of succinic dehydrogenase of the brain of mice, rats, guinea pigs and rabbits. *J. Histochem. Cytochem.*, 5:334, 1957.
905. Shimizu, N., Morikawa, N., and Okada, M.: Histochemical studies of monoamine oxidase of the brain of rodents. *Z. Zellforsch. Mikrosk. Anat.*, 49:389, 1959.
906. Shimizu, N., and Okada, M.: Histochemical distribution of phosphorylase in rodent brain from newborn to adults. *J. Histochem. Cytochem.*, 5:459, 1957.
907. Shuangshoti, S., and Netsky, M.G.: Human choroid plexus: morphologic and histochemical alterations with age. *Am. J. Anat.*, 128:73, 1970.
908. Siegel, S.: *Nonparametric Statistics for the Behavioral Sciences.* New York, McGraw-Hill, 1956.
909. Sigg, E.B., Gyermek, L., Hill, R.T., and Yen, H.C.Y.: Neuropharmacology of some harmane derivatives. *Arch. Int. Pharmacodyn. Ther.*, 149:164, 1964.
910. Singh, D.V., Narang, G.D., and Turner, C.W.: Effect of melatonin and its withdrawal on thyroid hormone secretion rate of female rats. *J. Endocrinol.*, 43:489, 1969.
911. Singh, D.V., and Turner, C.W.: Melatonin on endocrine DNA changes in female rats at increasing ages. *Acta Endocrinol. (Kbh.)*, 68:597, 1971.
912. Singh, D.V., and Turner, C.W.: Effect of melatonin upon thyroid hormone secretion rate in female hamsters and male rats. *Acta Endocrinol. (Kbh.)*, 69:35, 1972.
913. Skaug, O.E., Lingjaerde, P., and Malm, O.J.: P^{32} uptake in hypophysectomized rats. *Acta Endocrinol. (Kbh.)*, 29:315, 1958.
914. Skaug, O.E., Lingjaerde, P., and Malm, O.J.: P^{32} uptake in thymectomized hypophysectomized rats. *Acta Endocrinol. (Kbh.)*, 31:309, 1959.
915. Smith, A.R.: *Conditions Influencing Serotonin and Tryptophan Metabolism in the Epiphysis Cerebri of the Rabbit; a Fluorescence Histochemical, Microchemical and Electrophoretic Study.* Thesis, Purmerend, The Netherlands, Nooy's Drukkerij, 1972, p. 1.
916. Smith, A.R., Jongkind, J.F., and Kappers, J.A.: Distribution and quantification of serotonin-containing and autofluorescent cells in the rabbit pineal organ. *Gen. Comp. Endocrinol.*, 18:364, 1972.
917. Smith, B.: Monoamine oxidase in the pineal gland, neurohypophysis and brain of the albino rat. *J. Anat.*, 97:81, 1963.
918. Smith, M.L.: Effects of a purified pineal extract in unilaterally ovariectomized mice. *Anat. Rec.*, 169:432, 1971.
919. Smith, M.L., Jr., Orts., R.J., and Benson, B.: Effects of non-melatonin pineal factors in the PMS-stimulated immature rat. *Anat. Rec.*, 172:408, 1972.

920. Sneddon, J.M., and Keen, P.: The effect of noradrenaline on the incorporation of ^{32}P into brain phospholipids. *J. Neurochem.*, *19:*1297, 1970.

921. Snell, R.S.: Effect of melatonin on mammalian epidermal melanocytes. *J. Invest. Dermatol.*, *44:*273, 1965.

922. Snyder, S.: Development of enzyme activities and a circadian rhythm in pineal gland serotonin: evidence for a nonretinal pathway of light to pineal gland of newborn rats. *Adv. Pharmacol.*, *6A:*301, 1968.

923. Snyder, S., and Axelrod, J.: Influence of light and the sympathetic nervous system on 5-hydroxytryptophan decarboxylase (5-HTPD) activity in the pineal gland. *Fed. Proc.*, *23:*206, 1964.

924. Snyder, S.H., and Axelrod, J.: A sensitive assay for 5-hydroxytryptophan decarboxylase. *Biochem. Pharmacol.*, *13:*805, 1964.

925. Snyder, S.H., and Axelrod, J.: Circadian rhythm in pineal serotonin: effect of monoamine oxidase inhibition and reserpine. *Science*, *149:*542, 1965.

926. Snyder, S.H., Axelrod, J., Fischer, J.E., and Wurtman, R.J.: Neural and photic regulation of 5-hydroxytryptophan decarboxylase in the rat pineal gland. *Nature (Lond.)*, *203:*981, 1964.

927. Snyder, S.H., Axelrod, J., Smith, O.D., and Pucci, G.L.: Formation of methanol by an enzyme in an ectopic pinealoma. *Nature (Lond.)*, *215:*773, 1967.

928. Snyder, S.H., Axelrod, J., Wurtman, R.J., and Fischer, J.E.: Control of 5-hydroxytryptophan decarboxylase activity in the rat pineal gland by sympathetic nerves. *J. Pharmacol. Exp. Ther.*, *147:*371, 1965.

929. Snyder, S.H., Axelrod, J., and Zweig, M.: Circadian rhythm in the serotonin content of the rat pineal gland: regulating factors. *J. Pharmacol. Exp. Ther.*, *158:*206, 1967.

930. Snyder, S.H., Fischer, J., and Axelrod, J.: Evidence for the presence of monoamine oxidase in sympathetic nerve endings. *Biochem. Pharmacol.*, *14:*363, 1965.

931. Snyder, S.H., and Zweig, M.: Evidence for a non-retinal pathway of light to the rat pineal gland. *Fed. Proc.*, *25:*353, 1966.

932. Snyder, S.H., Zweig, M., Axelrod, J., and Fischer, J.E.: Control of the circadian rhythm in serotonin content of the rat pineal gland. *Proc. Nat. Acad. Sci.*, *USA*, *53:*301, 1965.

933. Soffer, L.J., Fogel, M., and Rudavsky, A.: The presence of a "gonadotrophin inhibiting substance" in pineal gland extract. *Acta Endocrinol. (Kbh.)*, *48:*561, 1965.

934. Solomon, S.S., Brush, J.S., and Kitabchi, A.E.: Divergent biological effects of adenosine and dibutyryl adenosine 3',5'-monophosphate on the isolated fat cell. *Science*, *169:*387, 1970.

935. Sorrentino, S.: Antigonadotropic effects of melatonin in intact and unilaterally ovariectomized rats. *Anat. Rec., 160:*432, 1968.
936. Spector, W.S. (Ed.): *Handbook of Biological Data.* Philadelphia, W.B. Saunders Co., 1956.
937. Sprince, H.: Indole metabolism in mental illness. *Clin. Chem., 7:*203, 1961.
938. Stefănescu-Gavăt, V.: Histochemical study of phosphatases in bovine pineal gland *(Bos taurus). Stud. Cercet. Endocrinol., 21:*329, 1970.
939. Steinman, A.M., Smerin, S.E., and Barchas, J.D.: Epinephrine metabolism in mammalian brain after intravenous and intraventricular administration. *Science, 165:*616, 1969.
940. Strada, S.J., Klein, D.C., Weller, J., and Weiss, B.: Effect of norepinephrine on the concentration of adenosine 3'5'-monophosphate of rat pineal gland in organ culture. *Endocrinol., 90:*1470, 1972.
941. Strassmann, G.S.: Iron deposits in the body and their pathologic significance. A Review. *Am. J. Clin. Pathol., 24:*453, 1954.
942. Straus, W.: Lysosomes, phagosomes and related particles. In Roodyn, D.B. (Ed.): *Enzyme Cytology.* London and New York, Academic Press, 1967, p. 239.
943. Studnitz, W.v.: Tryptophanhydroxylase im Corpus pineale beim Menschen. *Experientia, 23:*711, 1967.
944. Sturgeon, P.: Hemosiderin and ferritin. In Wolman, M. (Ed.): *Pigments in Pathology.* New York and London, Academic Press, 1969, p. 93.
945. Sturkie, P.D., and Meyer, D.: Circadian rhythm in blood and pineal levels of serotonin in chickens. *Fed. Proc., 31:*327, 1972.
946. Sturman, J.A., Rassin, D.K., and Gaull, G.E.: Relation of three enzymes of transsulphuration to the concentration of cystathionine in various regions of the monkey brain. *J. Neurochem., 17:*1117, 1970.
947. Sugiura, R.: Ratte shōka-sen no keitai-hassei narabi-ni sashiki-hasseigaku-teki kenkyū (Morphogenetic and histogenetic studies on the pineal gland of the rat). *Acta Anat. Nippon., 9:*409, 1936.
948. Supniewski, J., Misztal, S., and Marczyński, T.: Pharmacological properties of melatonin. *Acta Physiol. Pol., 11:*892, 1960.
949. Sutherland, E.W., and Rall, T.W.: The relation of adenosine 3',5'-phosphate and phosphorylase to the actions of catecholamines and other hormones. *Pharmacol. Rev., 12:*265, 1960.
950. Suzuki, Y.: Beiträge zur Anatomie des Epithalamus, besonders der Epiphyse, bei den Primaten. *Arb. Anat. Inst. Sendai, 21:*45, 1938.

951. Swaab, D.F., and Jongkind, J.F.: The hypothalamic neurosecretory activity during the oestrous cycle, pregnancy, parturition, lactation and persistent oestrous and after gonadectomy, in the rat. *Neuroendocrinology*, 6:133, 1970.

952. Swaab, D.F., and Jongkind, J.F.: Influence of gonadotropic hormones on the hypothalamic neurosecretory activity in the rat. *Neuroendocrinology*, 8:36, 1971.

953. Swislocki, N.I.: Decomposition of dibutyryl cyclic AMP in aqueous buffers. *Anal. Biochem.*, 38:260, 1970.

954. Swoboda, F.K.: A quantitative method for the determination of vitamin C in connection with determinations of vitamine in glandular and other tissues. *J. Biol. Chem.*, 44:531, 1920.

955. Szmuszkovicz, J., Anthony, W.C., and Heinzelman, R.V.: Synthesis of N-acetyl-5-methoxytryptamine. *J. Org. Chem.*, 25:857, 1960.

956. Takács, L., Kállay, K., and Karai, A.: Methodological remarks on Sapirstein's isotope indicator fractionation technique. *Acta Physiol. Acad. Sci. Hung.*, 25:389, 1964.

957. Takeuchi, T.: Histochemical demonstration of branching enzyme (amylo −1,4 → 1,6-transglucosidase) in animal tissues. *J. Histochem. Cytochem.*, 6:208, 1958.

958. Tallan, H.H.: Free amino acids in brain after administration of imipramine, chlorpromazine and other psychotropic drugs. In Holden, J.T. (Ed.): *Amino Acid Pools. Distribution, Formation and Function of Free Amino Acids*. Amsterdam, Elsevier Publ. Co., 1962, p. 465.

959. Tallan, H.H.: A survey of the amino acids and related compounds in nervous tissue. In Holden, J.T. (Ed.): *Amino Acid Pools. Distribution, Formation and Function of Free Amino Acids*. Amsterdam, Elsevier Publ. Co., 1962, p. 471.

960. Tannock, I.F.: A comparison of the relative efficiencies of various metaphase arrest agents. *Exp. Cell Res.*, 47:345, 1967.

961. Tapp, E., and Blumfield, M.: The weight of the pineal gland in malignancy. *Br. J. Cancer*, 24:67, 1970.

962. Tapp, E., and Huxley, M.: The weight and degree of calcification of the pineal gland. *J. Pathol.*, 105:31, 1971.

963. Taxi, J., and Droz, B.: Étude de l'incorporation de noradrenaline-³H(NA-³H) et de 5-hydroxytryptophane-³H (5HTP-³H) dans l'epiphyse et le ganglion cervical supériour. *C.R. Acad. Sci. [D] (Paris)*, 263:1326, 1966.

964. Taylor, A.N., and Farrell, G.: Facteur glomérulotrope. *Ann. Endocrinol. (Paris)*, 24:228, 1963.

965. Taylor, K.M., Gfeller, E., and Snyder, S.H.: Regional localization of histamine and histidine in the brain of the rhesus monkey. *Brain Res.*, 41:171, 1972.

966. Thiéblot, L., Alassimone, A., and Blaise, S.: Étude chromatog-

raphique et electrophorétique du facteur antigonadotrope de la glande pinéale. *Ann. Endocrinol. (Paris)*, 27:861, 1966.

967. Thiéblot, L., Bastide, P., Blaise, S., Boyer, J., and Dastugue, G.: De l'équipement enzymatique de la glande pinéale (Étude critique et expérimentale). *Ann. Endocrinol. (Paris)*, 26:313, 1965.

968. Thiéblot, L., Bastide, P., Blaise, S., Boyer, J., and Dastugue, G.: De l'équipement enzymatique de la glande pinéale. Étude critique et expérimentale. *Ann. Endocrinol. (Paris)*, 27:1, 1966.

969. Thiéblot, L., Berthelay, J., and Blaise, S.: Action de la mélatonine sur la sécrétion gonadotrope du Rat. *C.R. Soc. Biol. (Paris)*, 160:2306, 1966.

970. Thiéblot, L., and Blaise, S.: Principe anti-gonadotrope de la glande pinéale. *Rev. Roum. Endocrinol.*, 4:269, 1967.

971. Thiéblot, L., Blaise, S., and Alassimone, A.: Essai de caractérisation du principe anti-gonadotrope de la glande pinéale. *C. R. Soc. Biol. (Paris)*, 160:1574, 1966.

972. Thiéblot, L., Blaise, S., and Couquelet, J.: Recherche de dérivés indoliques dans les extraits de glande pinéale. *C. R. Soc. Biol. (Paris)*, 161:295, 1967.

973. Thompson, R.H.S.: The regional distribution of copper in human brain. In Kety, S. S., and Elkes, J. (Eds.): *Regional Neurochemistry. The Regional Chemistry, Physiology and Pharmacology of the Nervous System.* New York and Oxford, Pergamon Press, 1961, p. 102.

974. Tigchelaar, P.V., and Nalbandov, A.V.: Comparison of various commercial preparations of melatonin in immature rats. *J. Reprod. Fertil.*, 25:141, 1971.

975. Tinacci, F., and Fazzini, G.: Azione di un estratto di ghiandola pineale sulle cartilagini dell ratto in accrescimento. *Boll. Soc. Ital. Biol. Sper.*, 40:282, 1964.

976. Tingey, A.H.: The iron, copper and manganese content of the human brain. *J. Mental Science*, 83:452, 1937.

977. Tomatis, M.E., and Orias, R.: Changes in melatonin concentration in pineal gland in rats exposed to continuous light or darkness. *Acta Physiol. Lat. Am.*, 17:227, 1967.

978. Torack, R.M., and Barrnett, R.J.: Nucleoside phosphatase activity in membranous fine structures of neurons and glia. *J. Histochem. Cytochem.*, 11:763, 1963.

979. Torack, R.M., and Barrnett, R.J.: The fine structural localization of nucleoside phosphatase activity in the blood-brain barrier. *J. Neuropathol. Exp. Neurol.*, 23:46, 1964.

980. Toryu, Y.: Distribution of glycogen in the central and sympathetic nervous systems of the horse, with reference to histochemical analysis of the relation. *Sci. Rep. Res. Inst. Tohoku Univ. [Biol.]*, 12:1, 1937.

981. Traczyk, W.Z., Guzek, J.W., and Leśnik, H.: Distribution of antidiuretic substance in the diencephalon and mesencephalon of the dog. *Neuroendocrinology*, 6:56, 1970.
982. Trentini, G.P., De Gaetani, C.F., Botticelli, A., and Rivasi, F.: L'antagonismo epifisi-ipofisario. Modificazioni istomorfologiche ed istoenzimatiche epifisarie indotte dalla ipergonadotropinemia sperimentala nel ratto albino accecato. *Boll. Soc. Ital. Biol. Sper.*, 45:631, 1969.
983. Trentini, G.P., De Gaetani, G.F., Silva, C.B., and Rivasi, F.: Modificazioni istomorfologiche e microfluoroscopiche pinealiche indotte dalla splenectomia nella ratta albina prepubere e adulta. *Arch. De Vecchi Anat. Patol.*, 52:1, 1968.
984. Trueman, T., and Herbert, J.: The distribution of monoamines and acetylcholinesterase in the pineal gland and habenula of the ferret. *J. Anat.*, 106:406, 1970.
985. Tschiersch, B., and Mothes, K.: Amino acids: structure and distribution. In Florkin, M., and Mason, H.S. (Eds.): *Comparative Biochemistry*. New York, Academic Press, 1963, vol. V, part C.
986. Turkewitsch, N.: Die Entwicklung der Zirbeldrüse beim Rind (*Bos taurus* L.) *Gegenbaurs Morphol. Jahrb.*, 77:326, 1936.
987. Turkewitsch, N.: Eigentümlichkeiten der embryologischen Entwicklung des Epiphysengebiets des Schafes (*Ovis aries* L.). *Gegenbaurs Morphol. Jahrb.*, 79:305, 1937.
988. Turkewitsch, N.: Eigentümlichkeiten in der Entwicklung des Epiphysengebiets des Kaninchens (*Lepus cuniculus* L.). *Gegenbaurs Morphol. Jahrb.*, 79:634, 1937.
989. Uchida, K., Kadowaki, M., and Miyake, T.: Ovarian secretion of progesterone and 20α-hydroxypregn-4-en-3-one during rat estrous cycle in chronological relation to pituitary release of luteinizing hormone. *Endocrinol. Jap.*, 16:227, 1969.
990. Udenfriend, S., Bogdanski, D. F., and Weissbach, H.: Fluorescence characteristics of 5-hydroxytryptamine (serotonin). *Science*, 122:972, 1955.
991. Udenfriend, S., Witcop, B., Redfield, B. G., Weissbach, H.: Studies with reversible inhibitors of monoamine oxidase: harmaline and related compounds. *Biochem. Pharmacol.*, 1:160, 1958.
992. Udenfriend, S., Zaltzman-Nirenberg, P., and Nagatsu, P.: Inhibitors of purified beef adrenal tyrosine hydroxylase. *Biochem Pharmacol.*, 14:837, 1965.
993. Uemura, S.: Zur normalen und pathologischen Anatomie der Glandula pinealis des Menschen und einiger Haustiere. *Frankfurter Zeitschrift für Pathologie*, 20:381, 1917.
994. Urry, R. L., Barfuss, D. W., and Ellis, L. C.: Hydroxyindole-O-methyl transferase activity of male rat pineal glands following

hypophysectomy and HCG treatment. *Biology of Reproduction,*
6:238, 1972.

995. Vaisler, L., and Costiner, E.: The epiphyseal hormone—a liver pro-
tecting factor. *Stud. Cercet. Endocrinol., 14:*657, 1963.

996. Vaisler, L., Costiner, E., and Biner, S.: The action of vitamin B_{12}
and of epiphyseal hormone on the capacity of glucuronoconjuga-
tion of the injured liver in animals with experimental toxic
hepatitis. *Rev. Sci. Med., Acad. Repub. Pop. Roumaine, 8:*189,
1963.

997. van de Veerdonk, F.C.G.: Separation method for melatonin in pineal
extracts. *Nature (Lond.), 208:*1324, 1965.

998. van de Veerdonk, F.C.G.: A new separation procedure for melatonin
in extracts. In: *Symposium on Structure and Control of the
Melanocyte.* Berlin, Springer-Verlag, 1966, p. 82.

999. van de Veerdonk, F.C.G.: Demonstration of melatonin in amphibia.
*Curr. Mod. Biol., 1:*175, 1967.

1000. Vaughan, G.M., and Vaughan, M.K.: Effect of melatonin and other
pineal indoles on adrenal enlargement produced in male and
female mice by pinealectomy, unilateral adrenalectomy, castration and cold stress. *Anat. Rec., 172:*421, 1972.

1001. Vaughan, M., and Barchas, J.: Effects of melatonin and related compounds on the release of glycerol from rat adipose tissue *in
vitro. J. Pharmacol. Exp. Ther., 152:*298, 1966.

1002. Vaughan, M.K., Benson, B., and Norris, J.T.: Inhibition of compensatory ovarian hypertrophy in mice by 5-hydroxytryptamine and
melatonin. *J. Endocrinol., 47:*397, 1970.

1003. Vaughan, M.K., Benson, B., Norris, J.T., and Vaughan, G.M.: Inhibition of compensatory ovarian hypertrophy in mice by melatonin,
5-hydroxytryptamine and pineal powder. *J. Endocrinol., 50:*171,
1971.

1004. Vaughan, M.K., Reiter, R.J., and Vaughan, G.M.: Inhibition of compensatory ovarian hypertrophy by Altschule's pineal extract,
pineal indoles and vasopressin in mice and voles. *Am. Zool.,
11:*649, 1971.

1005. Vaughan, M.K., Reiter, R.J., Vaughan, G.M., Bigelow, L., and
Altschule, M.D.: Inhibition of compensatory ovarian hypertrophy in the mouse and vole: a comparison of Altschule's pineal
extract, pineal indoles, vasopressin, and oxytocin. *Gen. Comp.
Endocrinol., 18:*372, 1972.

1006. Vellan, E.J., Gjessing, L.R., and Stalsberg, H.: Free amino acids
in the pineal and pituitary glands of human brain. *J. Neurochem.,
17:*699, 1970.

1007. Venzke, W.G., and Gilmore, J.W.: Histological observations on the
epiphysis cerebri and on the choroid plexus of the third ventricle
of the dog. *Proc. Iowa Acad., Sci., 47:*409, 1941.

1008. Viveros, A.K., Arqueros, L., and Kirshner, N.: Release of catecholamines and dopamine-β-oxidase from the adrenal medulla. *Life Sci.*, *7:*609, 1968.

1009. Vlahakes, G.J., and Wurtman, R.J.: A Mg^{2+} dependent hydroxyindole O-methyltransferase in rat Harderian gland. *Biochim. Biophys. Acta*, *261:*194, 1972.

1010. Vogel, W.H., Orfei, V., and Century, B.: Activities of enzymes involved in the formation and destruction of biogenic amines in various areas of human brain. *J. Pharmacol. Exp. Ther.*, *165:*196, 1969.

1011. Volkman, P.H., and Heller, A.: Pineal N-acetyltransferase activity: effect of sympathetic stimulation. *Science*, *173:*839, 1971.

1012. Vollrath, L., and Schmidt, D.S.: Enzymhistochemische Untersuchungen an der Zirbeldrüse normaler und trächtiger Meerschweinchen. *Histochemie*, *20:*328, 1969.

1013. Volpe, J.J., and Laster, L.: Trans-sulphuration in primate brain: regional distribution of cystathionine synthase, cystathionine and taurine in the brain of the rhesus monkey at various stages of development. *J. Neurochem.*, *17:*425, 1970.

1014. von Bartheld, F., and Moll, J.: The vascular system of the mouse epiphysis with remarks on the comparative anatomy of the venous trunks in the epiphyseal area. *Acta Anat. (Basel)*, *22:*227, 1954.

1015. von Euler, U.S.: *Noradrenaline, Chemistry, Physiology, Pharmacology and Clinical Aspects.* Springfield, Illinois, Charles C Thomas Publ., 1956.

1016. von Euler, U.S.: Adrenergic neurotransmitter functions. *Science*, *173:*202, 1971.

1017. von Kup, J.: Über den Angriffspunkt der antigonadotropen Epiphysenwirkung. *Frankfurter Zeitschrift für Pathologie*, *54:*396, 1940.

1018. von Meduna, L.: Die Entwicklung der Zirbeldrüse im Säuglingsalter. *Z. Anat. Entwicklungsgesch.*, *76:*534, 1925.

1019. Voss, H.: Beobachtung dreier selbständiger juxtapinealer Konkrementkörperchen an einem menschlichen Gehirn sowie topochemische Untersuchungen an ihren Kalkkonkrementen und an Kolloidkugeln im benachbarten Nervengewebe. *Anat. Anz.*, *104:*367, 1957.

1020. Wackenheim, A., and Braun, J.P.: *Angiography of the Mesencephalon. Normal and Pathological Findings.* New York, Heidelberg, and Berlin, Springer-Verlag, 1970, p. 36.

1021. Wallace, R.B., Altman, J., and Das, G.D.: An autoradiographic and morphological investigation of the postnatal development of the pineal body. *Am.J. Anat.*, *126:*175, 1969.

1022. Wallen, E.P., and Yochim, J.M.: Pineal hydroxyindole-O-methyl transferase (HIOMT) and reproductivie cyclicity in the rat. *Fed. Proc.*, *30*:610, 1971.

1023. Walter, F.K.: Weitere Untersuchungen zur Pathologie und Physiologie der Zirbeldrüse, Z. *Gesamte Neurologie Psychiatrie*, *83*:411, 1923.

1024. Waltimo, O., and Talanti, S.: Histochemical localization of β-glucuronidase in the rat brain. *Nature (Lond.)*, *205*:499, 1965.

1025. Warren, P.J., Earl, C.J., and Thompson, R.H.S.: The distribution of copper in human brain. *Brain*, *83*:709, 1960.

1026. Wartenberg, H.: The mammalian pineal organ: electron microscopic studies on the fine structure of pinealocytes, glial cells and on the perivascular compartment. *Z. Zellforsch. Mikrosk. Anat.*, *86*:74, 1968.

1027. Wartenberg, H., and Gusek, W.: Elecktronenmikroskopische Untersuchungen über die Epiphysis Cerebri des Kaninchens. *Verh. Anat. Ges.*, *113*:173, 1964.

1028. Wartenberg, H., and Gusek, W.: Licht und elektronenmikroskopische Beobachtungen über die Struktur der Epiphysis Cerebri des Kaninchens. *Progr. Brain Res.*, *10*:296, 1965.

1029. Wartman, S.A., Branch, B.J., George, R., and Taylor, A.N.: Evidence for a cholinergic influence on pineal hydroxyindole O-methyltransferase activity with changes in environmental lighting. *Life Sci [I]*, *8*:1263, 1969.

1030. Webb, J.G., and Gibb, J.W.: Localization of tyrosine aminotransferase in brain. *J. Neurochem.*, *17*:831, 1970.

1031. Weber, W.W., Cohen, S.N., and Steinberg, M.S.: Purification and properties of N-acetyltransferase from mammalian liver. *Ann. N.Y. Acad. Sci.*, *151*:734, 1970.

1032. Weil-Malherbe, H., Axelrod, J., and Tomchick, R.: Blood-brain barrier for adrenaline. *Science*, *129*:1226, 1959.

1033. Weiss, B.: Differences in the stimulatory effects of norepinephrine (NE) and sodium chloride on adenyl cyclase (AC) of pineal gland and cerebellum. *Fed. Proc.*, *27*:752, 1968.

1034. Weiss, B.: Discussion of the formation, metabolism, and physiologic effects of melatonin. *Adv. Pharmacol*, *6A*:152, 1968.

1035. Weiss, B.: Similarities and differences in the norepinephrine-and sodium fluoride-sensitive adenyl cyclase system. *J. Pharmacol. Exp. Ther.*, *166*:330, 1969.

1036. Weiss, B.: Effects of environmental lighting and chronic denervation on the activation of adenyl cyclase of rat pineal gland by norepinephrine and sodium fluoride. *J. Pharmacol. Exp. Ther.*, *168*:146, 1969.

1037. Weiss, B.: Differential development of two cyclic nucleotide phosphodiesterases in the rat pineal gland. In Klein, D.C. (Ed.): *Pineal Gland: Proceedings of a Workshop*. New York, Raven Press, in press.

1038. Weiss, B., and Costa, E.: Effects of denervation and environmental lighting on norepinephrine-induced activation of adenyl cyclase of rat pineal gland. *Fed. Proc.*, 26:765, 1967.

1039. Weiss, B., and Costa, E.: Adenyl cyclase activity in rat pineal gland: effects of chronic denervation and norepinephrine. *Science*, 156:1750, 1967.

1040. Weiss, B., and Costa, E.: Selective stimulation of adenyl cyclase of rat pineal gland by pharmacologically active catecholamines. *J. Pharmacol. Exp. Ther.*, 161:310, 1968.

1041. Weiss, B., and Costa, E.: Regional and subcellular distribution of adenyl cyclase and 3′, 5′-cyclic nucleotide phosphodiesterase in brain and pineal gland. *Biochem. Pharmacol.*, 17:2107, 1968.

1042. Weiss, B., and Crayton, J.: Ovarian regulation of the norepinephrine-sensitive adenyl cyclase system of rat pineal gland. *Fed. Proc.*, 29:615, 1970.

1043. Weiss, B., and Crayton, J.: Gonadal hormones as regulators of pineal adenyl cyclase activity. *Endocrinology*, 87:527, 1970.

1044. Weiss, B., and Crayton, J.W.: Neural and hormonal regulation of pineal adenyl cyclase activity. In Greengard, P., and Costa, E. (Eds.): *Role of Cyclic AMP in Cell Function*. New York, Raven Press, 1970.

1045. Weiss, B., Lehne, R., and Strada, S.: Rapid microassay of adenosine 3′, 5′-monophosphate phosphodiesterase activity. *Anal. Biochem.*, 45:222, 1972.

1046. Weissbach, H., and Axelrod, J.: The enzymatic biosynthesis of melatonin. *Fed. Proc.*, 19:50, 1960.

1047. Weissbach, H., Redfield, B.G., and Axelrod, J.: Biosynthesis of melatonin: enzymatic conversion of serotonin to N-acetylserotonin. *Biochim. Biophys. Acta*, 43:352, 1960.

1048. Wells, J.W.: Steroids in the pineal gland of the domestic fowl (*Gallus domesticus*): cholesterol and its biosynthesis. *Comp. Biochem. Physiol.*, 40B:723, 1971.

1049. Wells, S.A., Jr., Wurtman, R.J., and Rabson, A.S.: Viral neoplastic transformation of hamster pineal cells *in vitro*. Retention of enzymatic function. *Science*, 154:278, 1966.

1050. West, G.B.: The comparative pharmacology of the suprarenal medulla. *Q. Rev. Biol.*, 30:116, 1955.

1051. Whitby, L.G., Axelrod, J., and Weil-Maherbe, H.: The fate of H³-norepinephrine in animals. *J. Pharmacol. Exp. Ther.*, 132:193, 1961.

1052. Winbury, M.M., Kissil, D., and Losada, M.: Approaches to the study of nutritional blood flow—extraction of Rb⁸⁶ by the heart and hind limb. In Roth, L.J. (Ed.): *Isotopes in Experimental Pharmacology*. Chicago and London, The University of Chicago Press, 1965, p. 229.

1053. Wislocki, G.B., and Dempsey, E.W.: The chemical histology and cytology of the pineal body and neurohypophysis. *Endocrinology, 42:*56, 1948.

1054. Wislocki, G.B., and Leduc, E.H.: Vital staining of the hematoencephalic barrier by silver nitrate and trypan blue, and cytological comparisons of the neurohypophysis, pineal body, area postrema, intercolumnar tubercle and supraoptic crest. *J. Comp. Neurol., 96:*371, 1952.

1055. Witebsky, E., and Reichner, H.: Die serologische Spezifität der Epiphyse. *Zeitschrift für Immunitätsforschung und experimentelle Therapie, 79:*335, 1933.

1056. Wolfe, D.E.: The epiphyseal cell: an electron-microscopic study of its intercellular relationships and intracellular morphology in the pineal body of the albino rat. *Progr. Brain Res., 10:*332, 1965.

1057. Wolfe, D.E., Axelrod, J., Potter, L.T., and Richardson, K.C.: Localization of norepinephrine in adrenergic axons by light-and electron-microscopic autoradiography. *Electron Microscopy.* New York, Academic Press, 1962, vol. 2.

1058. Wolfe, D.E., Potter, L.T., Richardson, K.C., and Axelrod, J.: Localizing tritiated norepinephrine in sympathetic axons by electron microscope autoradiography. *Science, 138:*440, 1962.

1059. Wolman, M. (Ed.): *Pigments in Pathology.* New York, Academic Press, 1969.

1060. Wolstenholme, G.E.W., Knight, J. (Eds.): *The Pineal Gland.* Edinburgh and London, Churchill Livingstone, 1971.

1061. Wong, P.Y., and Fritze, K.: Determination by neutron activation of copper, manganese, and zinc in the pineal body and other areas of brain tissue. *J. Neurochem., 16:*1231, 1969.

1062. Wong, R., and Whiteside, C.B.C.: The effect of melatonin on the wheel-running activity of rats deprived of food. *J. Endocrinol., 40:*383, 1968.

1063. Wood, J.G.: Cytochemical localization of 5-hydroxytryptamine (5-HT) in the central nervous system (CNS). *Anat. Rec., 157:*343, 1967.

1064. Woolley, D.W.: *The Biochemical Bases of Psychoses or the Serotonin Hypothesis about Mental Diseases.* New York, John Wiley and Sons, Inc., 1962.

1065. Woolley, D.W., and van der Hoeven, T.: Serotonin deficiency in infancy as one cause of a mental defect in phenylketonuria. *Science, 144:*866, 1964.

1066. Woolley, D.W., and van der Hoeven, T.: Prevention of a mental defect of phenylketonuria with serotonin congeners such as melatonin or hydroxytryptophan. *Science, 144:*1593, 1964.

1067. Wragg, L., Machado, C., and Machado, A.: Serotonin rhythm independent of sympathetic nerves in the pineal body of the immature rat. *Anat. Rec., 160:*453, 1968.

1068. Wragg, L.E., Machado, C.R.S., Snyder, S.H., and Axelrod, J.: Anterior chamber pineal transplants: their metabolic activity and independence of environmental lighting. *Life Sci.*, 6:31, 1967.

1069. Wurtman, R.J., Altschule, M.D., Greep, R.O., Falk, J.L., and Grave, G.: The pineal gland and aldosterone. *Am. J. Physiol.*, 199:1109, 1960.

1070. Wurtman, R.J., Altschule, M.D., and Holmgren, U.: Effects of pinealectomy and of bovine pineal extract in rats. *Am. J. Physiol.*, 197:108, 1959.

1071. Wurtman, R.J., and Axelrod, J.: The formation, metabolism, and physiologic effects of melatonin in mammals. *Progr. Brain Res.*, 10:520, 1965.

1072. Wurtman, R.J., and Axelrod, J.: Effect of chlorpromazine and other drugs on the disposition of circulating melatonin. *Nature (Lond.)*, 212:312, 1966.

1073. Wurtman, R.J., and Axelrod, J.: A 24-hour rhythm in the content of norepinephrine in the pineal and salivary glands of the rat. *Life Sci.*, 5:665, 1966.

1074. Wurtman, R.J., Axelrod, J., and Antón-Tay, F.: Inhibition of the metabolism of H³-melatonin by phenothiazines. *J. Pharmacol. Exp. Ther.*, 161:367, 1968.

1075. Wurtman, R.J., Axelrod, J., and Barchas, J.D.: Age and enzyme activity in the human pineal. *J. Clin. Endocrinol. Metab.*, 24:299, 1964.

1076. Wurtman, R.J., Axelrod, J., and Chu, E.W.: Melatonin, a pineal substance: effect on the rat ovary. *Science*, 141:277, 1963.

1077. Wurtman, R.J., Axelrod, J., and Chu, E.W.: The relation between melatonin, a pineal substance, and the effects of light on the rat gonad. *Ann. N.Y. Acad. Sci.*, 117:228, 1964.

1077a. Wurtman, R.J., Axelrod, J., Chu, E.W., and Fischer, J.E.: Mediation of some effects of illumination on the rat estrous cycle by the sympathetic nervous system. *Endocrinology*, 75:266, 1964.

1078. Wurtman, R.J., Axelrod, J., Chu, E.W., Heller, A., and Moore, R.Y.: Medial forebrain lesions: blockade of effects of light on rat gonads and pineal. *Endocrinology*, 81:509, 1967.

1079. Wurtman, R.J., Axelrod, J. and Fischer, J.E.: Melatonin synthesis in the pineal gland: effect of light mediated by the sympathetic nervous system. *Science*, 143:1328, 1964.

1080. Wurtman, R.J., Axelrod, J., and Kelly, D.E.: *The Pineal*. New York, Academic Press, 1968.

1081. Wurtman, R.J., Axelrod, J., and Phillips, L.S.: Melatonin synthesis in the pineal gland: control by light. *Science*, 142:1071, 1963.

1082. Wurtman, R.J., Axelrod, J., and Potter, L.T.: The uptake of H³–melatonin in endocrine and nervous tissues and the effects of constant light exposure. *J. Pharmacol. Exp. Ther.*, 143:314, 1964.

1083. Wurtman, R.J., Axelrod, J., Sedvall, G., and Moore, R.Y.: Photic and neural control of the 24–hour norepinephrine rhythm in the rat pineal gland. *J. Pharmacol. Exp. Ther., 157*:487, 1967.

1084. Wurtman, R.J., Axelrod, J., Snyder, S.H., and Chu, E.W.: Changes in the enzymatic synthesis of melatonin in the pineal during the estrous cycle. *Endocrinology, 76*:798, 1965.

1085. Wurtman, R.J., Axelrod, J., and Roch, R.: Demonstration of hydrox-yindole-O-methyl transferase, melatonin and serotonin in a metastatic parenchymatous pinealoma. *Nature (Lond.), 204*:1323, 1964.

1086. Wurtman, R.J., and Kammer, H.: Melatonin synthesis by an ectopic pinealoma. *N. Engl. J. Med., 274*:1233, 1967.

1087. Wurtman, R.J., Larin, F., Axelrod, J., Shein, H.M., and Rosasco, K.: Formation of melatonin and 5-hydroxyindole acetic acid from ^{14}C-tryptophan by rat pineal glands in organ culture. *Nature (Lond.), 217*:953, 1968.

1088. Wurtman, R.J., Rose, C.M., Chou, C., and Larin, F.: Daily rhythms in the concentrations of various amino acids in human plasma. *N. Engl. J. Med., 279*:171, 1968.

1089. Wurtman, R.J., Rose, C.M., Matthysse, S., Stephenson, J., and Baldessarini, R.: L-Dihydroxyphenylalanine: effect on S-adenosylmethionine in brain. *Science, 169*:395, 1970.

1090. Wurtman, R.J., Shein, H.M., Axelrod, J., and Larin, F.: Incorporation of ^{14}C-tryptophan into ^{14}C-protein by cultured rat pineals:stimulation by L-noradrenaline. *Proc. Nat. Acad. Sci., USA,62*:749, 1969.

1091. Wurtman, R.J., Shein, H.M., and Larin, F.: Mediation by β-adrenergic receptors of effect of norepinephrine on pineal synthesis of $[^{14}C]$ serotonin and $[^{14}C]$ melatonin. *J. Neurochem., 18*:1683, 1971.

1092. Yagihara, Y., Salway, J.G., and Hawthorne, J.N.: Incorporation of ^{32}P *in vitro* into triphosphoinositide and related lipids of rat superior cervical ganglia and vagus nerves. *J. Neurochem., 16*:1133, 1969.

1093. Yamada, H.: Beiträge zur Anatomie des Epithalamus, und zwar der Epiphyse bei der Echidna. *Arbeiten aus dem Anatomischen Institut der Kaiserlich–Japanischen Universität zu Sendai, 21*:149, 1938.

1094. Yamamoto, M., Diebel, N.D., and Bogdanove, E.M.: Radioim-munoassay of serum and pituitary LH and FSH levels in intact male rats and of serum and pituitary LH in castrated rats of both sexes—apparent absence of diurnal rhythms. *Endocrinology, 87*:798, 1970.

1095. Yamamura, Y.: Inhibitory effect of ubiquinone' on biosynthesis of aldosterone in rat adrenal *in vitro. Endocrinol. Jap., 17*:143, 1970.

1096. Yang, H.-Y.T., Goridis, C., and Neff, N.H.: Properties of monoamine oxidases in sympathetic nerve and pineal gland. *J. Neurochem.*, *19:*1241, 1972.

1097. Zieher, L.M., and Pellegrino de Iraldi, A.: Central control of noradrenaline content in rat pineal and submaxillary glands. *Life Sci.*, *5:*155, 1966.

1098. Zweens, J.: Influence of the oestrous cycle and ovariectomy on the phospholipid content of the pineal gland in the rat. *Nature (Lond.), 197:*1114, 1963.

1099. Zweens, J.: *The Pineal Lipid Content in Rat and the Involvement of the Epiphysis Cerebri in the Hypophyseo-gonada Interrelation.* Thesis. Groningen, The Netherlands, Rijksuniversiteit te Groningen, 1964, p. 1.

1100. Zweens, J.: Alterations of the pineal lipid content in the rat under hormonal influences. *Progr. Brain Res., 10:*540, 1965.

1101. Zweig, M., and Axelrod, J.: Relationship between catecholamines and serotonin in sympathetic nerves of the rat pineal gland. *J. Neurobiol., 1:*87, 1969.

1102. Zweig, M.H., and Snyder, S.H.: The development of serotonin and serotonin-related enzymes in the pineal gland of the rat. *Communications in Behavioral Biology,* [A], *1:*103, 1968.

1103. Zweig, M., Snyder, S.H., and Axelrod, J.: Evidence for a nonretinal pathway of light to the pineal gland of new born rats. *Proc. Nat. Acad. Sci., USA, 56:*515, 1966.

INDEX

A

Accessory optic system (*see* Optic tracts)
Acervuli (*see* Corpora arenacea)
Acetal phosphatides, pineal content, 92, 99, 102
Acetylcholine (ACh)
  biosynthesis, 261
  metabolism, 262
  neurotransmitter function, 266
Acetylcholinesterase (AChE, E.C. 3.1.1.7), 266–267
  in pineal, 266–267
N-Acetylglucoseamine, pineal uptake in glycoprotein, 297
Acetylsalicyclic acid esterase (E.C. 3.1.1.b), 268
N-Acetylserotonin, 140–143, 145–146
  assay, 146
  pineal concentrations, 145–146
  separation, 141–143
  structure (*Fig.*), 140
N-Acetylserotonin-O-methyltransferase (*see* Hydroxyindole O-methyltransferase)
N-Acetyltransferase of pineal gland
  circadian rhythm, 160
  development, 163–165
  effect of
    dibutyryl cyclic-AMP, 160
    harmine, 160
    norepinephrine, 160
      mediation by cyclic-AMP, 160
    sympathetic stimulation, 161
Acid hematein-positive (Type II) cells, 74, 76, 88–90
Acid hematein reaction, 76–77, 102
Acid phosphatase (E.C. 3.1.3.2), 269–271
Aconitase (E.C. 4.2.1.3), 279
Aconitate hydratase (E.C. 4.2.1.3), 279
Actinomycin D, effect on pineal 5-HT, 183
Activation of pineal, timing and mechanisms, 324–331
ACTH, effect on

melatonin's actions, 190
pineal,
  lipid, 85
  ^{32}P inorganic phosphate uptake, 53
Acylcholine acyl-hydrolase (E.C. 3.1.1.8), 267
Acyltransferases, 260–263
Adenosine
  effects in pineal gland, 224–225
  structure (*Fig.*), 225
Adenosine 3′,5′-monophosphate (c-AMP), 225, 227–231, 240, 271, 296–297
  actions, 227–231, 240, 271, 296–297
  dependent protein kinase in pineal, 228, 265
  effects on in pineal by hormones and neurotransmitters, 229–231, 240
  pineal content, 228
    circadian rhythm in, 228, 240
  structure (*Fig.*), 225
  synthesis, 229, 240
Adenosine 3′,5′-monophosphate phosphodiesterase (E.C. 3.1.4.c), 271–272
Adenosine triphosphate (ATP), 225–227,

  measurement, 226
  pineal content, 226
    effect of light, 226
  structure (*Fig.*), 225
S-Adenosylhomocysteine (SAH), 126, 129, 161, 231
  inhibition of
    HIOMT, 161
    transmethylations, 231
  routes of formation, 231
S-Adenosylmethionine (SAMe), 126–129, 225, 231–233, 240
  biosynthesis, 225, 231
  effects on tissue levels by
    methionine, 128
    pyrogallol, 128

407